Exploring Best Child Development Practices in Contemporary Society

Nava R. Silton
Marymount Manhattan College, USA

A volume in the Advances in Medical Education, Research, and Ethics (AMERE) Book Series

IGI Global
DISSEMINATOR OF KNOWLEDGE

Published in the United States of America by
IGI Global
Medical Information Science Reference (an imprint of IGI Global)
701 E. Chocolate Avenue
Hershey PA, USA 17033
Tel: 717-533-8845
Fax: 717-533-8661
E-mail: cust@igi-global.com
Web site: http://www.igi-global.com

Library of Congress Cataloging-in-Publication Data

Names: Silton, Nava R., 1981- editor.
Title: Exploring best child development practices in contemporary society / Nava R. Silton, editor.
Description: Hershey, PA : Medical Information Science Reference, [2020] | Includes bibliographical references and index. | Summary: "This book explores current research-based approaches on raising happy, healthy, and successful children from varying backgrounds, abilities, and preferences"--Provided by publisher.
Identifiers: LCCN 2019046411 (print) | LCCN 2019046412 (ebook) | ISBN 9781799829409 (hardcover) | ISBN 9781799829416 (ebook)
Subjects: MESH: Child Development | Child Rearing | Parent-Child Relations | Parenting
Classification: LCC LB1048.5 (print) | LCC LB1048.5 (ebook) | NLM WS 105 | DDC 649/.68--dc23
LC record available at https://lccn.loc.gov/2019046411
LC ebook record available at https://lccn.loc.gov/2019046412

This book is published in the IGI Global book series Advances in Medical Education, Research, and Ethics (AMERE) (ISSN: 2475-6601; eISSN: 2475-661X)

British Cataloguing in Publication Data
A Cataloguing in Publication record for this book is available from the British Library.

Advances in Medical Education, Research, and Ethics (AMERE) Book Series

ISSN:2475-6601
EISSN:2475-661X

MISSION

Humans are living longer now than ever as a result of advances in the medical field. Having the tools available to train knowledgeable and ethical future generations of doctors and medical researchers is essential to continuing to advance our understanding of the human body and develop new ways of treating and curing sickness and disease.

The **Advances in Medical Education, Research, and Ethics (AMERE)** book series highlights publications pertaining to advancements in pedagogical practice for developing future healthcare professionals, research methods, and advancements in the medical field, as well as moral behavior and practice of healthcare professionals, students, and researchers. Featuring research-based book publications that are highly relevant to the healthcare community, this series is ideally designed for library inclusion at medical universities and research institutions as well as personal use by medical professionals, researchers, and upper-level students entering the field.

COVERAGE

- Clinical Research
- Conflicts of Interest
- Ethics in Medicine
- Healthcare Pedagogy
- Medical Curricula
- Medical Simulation
- Patient Data
- Professional Development
- Research Methods
- Scientific Misconduct

IGI Global is currently accepting manuscripts for publication within this series. To submit a proposal for a volume in this series, please contact our Acquisition Editors at Acquisitions@igi-global.com or visit: http://www.igi-global.com/publish/.

The Advances in Medical Education, Research, and Ethics (AMERE) Book Series (ISSN 2475-6601) is published by IGI Global, 701 E. Chocolate Avenue, Hershey, PA 17033-1240, USA, www.igi-global.com. This series is composed of titles available for purchase individually; each title is edited to be contextually exclusive from any other title within the series. For pricing and ordering information please visit http://www.igi-global.com/book-series/advances-medical-education-research-ethics/132365. Postmaster: Send all address changes to above address.

Titles in this Series

For a list of additional titles in this series, please visit:
http://www.igi-global.com/book-series/advances-medical-education-research-ethics/132365

Handbook of Research on the Efficacy of Training Programs and Systems in Medical Education
Ruth Gotian (Weill Cornell Medicine, USA) Yoon Kang (Weill Cornell Medicine, USA) and Joseph Safdieh (Weill Cornell Medicine, USA)
Medical Information Science Reference • © 2020 • 566pp • H/C (ISBN: 9781799814689) • US $365.00

Gender Equity in the Medical Profession
Maria Irene Bellini (Belfast Health and Social Care Trust, UK) and Vassilios E. Papalois (Imperial College London, UK)
Medical Information Science Reference • © 2020 • 339pp • H/C (ISBN: 9781522595991) • US $265.00

Preparing Physicians to Lead in the 21st Century
Valerie Anne Storey (University of Central Florida, USA) and Thomas Edward Beeman (University of Pennsylvania Health System, USA)
Medical Information Science Reference • © 2019 • 245pp • H/C (ISBN: 9781522575764) • US $245.00

Optimizing Medical Education With Instructional Technology
Erdem Demiroz (Trakya University, Turkey) and Steven D. Waldman (University of Missouri – Kansas City School of Medicine, USA)
Medical Information Science Reference • © 2019 • 291pp • H/C (ISBN: 9781522562894) • US $215.00

Exploring the Pressures of Medical Education From a Mental Health and Wellness Perspective
Christina Ramirez Smith (University of the Bahamas, Bahamas)
Medical Information Science Reference • © 2018 • 349pp • H/C (ISBN: 9781522528111) • US $225.00

IGI Global
DISSEMINATOR OF KNOWLEDGE

701 East Chocolate Avenue, Hershey, PA 17033, USA
Tel: 717-533-8845 x100 • Fax: 717-533-8661
E-Mail: cust@igi-global.com • www.igi-global.com

Editorial Advisory Board

Table of Contents

Detailed Table of Contents

on infusing life with positive qualities. Other topics concerning happiness stem from positive psychology. It is imperative to understand them and consider them throughout a child's life. Children's minds are constantly developing to understand new things around them. Children aren't going to be happy at all times, and there will be moments when they throw tantrums or have other issues. When these moments occur, it is important for parents, teachers, and other adults to handle them the right way.

In recent years, there has been widespread interest across both the research and public sectors in understanding how to promote children's lifelong success in a range of domains. While a focus on promoting success in children remains salient, equally salient in the research is how children fail—specifically, how children prevail in the face of failure, adversity, and other challenges over time. The chapter explores parenting and family factors that predict grit. This chapter investigates a range of parenting and family factors, including demographic characteristics, parenting behaviors and styles, and family cultural and environmental factors. Based on this research, the chapter provides overarching recommendations to researchers seeking to understand grit in a family context.

This chapter explores interpersonal relationships in family dynamics and romantic relationships as they pertain to grit, goal setting, and social support. Individuals in various types of relationships will be explored, such as married and non-married couples, couples with children, and couples without children. In addition, this chapter will examine the influence that partners and family members have on one another and the several outcomes that result in different kinds of family and relational supports. The chapter will also explore the importance of using all three methods (grit, goal setting, social support) in conjunction with one another, since the three are vital to long-term success in interpersonal relationships and positive family dynamics, regardless of environmental or socio-economic differences in each case. Examples with evidentiary and anecdotal support will be used to explain the benefits or detriments of having or not having these traits in interpersonal relationships and family dynamics. These examples were selected to be inclusive and to relate to family, parental, and spousal relationship structures.

Foreword

When I gave birth to my son in 2004, there was no shortage of places to turn to for advice. I could look to my own parents or in-laws, but they might be disappointed if I ignored them. I could ask his pediatrician, but unless there was significant bleeding involved, I would have to wait until my call was returned. Online, mommy bloggers became my haven and primary resource for advice. This communal and somewhat anonymous connection would become the inspiration for my own research.

Fifteen years later, the amount of advice and guidance has exploded thanks in part to social media, which allows people to be only a friend click away. With all this information at our fingertips, the glut of parental information has confused people on where to seek reliable advice, what to consider suspect, and what to forward to other new parents. In parallel fashion scholarly research also has burgeoned in this arena. While I once had to explain to people what "motherhood research" is and why it is needed, now research on parenting transects several fields. It is important progress that scholars value the study of parenting systematically within psychology, anthropology, sociology, and communication, among other disciplines. However, a myriad of research on parenting across these fields needs to be synthesized and assessed for patterns. This is where Dr. Nava Silton's edited collection *Exploring Best Child Development Practices in Contemporary Society* comes in.

In this book, Dr. Silton weaves together both theoretical and practical research, leaving doors open for possible avenues of future study. While parenting was once treated as a monolithic experience, Dr. Silton explores it not as one-size-fits-all but as a specialized experience through a cross section of research in development, personality, upbringing, and other topics. An innovation in this collection is the unexpected connections made between different related areas of research. Studies on kindness and emotional intelligence are paired with research on parenting children with disabilities and studies on health, diet, and development. Readers can draw their own links between subjects. The draw of this collection is its up-to-date review of research in specialized fields along with offering windows into what might, or should be, the next areas of research.

This collection acknowledges the plethora of research on parenting while helping to establish parenting research as a distinct field of study. Parenting research long has been present but couched within the larger fields of family, gender, and psychology studies. Dr. Silton's newest collection offers an important window into how studies in parenting benefit from a variety of approaches from different fields. I look forward to re-visiting my own studies while thinking about future possibilities for cross-disciplinary approaches.

Laura Tropp
Marymount Manhattan College, USA

Laura Tropp *is the author of A Womb with a View: America's Growing Interest in Pregnancy, Praeger, 2013; Grandparents in a Digital Age: The Third Act, Lexington Books, 2019; and the co-editor of Deconstructing Dads: Changing Images of Fathers in Popular Culture, Lexington Books, 2015.*

Preface

In an impassioned discourse on achieving peace, the sages of the Babylonian Talmud (around 500 C. E.) in *Brachot* 64A, suggest that our children are integral to the world. They wrote, "The disciples of the sages increase peace in the world… great shall be the peace of your children. Do not read *banayich*, (your children) but *bonayich* (your builders)" And in Tractate *Shabbat*, "The world does not exist but for the breath of schoolchildren," perhaps because the children need adult models of creative learning.

Today there is no less a conviction that our children will shape the future. Books about parenting fill yards of shelving in libraries and bookshops, not to mention internet sources and blogs. Pediatrician Dr. Benjamin Spock wrote the bestselling *Baby and Childcare* in 1945 for new parents. It was and still is (after dozens of printings) an encyclopedic guide with emphasis on convincing these neophyte parents that they should trust themselves and carefully follow his medical and developmental guidelines. In 2004, Ann Douglas wrote *The Mother of All Parenting Books,* the ultimate guide for raising a happy child from the preschool to pre-teen age bracket. She tried, she said, to pen a book that boasts pooled knowledge and shared experiences-- one that would keep parents involved well after the preschool years. For parents with limited time but lofty aspirations for their growing children, more recently (2010), Ellen Galinsky's *Mind in the Making,* offers seven essential life skills every child needs: 1) Focus and self-control, 2) Perspective-taking, 3) Communicating, 4) Making connections, 5) Critical thinking, 6) Taking on challenges, and 7) Self-directed, engaged learning -well researched insights into early childhood learning. But the prize for the slimmest volume and the most worn out pages (in a local library) goes to Erica Reischer's *What Great Parents Do: 75 Simple Strategies for Raising Kids Who Thrive.* The brief chapters (1-2.5 pgs. each) comprise succinct, achievable challenges for parents and kids in a handbook-like format.

Aligned with these helpful resources, this text uniquely contributes to the parenting world, by offering contemporary research on how to best raise happy, healthy and successful children. The text begins with discussions of flow and happiness and then discusses the critical importance of grit, emotional intelligence and kindness for nurturing productive and successful citizens of the world. Moreover, it then delves into best practices for parenting children with a variety of challenges. Whether it be children who are confronting eating disorders, behavioral disorders, like conduct disorder and oppositional defiant disorder, or autism spectrum disorders, this book not only offers comprehensive information about the disorders, but about how best to address them, as well. Finally, the book concludes with chapters pertaining to the importance of strong early attachment patterns and of ensuring that children are protected throughout the world.

Tatiana and Stephanie Valencia are sisters. Tatiana is a dancer and works at the Counseling and Wellness Center at Marymount Manhattan College. Stephanie teaches art to middle school students in a Bronx public school. Their chapter on *Cultivating Flow and Happiness in Children* stems from each of their unique experiences in the dance and art worlds, respectively. The work is also inspired by research into the inner workings of the NY Public School System They demonstrate how the three concepts of flow, creativity and happiness are closely related and how to cultivate this dreamlike flow into one's own grown-up life and then to model it for one's children. Tatiana is especially focused on the dangers and impact of stress and finds that flow can effectively enhance "an individual's efficacy and personal development."

In *The Pursuit of Happiness*, Jaclyn Kell worries that those who struggle to achieve happiness will have a stress-filled life and will have difficulty forging relationships. She shines a wide lens on the attainment of happiness in multiple ways, citing often the seminal work of Martin Seligman on Positive Psychology. Kell touches on how essential it is that parents and teachers take time to try to understand their charges, offer positive facial cues, manage tantrums, and keep children safe. This article brings to mind the helpful insights of the late Haim Ginott who wrote *Teacher and Child*, published in 1972 (among countless other publications). Here are just a few insights from Ginott: "Treat a child as though he already is the person he's capable of becoming… While parents possess the original key to their offspring's experience, teachers have a spare key. They, too, can open or close the minds and hearts of children." And finally, "If you want your children to improve, let them overhear the nice things you say about them to others."

But what if a child fails and there's nothing amazing to report? The self-esteem movement of the 80's and 90's would have jumped in with all manner of approbations to shore up such a child, but the newest studies on "grit," effortful perseverance and passion for long-term goals, predict better outcomes for young people who have encountered challenges, adversity and failure and pressed on despite these obstacles. In earlier volumes, Emily Hotez Ph.D., a project scientist for the Life Course Intervention Research Network at the UCLA Center for Healthier Children, Families and Communities, has researched parent-child relationships, autism and families in poverty. In this volume she addresses grit which developed from her work with diverse college students and from "numerous findings that link grit to achievement." She also explores which parenting styles, demographics, cultural and environmental factors are most closely associated with grit.

Can grit power through interpersonal relationships, family dynamics and even romantic relationships? Valerie Blanchard McGehee, who holds a doctorate in higher education, leadership, management and policy from Seton Hall University, considers that challenge and evaluates grit, goal setting and social support and their roles in completing a doctorate. Additionally, Dr. Blanchard-McGehee has combined her careers as educator, entrepreneur and salesperson to become a client partner at Franklin Covey where she became a certified facilitator for "The Seven Habits of Highly Effective People" and "The Seven Habits of Highly Effective Families."

While the topic of grit is relatively new, emotional intelligence is alluded to as early as the 1920's. Amanda Anzovino who earned a B.A. in Psychology with minors in Forensic Psychology, Social Work and Sociology, and I (Nava R. Silton, Ph.D.), an Associate Professor of Psychology at Marymount Manhattan College, describe the history and components of emotional intelligence and explain the differences between EQ (the emotional quotient) and IQ (the intelligence quotient) "in terms of predicting future life success." Though it may seem premature for a new parent to consider these notions, Anzovino and I consider strategies for becoming an emotionally intelligent parent and for promoting such strategies in a child's early years in the home.

Flow, happiness, grit and emotional intelligence are so integral to the life success of a child. However, if you identify with Mr. Rogers, you might add one more ingredient to that list. Mr. Rogers suggests that there are "three ways to ultimate success: The first way is to be kind. The second way is to be kind and the third way is to be kind." In our *Kindness Makes a Difference Chapter*, Patrick Riley, Amanda Anzovino and I employ high quality interventions "wherein stories, role-plays and other media…promote more positive intergroup attitudes especially with regard to enhancing the attitudes, intentions and interests of typical children toward their peers with differences." As a developmental psychologist (who received my B.S. at Cornell University and my M.A. and Ph.D from Fordham University), I have always been intrigued by how deeply children can show kindness and empathy to others once they better understand them, their intentions, their differences and strengths. As someone who worked at Nickelodeon, Sesame Workshop and Mediakidz and consulted for Netflix and the Autism Seaver Center, I also see the power and potential of media in disseminating these important developmental messages to parents and children alike. Patrick Riley, a Psychology and Public Health Major at Marymount Manhattan College and my revered lead student researcher for the last three years on Addy & Uno and Realabilities Projects, uses his internships at Quad Preparatory School (which caters to twice exceptional children) and at the Child Mind Institute (which caters to children with ADHD among other populations) to enhance each project we pursue. Finally, it was through Amanda Anzovino's efforts that we were able to assess our *Realabilities Educational Materials* with individuals with disabilities, directly. *Kindness Makes a Difference* is chockful of creative products to help imbue kindness and empathy in children, and it offers detailed statistics on the outcomes of applying these various forms of media (a comic book series and an off-Broadway Musical) to reduce bullying children with disabilities and mental health disorders and to promote kindness, empathy and sensitivity in and out of the schools.

While our *Realabilities Comic Book Series* and *Addy & Uno Off-Broadway Musical* don't require screen-time, parents the world over are staggering under the weight and guilt of allowing their children of all ages to watch endless hours of television and often inappropriate programs. The subsequent chapter is fascinating in that "it addresses the diverse ways children consume both food and media… and how these two variables can be related and have reciprocal effects." Lauren Ashbrook, a graduate of Marymount Manhattan College with B.A.s in Psychology and Business, focuses on eating disordered eating and the negative effects of various marketing techniques on consumers. Thankfully, she also includes best practices for formulating an overall healthy food and media diet for children.

In addition to the challenges of managing eating disorders and healthy food and media diets, Conduct Disorder (CD) and Oppositional Defiant Disorder (ODD) are especially challenging behavioral disorders to address. Ingrid Brussier is a French International Psychology student, who has been recognized on the Dean's List each year at Marymount Manhattan College. She is already involved in research and translation projects to aid the Psychology department's faculty. In this chapter, Brussier considers the symptoms of each of these behavioral disorders, their effect on social and biological development and their consequences. She also discusses treatments/therapy options and considers their efficacy.

Moreover, a very challenging set of disorders to address and manage are Autism Spectrum Disorders. Giulia Perasso, a psychologist and Ph.D. candidate at the University of Pavia (Italy), who works at the Department of Brain and Behavioral Science, focuses on the issues and the strengths that ASD children's mothers and fathers experience in everyday life. Her partner, Jacopo DeAngelis, a psychologist and Ph.D. candidate at the University of Milano, delves deeply into social cognition and autism. In addition, he studies pain perception and empathy in individuals with ASD, describes diagnostic tools and strives to increase the quality of parent-mediated interventions. Since children with ASD display strong impairment in social and communication skills, it is difficult for parents to interpret their children's needs and emotions.

In typical children, attachment to the mother will look different from children on the spectrum, but the diverse styles that present even among typical children can have lasting impacts on a child's social life. Erika Nolan, a B.A. candidate at Marymount Manhattan College, majors in Psychology and minors in Music and Theater. She is eager to learn what behaviors yield which attachment behaviors. As an art teacher for children ages 4 to 10, her fascination with attachment theory has increased and deepened. As a musician, she has studied the effects of music on the moods of college students and hopes to become a music therapist. We hope to hear from Erika again and again. She's young, talented and devoted to her research on children. It seems that she's already realized that music is magical—especially for children.

What else is magical for children? Recently I stumbled across *How Eskimos Keep Their Babies Warm and Other Adventures in Parenting (from Argentina to Tanzania and Everything in Between).* The author, Mei -Ling Hopgood, hopes to glean nuggets of best practices as she observes parents in diverse cultures caring for their babies and young people. For example, "An !Kung San woman of Botswana…carries her baby at all times. She lets the baby breastfeed…on demand. A San child would never be left to sleep alone…" But Dr. Poloko Nuggert Ntshwarang and Odireleng Mildred Shehu cast a wider net and are concerned with legal reforms in Botswana. In our last chapter, they adopt a critical discourse analysis (CDA) to examine how Botswana's Children's Act of 2009 informs children's policy and parenting behaviors. Both women are concerned with social protection for children and caregiving.

None of the studies we've described, nor their authors, promise that the work of raising independent, compassionate, competent happy kids is intuitive or simple. In most cases, parents need to model CONSISTENTLY the behaviors they hope to ingrain in their children. Much easier said or written than done. A dramatic case in point can be seen in the Book of Genesis which is rife with parenting missteps and children who encounter multiple obstacles. Nowadays, the epidemic of screen overload is tangentially treated in Lauren Ashbrook's chapter on media and food diets, but its omnipresence may impact the screen-addicted parent (who cannot pay enough attention) even more than the child. Even a very young child, from her perch in a highchair is observing, hearing and internalizing the ruckus around her.

We end with more sage advice from Proverbs 22:8. "Train up a child in the way he should go, and when he is old, he will not depart from it."

If you not only teach flow, happiness, grit, emotional intelligence, kindness, empathy and sensitivity to your children, but consistently model these skills in your own actions and life pursuits, your children will most surely glean the utmost from their interactions with and attachments to their astute caregivers.

Nava R. Silton
Marymount Manhattan College, USA

Acknowledgment

This text would not have been possible without a wonderful meeting of minds. First and foremost, I want to gratefully acknowledge all of the esteemed authors who shared their latest engrossing findings in the exciting, diverse and evolving areas of Child Development and Parenting.

I look forward to our future correspondence and collaboration.

Secondly, I'd like to graciously thank the peer reviewers who meticulously evaluated the relevance of content, syntax and empirical rigor of each chapter. Thank you.

Marymount Manhattan College (MMC) students, Patrick Riley '20 and Regina Colie '22 graciously offered their assistance in the early stages of this project. It did not take long before they were inspired and enthused by the innovative research in this area. Marymount Manhattan College (MMC) is one of the most creative and refreshing institutions I have ever had the pleasure of being affiliated with and I thank the whole MMC Community for their constant support and encouragement.

Additionally, I am grateful to Jan Travers, Josh Christ, Eric Whalen, Morgan Brajkovich, and Carlee Nilphai for their assistance during the editing process. They were always prompt, comprehensive, patient and gracious in their responses.

Moreover, I would like to thank my incredible husband, Ariel, and my charming and hilarious little men and lady, Judah Lior, Jonah Gabriel, Jacob Zeke, and Jordana Leah, for their warmth, humor, inspiration and patience throughout this endeavor. I want to acknowledge my father, Rabbi Paul Silton and my wonderful siblings, Elana, Michal, Akiva, Tamar, Aviva, and my twin sister Shira for their constant encouragement and support. Finally, I owe the largest debt of gratitude to my own dear mother, who made my childhood so delightful and memorable and continues to nurture my interests, ambitions and passions. She is a consummate renaissance woman, who is not only brilliant, creative and wise, but patient, kind and beyond generous with her time and guidance. I will cherish this text all the more since her beautiful mind and loving hands painstakingly reviewed its contents.

I want to extend a final note of gratitude to all of the educators, academics, and professionals who not only research best practices for healthy Child Development and Parenting, but who practice it each day with their own children or with those they teach or mentor.

Nava R. Silton
Marymount Manhattan College, USA

Chapter 1
Cultivating Flow and Happiness in Children

Tatiana Camila Valencia
Marymount Manhattan College, USA

Stephanie Johan Valencia
Parsons School of Design, USA

ABSTRACT

This chapter emphasizes the interrelatedness of three important concepts: flow, creativity, and happiness. In positive psychology, "flow" is identified as a state of consciousness that involves an energized focus as one presently engages in an enjoyed activity. This chapter will help readers understand how to cultivate flow and creativity in their everyday lives and explain why doing so can lead to an enhancement in wellbeing and personal development. The important role of parenting in a child's life will also be addressed as children absorb a vast amount of information from their parents who innately are their first mirroring role models. The authors will also provide insight into personal and societal barriers that may hinder creative expression and the sustainment of happiness.

INTRODUCTION

Happiness has been a prevalent topic for years. It is seen all around the world in various realms: marketing, health, success, relationships, governmental policymaking, etc. In psychology, happiness has been referred to as "subjective well-being" which describes individuals' various opinions on the definition of happiness and what brings them happiness. What is certain, however, is that happiness is strongly sought

DOI: 10.4018/978-1-7998-2940-9.ch001

after. Happiness is frequently conceived of as a stamp to enhance the quality of life as described in Gruber and Mauss, and Tamir (2011), "Happiness facilitates the pursuit of important goals, contributes to vital social bonds, and broadens our scope of attention to enable processing of new ideas and stimuli in the environment" (pp.229). While happiness may appear to be an elusive topic, research shows that its effects are complex and worth pursuing. Research from 255 studies on happiness reveals that happier people make better use of their time at work, have higher paying jobs and superior roles, have more friends and social support, are better leaders, are more likely to have a fulfilling marriage, are healthier, live longer and are more resilient than unhappy people (Diener and King and Lyubomirsky, 2005). This chapter will aim to address how children can delve into the richness of life through two facilitators of happiness: flow and creativity.

Creativity is often viewed as the use of the imagination to create something original, but creativity also requires the willingness to try, fail, see life in a different way or experience challenge (Csikszentmihalyi, 1996). It is also about translating creative endeavors into one's personal life by planning and most importantly, believing one is capable of experiencing novelty. Similarly, flow isn't just merely a state of pleasurable feelings and spontaneous moments of contentment. Flow's greater purpose is to build perseverance and discipline; both qualities that challenge many aspects of the human condition that otherwise would remain dormant. Also explored in this chapter, are the benefits parents produce by joining in on their child's creative adventures, as well as perceiving their own contentment as equally important to that of their child.

Flow is recognized as an experience of full investment in the present moment while engaging in an activity that brings both enjoyment and energized concentration. Structured disciplines that offer consistent challenges and engagement are areas in which people are most receptive to experiencing flow: rock climbing, dancing, painting, sports, reading and martial arts, for example. Mihaly Csikszentmihalyi, describes that the experience of flow as the state of mind in which an individual feels fully alive, competent and creative is often the result of combining optimal experience with a challenge and skill balance. Unlike feeling pleasurable moments, in flow, skills are always held accountable to the growing challenge. Pleasurable moments also known as "peak experiences" are bursts of enjoyment that are often fleeting and as seen in Delle Fave (2009) free of the "…cognitive, motivational and emotional components" that coexist in flow (p.1). The process and purpose driven nature of a flow activity is a key component of this experience since it allows the individual to internally grow with his/her external world, which in turn can lead to psychological and societal growth (Csikszentmihalyi, 1990).

Previously, flow has been linked to self-determination (Deci & Ryan, 2000) and as shown in Snyder and Lopez (2009) "commitment and achievement during high school years (pp.199)". Csikszentmihalyi and Nakumara (2009) also present studies showing that students who experienced more flow and less anxiety had participated in school-related activities and persisted in their respective talents (Csikszentimihalyi et al., 1993). Flow has also been associated with a greater perceived competence and relatedness to others (Deci & Ryan, 2000). Moreover, Csikszentmihalyi & Nakumara (2009) noted that flow leads to diminished delinquency in students who experienced high adversity in the household and/or in school settings. The subjective nature of these concepts- flow, happiness and creativity and the way they positively influence prevalent issues of modern society, makes this relationship an interesting one to examine.

HAPPINESS

A Brief History of Happiness

Many philosophers have shared their own take on what happiness is and have juggled its various and distinct meanings. Some ancient Greeks for instance, perceived happiness as a random occurrence, only something felt out of good fortune or the gift of God (Lenoir, 2013). Another happiness belief was seen in the 19th century that claimed that it was actually unhappiness that deserved greater respect, since it was perceived to show the raw authenticity of humanity (Lenoir, 2013). In contrast, Kant believed that happiness was a reward granted by God and hence could only be found after death (Lenoir, 2013).

Later, Greek philosophers Aristotle, Plato and Socrates used the term *Eudaimonia* to refer to living and doing well and believed that happiness was directly connected to good virtues (Lenoir, 2013). In the Eastern World, multiple philosophical systems embedded the belief that establishing mind and body techniques such as yoga, meditation and deep breathing could also lead to a happier and healthier life (Csikszentmihalyi, 1990).

To continue shining the light on meaning as opposed to short-lived pleasures, Buddha paved the way to a very important role in happiness—the power of our minds and our ability to connect to our human nature. This is seen in a recent interview with the 14th Dalai Lama (Tenzin Gyatso), a Buddhist monk who is widely respected for his human/divine nature and advocacy in helping others. The Dalai Lama states, "...the conclusion is that affection and concern for others' well-being is the best way to achieve your own happy life, healthy body, and longer life. You don't need drugs or tranquilizers if you keep affection in your heart" (McLeod, 2018). He also expresses the dangers of thinking only about oneself, "...having a self-centered attitude- creates a lot of anxiety, loneliness, fear, and anger" (McLeod, 2018). In this statement, he stresses that spreading compassion and affection to others is a mutual and effective generator of happiness since such qualities create connection and unity, fundamental to our social nature. The yogic philosophy in Hinduism also seeks to merge self-transformation with the universal spirit (Galantino and Quinn, 2008). Some leading thinkers began viewing happiness in a broader, more worldly perspective; so much so that the Declaration of Independence clearly states that happiness is a *total* right.

Fast forward to today and Positive Psychology, an entirely new realm in psychology exists where happiness is a prevalent topic of research. This branch is focused on questioning what makes life worth living rather than concentrating on the pathology or issues of mental health. More research, therefore, brings light to preventative measures that can function to not only avoid illnesses from occurring in the first place, but to implement habits that enable humans to thrive in health and self-development. Clearly happiness has been dissected, argued, and portrayed in different realms through multiple perspectives, across cultures and generations. One could argue that the direction happiness has now led people to find empowerment in personal accountability.

Humanistic psychologist Abraham Maslow, who introduced the Hierarchy of Needs, demonstrates that unless people have their physiological, safety, sense of belonging, love and esteem needs met, they cannot reach the top of the pyramid where self-actualization resides. The term self-actualization refers to meeting one's fullest potential to freely express creativity and life's deepest personal pursuits. Maslow argues that if these needs are not yet met, energy is constantly diminished whether consciously or subconsciously to fill such missing needs and desires. Similar to any healthy relationship, if a person has not invested time and effort in self-development as it relates to building self-esteem, setting personal values, morals and establishing boundaries, it becomes difficult to develop any relationship. Before engaging with the environment, a foundation must be solid and that fundamental base starts with the self.

Common Misconceptions of Happiness

As theories and ideas begin to be explored through various individuals, societies and cultures, false beliefs about happiness also accrue. A misconception about what can bring people lasting happiness is an abundance of material goods, reputation and economic status, which are all derived from external motivations. However, research has shown that although these characteristics can facilitate or improve life in some way, they quickly lose their value. Research on hedonic adaptation, shows that we are masters at adapting to both good and bad events. Take one's dream job, car or house for instance- these external factors accumulate desired momentum in the mind for a while and then lose their thrill once adaptation takes over and the experience becomes familiar. For example, previous research has shown that human beings have a happiness set-point that marks their average genetic happiness level. To explain this concept, the Hedonic Treadmill was termed by Bickman and Campbell (1971), who observed how quickly people's happiness would return to original set-points soon after a negative or positive event took place.

As supported in Diener and Lucas and Scollon (2006) "...The treadmill theory explained the observation that people with substantial resources are sometimes no happier than those with few resources and that people with severe problems are sometimes quite happy" (p.2). However, new research has found that human adaptation is more malleable than we think, implying that we shouldn't automatically discard all efforts to increase well-being in the long-term (Diener, et al., 2006). For instance, cultivating gratitude for possessions and relationships that one already has is a key component to sustaining happiness as seen in Larsen and McKibban (2008), "...the effect of possessions, on well-being depends on how people value those possessions, a finding that speaks to the subjectivity of well-being" (pp.375).

How Much Responsibility Do We Actually Have?

According to Sheldon and Schkade and Lyubomirsky (2005), approximately 50% of our happiness is dependent on genetic makeup, 40% is influenced by our life experiences and 10% is influenced by life circumstances. Although 50% of genetics account for a large percentage of uncontrollable factors, life experiences and circumstances are greatly impacted by our personal choices and behaviors. Life circumstances seem to spontaneous and uncontrollably affect people's lives. However, people often undermine or fail to recognize in the first place that the way one perceives such circumstances and chooses to cope, can actually influence our happiness more heavily than the circumstance itself. The authors therefore, suggest that human beings have a lot of responsibility towards achieving their own happiness.

The societal identity of happiness is currently shifting in a direction that honors and respects the pursuit towards happiness as a means rather than as an end, a process as opposed to a product or final outcome such as a job promotion, a luxury car, a bigger home, etc. Happiness is very rarely seen as a work in progress and is thought of even less, as a difficult process, filled with challenges and grit. For this reason this chapter provides tools for ways to experience happiness through creativity and flow. This version of happiness requires effort, personal responsibility and active attention in exchange for sustainable happiness. Since stress is a normal part of life but is often perceived as a main inhibitor of happiness, a study questioning the relationship of perceived stress and flow is presented.

Perceived Stress and Flow

A study on a diverse group of physically active people was conducted to see whether there is a correlation between perceived stress and flow experiences in participants. The author predicted that participants' greater levels of flow would correlate with a lower level of perceived stress. Specifically, the author suggested that confronting life stressors the way one confronts a challenge in their favorite flow activity, with curiosity, patience and eagerness, leads to better coping. Lastly, the researcher explored whether general levels of self-efficacy are associated with perceived stress and engagement in flow. Since stress plays a vital role in pathology and life dissatisfaction, this study will examine whether flow can decrease perceived stress and increase psychological well-being.

Perceived Stress

Similar to the challenge and skill balance found in flow, confronting daily stressors also leads one to assess their skills in relation to the external challenge. Perception plays a vital role in the way people experience life. For instance, a certain perception of stress is formed depending on how much one believes he/she has the sufficient number of skills to meet the challenge at hand. Perception is constantly being informed by the thoughts playing before, during and after an experience. Dr. Bruce H. Lipton, a developmental biologist best known for promoting the controversial idea that genes and DNA can be manipulated by a person's beliefs, once wrote, "The moment you change your perception, is the moment you re-write the chemistry of your body." Since thoughts can manipulate the chemistry of internal states, the researcher suggests that the way in which people perceive themselves (skills) and the world around them (stressors) has a significant influence on wellbeing and overall life satisfaction. Knowing this, it is especially important to remember that for the most part, people are in control of their thoughts and have the ability to change them when and how they want. Flow has the potential to build psychological resilience by training the mind to facilitate a balance of skill and challenge, develop a love of approaching problems, adopt multiple ways of solving problems and acquire a thick skin that is tolerant of risk and resilient to failure (Csikszentmihalyi and Montijo and Mouton, 2018). This perseverance muscle used in flow can therefore have a positive impact on mental health and on self-determination (Deci & Ryan, 2000).

There are eight dimensions that are present in the flow state. Both flow and the perception of stress are multifaceted concepts, yet they possess various similarities most of which can be highlighted through the eight dimensions of flow: 1. challenge and skill balance, 2. action-awareness merging, 3. Clear goals, 4. unambiguous feedback, 5. concentration on task at hand, 6. sense of control, 7. loss of self-consciousness and 8. transformation of time.

THE 8 DIMENSIONS OF FLOW AS THEY RELATE TO STRESS

Challenge-Skill Balance

Having a challenge and skill balance is essential to the flow experience. If skills are too low in comparison to the challenge at hand, what results is anxiety and if skills are too high in comparison to the challenge, boredom occurs. Csikszentmihalyi (1900) states that anxiety and boredom are the two primary obstacles that impede the enjoyment of life. When a balance forms between one's internal capacity (skills) and an external stimulus (challenges), there is enough ease to enjoy the activity and just the right amount of motivating pressure to overcome the presented challenge. As the challenge increases, so does the individual's skills and as a result, this generates a sense of positive reinforcement that can develop personal complexity and growth.

A good example of this is seen in Csikszentmihalyi's (1988) text, which describes Indian tribes of British Columbia where the elders sought new experiences after agreeing that their world had become too predictable. The entire population of elders would collectively decide that they would move to a different part of *Shushwap* every 25-30 years in order to attract new challenges, "...there were new streams to figure out, new game trails to learn, new areas where the balsamroot would be plentiful. Now life would regain meaning and be worth living. Everyone would feel rejuvenated and healthy." This example shows just how much challenge is desired and necessary for the evolution of the human race as Buettner (2017) quotes Csikszentmihalyi, "People need to be challenged. It's in our genes. We develop self-confidence through adversity. They're the building blocks to happiness."

Merging of Action and Awareness

The second dimension of flow is a merging of actions and awareness, which means that one's attention is channeled through the activity at hand, giving way to fluency of internal and external communication. Often people can seem to be engaged with the activity that they are participating in when in reality their attention is elsewhere. For example, a swimmer can appear to be receiving instructions from his/her coach but is actually visualizing his/her next meal in great detail. If this swimmer is then told to execute a difficult swim combination but remains distracted with thoughts that do not pertain to the activity, his/her performance will certainly suffer.

Concentration on Task at Hand

The third dimension is categorized as the focus on the task at hand, referring to deep concentration in the present moment where distractions are excluded from consciousness. For example if a yoga student is in a pose and starts becoming disturbed by latecomers, a reoccurring cough or someones phone going off, the pose can suddenly become mindless and even more difficult since the mind now has to work harder to regain equilibrium with the body.

Loss of Self- Consciousness

People who engage in flow activities must also lose their self-consciousness in order to perform to the best of their ability. If they fail to do so, important energy is taken away to attend to self-doubts, anxieties and insecurities rather than to what really matters- mindful engagement in performance. For example, a dancer that appears to be grasping the choreography being taught can actually be preoccupied by what surrounding classmates might be thinking of his/her movement. Growing within one's talent often depends on whether an individual is willing to face the challenges that come with wanting to protect the ego. If this mindset is successfully achieved, individuals can even come to find as quoted by Csikszentmihaly, 1996, "Paradoxically, the self expands through acts of self-forgetfulness." After total involvement in flow, individuals have a stronger self-concept since they have pushed passed self-inflicted boundaries and in turn may feel a part of something greater than themselves.

Clear Goals

In the flow state, challenges spur continuous goals through which the individual is pushed to enhance his/her skills in order to find a balance within the activity again. Clear goals (whether set in advance or developed during involvement), allow the participant to know exactly what needs to be done, at which moment and how. For example, a swimmer in a race must know he/she needs to swim 10 laps of freestyle and make the least amount of time compared to his/her competitors. After knowing this he/she may go even further to also know when to begin slowing down or speeding up. Without a clear goal there is no orientation in flow, internal and external energy become stagnant and the challenge and skill dynamic is disrupted.

Unambiguous Feedback

The immediate and clear feedback when engaging in an activity allows individuals to know whether they are succeeding in a goal (Csikszentmihaly, 2014). Without confusion about how one is doing in relation to the external activity, the self is able to connect and grow with its environment. An example, of unambiguous feedback is for dancers to know they have landed a clean double pirouette (turn) because they did not hop on their leg or distort their placement. Another example is soccer players who know they made a good decision because the quick pass they made to their teammate resulted in a goal.

Sense of Control

Sense of control does not necessarily mean being in control but rather is the belief that one has the *potential* to exercise control at any given moment, especially in difficult situations (Csikszentmihaly, 2014). This empowers the individual to feel efficient since his/her skills may overcome difficult challenges. During a race, a runner must feel a sense of control over his/her mind/body in relationship to the goal at hand. If not energy is constantly being spent (often in the form of stress) trying to gain this sense of control back.

Transformation of Time

In flow, the perception of time is altered through a faster or slower lens. Time can appear to slow down, as often happens when one engages in deep thinking (writing) or speed up as can occur in a fun dance class for example. Alternatively, what may also arise is the irrelevance of time as an existing factor in one's awareness (Csikszentmihaly, 2014). This suggests that flow encompasses unconventional perceptions of time that are typically inaccessible to the human experience.

Method

The current study investigates whether there is a negative correlation between perceived stress and engagement in flow. Although real-life challenges (often stressors) are not nearly as interesting or fun as a favorite flow activity, they are nonetheless, still a challenge. In flow, resilience is bound to increase as one repeatedly faces challenges and is pushed to increase his/her skills within his/her preferred activity. Similarly, while confronting daily stressors one has to assess skills in relation to the external challenge. The researcher's hypothesis states that people who engage in flow activities are more likely to have a lower perceived stress level. To expand on this hypothesis, the researcher also predicted that if individuals approached real-life situations the way they approach flow -with curiosity, patience and eagerness- people would confront stressful situations with a similar sense of determination. In addition, the researcher will explore whether participants' general self-efficacy (GSE) levels are also influencing factors on perceived stress and engagement in flow.

Population

A total of 73 physically active people participated in this study from a wide variety of athletic disciplines such as Yoga, Dance, Sports, Martial Arts, etc. Surveys were distributed to students at various colleges in New York. The population in this study was evenly distributed among a diverse range of race/ethnic backgrounds, Hispanic/ Latino (41.1%), Black or African American (24.7%), White (32.9%) and Asian (1.4%) people. Thirty-nine participants were female and 33 participants were male. The age range was 34 with a mean age of 23.38 (minimum of 18 and a maximum of 52 years of age).

Measures

- *Perceived Stress Scale:* (Cohen & Williamson, 1988) is the most common psychological instrument used for measuring participants' perception of stress. The researcher used the PSS because perception plays a vital role in the way people experience life. Studies have shown that the way thoughts and external daily occurrences are perceived can predict a wide array of health outcomes. In this questionnaire, participants were asked how random, uncontrollable, and overwhelming they find their lives to be. The questions in the PSS ask about feelings and thoughts during the last month, which were compared with the way participants, responded to their flow engagement.
- *Flow-Short Scale* (Rheinberg, Vollmeyer, & Engeser, 2003) is often used to get a typical flow score for potential flow state scenarios. The flow items in this survey were separated into two factors: (1) fluency of performance (items 2, 4, 5, 7, 8, 9) and (2) absorption by activity (items 1, 3, 6, 10). The additional items (11-13) were used to measure worry or level of importance.
- *The General Self-Efficacy Scale* (Schwarzer & Jerusalem, 1995) is correlated to positive emotions and positivity while negative factors were found for stress and health complaints. This measure is being used to see if there is a correlation among self-efficacy, perceived stress and engagement in flow.

Results

Results indicated that there was no significant correlation between self-efficacy and flow. However, significance was found at the .001 and .05 levels for all of the other correlations. For instance, there was a negative correlation between flow and perceived stress as well as self-efficacy and stress. Another negative correlation was found between age and perceived stress, meaning that older individuals showed lower levels of perceived stress than younger individuals. A positive correlation was also found between age and flow, showing that older individuals had higher levels of flow. Aligned with numerous previous studies, females also showed a higher level of perceived stress than men. Tables and charts highlighting these correlations can be found in the Appendix. In addition, the qualitative research conducted found supporting evidence that flow activities help individuals feel less stressed.

Conclusion of Study

One's level of perceived stress and whether or not one engages in flow is dependent on a number of different factors such as personality, socioeconomic status, access to resources and social support. However, high perceived stress and younger age appear to be the most predominant inhibitors of the flow experience. The researcher suggests that the negative correlation between age and stress could be due to the greater level of understanding and introspection people experience, as they get older. As a result, older people may have a more developed coping ability towards stress as well as greater receptiveness and maturity to experience flow. As the researcher predicted, results indicate that if someone has low self-efficacy, he/she is more likely to experience a high perception of stress in his/her life. For this reason, interventions and workshops on stress management and empowerment should be implemented at all levels of schooling, with a focus on adolescents and college students. College is often a time when previous engagement in physical activities decreases, while stress levels increase.

Previous studies and research on flow align with our results indicating that a higher flow score is directly correlated with a lower perception of stress. This could be due to the active participation of a flow activity which can de-stress the mind/body, also suggesting that flow is a potential role-model that helps people translate this organized consciousness experience (flow) into the way one copes with stress in everyday life.

Discussion Points of Study

Stress is a common factor that influences everything from our daily mood to our overall happiness and health. However, this study aims to show that stress very often must cross our perception barrier before it can be experienced. This means that the ways in which we perceive or respond to stress are not permanent, but are rather malleable.

Flow helps individuals and society in a diverse range of ways from preventing pathology to stimulating a mundane work life. Csikszentmihalyi, et al. (2018) shows that flow can be applied to different domains like psychology, education, business management, athletics and neuroscience. It also creates mental order in our consciousness, which helps reduce anxiety, positively challenges the mind/ body connectivity, and even strengthens the relationship between the self and the environment.

Happiness in Children

Children are around parents, caregivers and peers throughout the day, so it is essential to understand just how important social bonds are to their integral health. As seen in Diener and Oishi (2005), research on social psychology and well-being shows that social relationships are more important than material prosperity. Now, understanding how motivators that stem from external sources do not necessarily lead to long-term happiness, the following examples show ways both parents and children can bring more flow, creativity and happiness into their lives through intrinsic motivation.

Involvement in activities that provide a good "fit" with the child's personality, culture, and social support system, show greater intrinsic motivation to begin and sustain an activity (Lyubomirsky, 2012). Therefore, participating in play-like activities that both the child and parents enjoy and can engage in together can strengthen social bonds and increase happiness. Activities parents and children can participate in together can include, active reading, interactive outside play, yoga, bike riding, swimming or even meditation. A study on yoga suggested that the decrease in breath rate detected in children participating in a 6-month yoga program was due to yoga's ability to calm the nervous system enough to reduce anxiety and fear (Galantino and Quinn, 2008).

Mindfulness and meditation are two other respected practices that have gained wide-spread recognition throughout the years as a flexible state of mind where one is consciously present in the moment with a sharp attention to surroundings and respective feelings. Mindfulness is different from mindlessness and distraction as Langer (2000) clearly states, "When we are mindless, our behavior is rule and routine-governed; when we are mindful, rules and routines may guide our behavior, rather than pre-determine it" (p.1). Both mindfulness and meditation practices show various cognitive and behavioral benefits that can facilitate children's approach in awakening their interest in creativity and later sustain their involvement once engaged.

A study consistent with past research on the effects of Transcendental Meditation (TD) found that middle school students practicing this technique showed improved social emotional learning and reduced emotional problems (Valosek, Nidich,Wendt and Grant, 2019). Enhancing learning ability and decreasing psychological distress speaks to how children can use meditation as a gateway toward flow and creativity. Meditation can help students become more self-aware, a quality helpful in creative pursuits and can also help them self-manage, a skill helpful for inducing flow where qualities like patience and discipline are necessary. In this study students practiced for a short period of time (10 minutes total) and received numerous benefits to their well-being. This shows that parents only need a small amount of quiet, alone time or time with their children to feel a difference in everyday experience as Valosek et al. (2019) notes, "These transformations in inner experience and in brain functioning could positively change how one interacts with one's social environment and how one meets challenges in life." With frequent practice in meditation, children can become less reactive to external stimuli and more in control of their experiences. This can be helpful in moments where children have to work together and practice social skills such as sharing, taking turns and showing compassion or when a child has to accept responsibility for his/her actions, pay attention, follow advice or have patience in a project (Valosek et al., 2019).

Mindful Parenting Theory

This leads into the necessary discussion on parental care and the importance of parents building a healthy relationship with their children as well as facilitating their children's relationships with others. Relationships and family bonds are one of the most important factors that play into a child's resilience when dealing with any disorder. Attention-Deficit Hyperactivity Disorder (ADHD) is highly prevalent, affecting approximately 5% of children worldwide (Polanczy GV et al as cited in Evans, 2018, p. 10). This neurobiological disorder is characterized by symptoms of disengagement and/or hyperactivity/impulsivity (Polanczy GV et al as cited in Evans, 2018, p. 10). Parents assume numerous challenges when managing children's ADHD symptoms and associated stigmas. This often leads to an increase in parental stress when compared to the general population. Therefore, it is imperative when considering treatment that the broader social fabric of children with ADHD is accounted for, since parents are both negatively impacted by their children's challenging behaviors and may also create a continuing negative feedback loop that allows for the symptoms to persist and/or worsen.

Children are reporting higher stress levels today than ever before. The effects of experience compellingly influence brain development through the formation of synaptic circuits. Evidence shows that positive and negative experiences demonstrate their impact on the wiring of the brain. It is important to note that the nature of the experience itself, coupled with the maturity of the brain at the time of the experience, will determine or at least influence whether the resulting neural change is beneficial or destructive to the child (Evans, 2018, p. 57).

Prioritizing mindful meditation breaks has been shown to make lasting impacts on disease prevention and treatment. According to the American Academy of Pediatrics (AAP), meditation can help with "...anxiety, depression, school performance, sleep, behavior problems and eating disorders" (2016). Other studies have highlighted physical benefits. Meditation is known to have calming effects on the nervous system and decreases stress hormones circulating in the body. Such physical benefits show improvements in gastrointestinal symptoms, obesity, headaches, high blood pressure, pain sensitivity and immune function (AAP, 2016). Studies have also found that involving parents in meditation-based interventions is likely to address parent stress, parent psychopathology as well as maladaptive parenting- all of which reinforce the child's symptoms (Evans, 2018, p. 10). Mindful Parenting Theory suggests that mindful practices allow parents to positively respond rather than react to their child's behavior and ultimately allows for more enduring enjoyment in the parent-child relationship (Evans, 2018. p. 11). This reinforces that the child and parent dynamic only thrives when they interact harmoniously, as they directly affect one another.

Living in the digital age, it has become difficult to detach and disconnect from the social normalcy of technology use. Therefore, to help children manage this digital generation, AAP recommends setting limits on how long children use technology. Finding time to co-play with children can also help mend social isolation by stimulating bonding and demonstrating interest in what children find entertaining.

Smart phones, tablets, digital watches and all other types of gadgets available today have successfully integrated into daily living with alarming ease. Even more essential is an awareness of the ways in which technology availability and accessibility can seamlessly serve as an emotion pacifier. Adults often use technology as a coping mechanism, a way to "pass time" which can serve as a distraction from facing strong emotions. Parents can model open communication by asking children what they feel or how their day went at school. Although media can help keep children still and quiet for long periods of time, AAP states that "children need to be taught how to identify and handle strong emotions, come up with activities to manage boredom or calm down through breathing, talking about ways to solve the problem, and finding other strategies for channeling emotions (2018).

One way children can manage boredom and release stressors of daily life is through physical activity. According to AAP (2003), 1 in 3 children are overweight or obese in the U.S. It is imperative for children to find activities that they enjoy so that they are more internally motivated to consistently engage in them. Parents can help facilitate this personality-activity match by exposing their children to different sports and disciplines that they can then choose from. Aside from parents acting as effective role models to their children by engaging in physical activity themselves, parents can also be their children's first influence in learning time-management. Often physical activity gets pushed to the back burner as other responsibilities begin to take over. When parents show effort in planning ahead and making time for physical activity, their children will enjoy the potential benefits of flow, exercise and most importantly, learn to make time for what matters to them.

Engagement in flow-inducing activities such as meditation and yoga can cultivate independence, confidence, self-efficacy and decrease stress. While greatly beneficial for personal growth, these character strengths can later translate into the development of positive social relationships with others.

OVERCOMING PERSONAL AND SOCIETAL BARRIERS

Personal Barriers

One common personal obstacle is the waste of free time. When there is no external force demanding that we concentrate, mental chaos takes over (Csikszentmihalyi, 1996). Therefore, taking charge of our schedule is important or we are bound to become anxious or bored. A great way to structure time is by setting goals and engaging in hobbies that demand skill. Taking time to unwind is essential to maintaining balance, but often when people become overworked, they tend to rest in a passive state. Resting does not always have to be inactive and empty; It can involve a change in activity that awakens another area of the brain or body (Csikszentmihalyi, 1996). Now if adults crave rest or a change in routine, imagine how much a vibrant, energy-filled child might need these same shifts in experience. The Danish government understands that their people will work their best, when they feel their best. Their society and lifestyle allows them to do what they love. The country's government and social values show that the Danes have a great awareness of what can bring them authentic self-fulfillment. Aside from financial well-being and community engagement, they find meaning and purpose in their everyday activities as quoted in Butner (2017), "The Danish society, it seems, encourages the kind of balance between engaging work and rewarding play" (p. 49). If the education system allocated more of its curriculum to free time between learning for creative tasks, free play and thinking, a child could function more effectively. Flow can be experienced during free time or moments in the day specifically dedicated for play. As seen in Carey (2014), spaces in between learning are not only a fun time for growth and exploration, it is also necessary for a child's retention and overall learning process.

Another way of structuring time is by investing time and effort into creating habits that allow one's personal interests to be expressed (Csikszentmihalyi, 1990). By doing so, free time is molded and under one's control. Nonetheless, this can only be achieved by manifesting inner discipline and internal motivation. For instance, dancers benefit from perseverance when they find themselves struggling with a certain technique. Perseverance helps them sustain their efforts enough to get past the "difficult phase." If commitment during this challenging phase did not occur, dancers would not be able to experience the enjoyment of dancing with both artistry and technicality. When one lacks personal motivation, social support in the form of verbal and physical encouragement (through affection) is crucial in creating positive reinforcement in a child's experience.

Societal Barriers

Education

Society, under ideal conditions, values the developmental process of children becoming adults. Montessori theory embodies the understanding that "Playfulness and seriousness correspond to the balance between freedom and discipline" (Kahn, D. 2003). This harmonious paradox is one the current education system seems to be failing to master. The challenges in child development cannot be fully understood without recognizing the limitations of society's education system.

One could argue that a child's initial rite of passage into society is his/her *first* day of school. School is a social space where knowledge, societal norms, values and traditions are disseminated over time. Since school is such a respected social norm that develops into our culture, the underlying flaws of this complex system very easily go unnoticed. Ken Robinson states, "The most fundamental question is, *what is education for*?" (Robinson, 2015 pp. xix). The answer to that question is as complex as the population that it serves, in the classrooms of America. The purpose of that question is meant to merely scratch the surface and highlight how vastly complex education reform is. Systems Theory suggests that, "The least obvious part of a system is identifying its function or purpose, and it is often the most crucial determinant of the system's behavior" as seen in Meadows, D. H. 2008. p. 188. Therefore, if a system is no longer behaving the way it once did at its conception, it is safe to say that its purpose has changed. A system's original purpose can change due to the complexity of all of its different stakeholders (policy makers, superintendents, chancellors, teachers, parents, etc.), who possess varying degrees of expertise, motivation and accountability. This implies that if the purpose of a system is ambiguous and chaotic, behavior is likely to be chaotic, as well. Traditional education is criticized for being outdated, stuck in patterns that were designed for the industrial age (Robinson, 2015). These patterns once filled the needs for that era, but in the long term it has stunted growth and potential to adapt to changing times.

Michelle A. Rhee, an American educator and advocate for education reform was Chancellor of District of Columbia Public Schools. She boldly states, "There's this unbelievable willingness to turn a blind eye to the injustices that are happening every day in our schools in the name of harmony amongst adults" (Chilcott & Guggenheim, D. 2010). Power structures within the education system reinforce control and the lack of it among both children and adults.

Leaders who actively ignore the education systems' faults just because they are hard to investigate and quantify, develop faulty models. Today's educational system is designed to collect data that is easily measured, rather than cultivating and assessing the conditions for a child's happiness, self-efficacy, and resilience- all qualities that lead to personal growth. These constructs are not easy to define or measure; yet they are some, if not the most important concepts towards living a meaningful life. No one can easily define or measure such values but if our education system isn't designed to produce these qualities, and if society as a collective does not justify their presence, they will cease to exist (Meadows, D. H. 2008, p. 176). This simple input/output equation clearly exemplifies our current working structure, "If you run an education system based on standardization and conformity that suppresses individuality, imagination, and creativity, don't be surprised if that's what it does" (Robinson, 2015, p. xxii).

The root of the problem with enormous structural systems like education comes down to what Don Michael calls, "error-embracing." It takes a lot of courage for a system vital to an economy's health to embrace, let alone admit to errors. However, when one addresses complex social issues, feigning "success" or better yet, "sustainable success," can result in decreasing the system's credibility and ability to learn. Therefore, error embracing is integral for learning (Meadows, D. H. 2008, p. 181). The societal vulnerability of uncertainty creates the right conditions for an iterative approach that encourages reinvention and builds resiliency within a system. Being honest and making clear distinctions between what works for adults and how that might not align with what works for children is a step in the right direction. A vision for our education system needs to be organized in such a manner in which previous mistakes can be learned from and those lessons can then be adapted to meet society's ever-changing needs. Typically vulnerabilities in a system are kept hidden, but it is up to education leaders to break the cycle and to be transparent about what works and what doesn't in today's twenty-first century classrooms.

The Education System was created in the middle of the 19th century due to the major labor demands of the Industrial Revolution. It was built on the principles of mass production and efficiency. Today we have limitless opportunities to engage young people's imaginations and to provide forms of teaching and learning that are highly customized to them (Robinson, 2015). Yet we haven't fully harnessed all of that power in order to deliver the service that is education to its capacity.

It is important to distinguish the difference between symptoms and causes. There are several symptoms to the problems of education, which could not be fully understood unless the underlying systems that allow them to exist and flourish are identified (Zhao, Y. 2017). On the 2015 Programme for International Student Assessment (PISA), the U.S. continued to register mediocre scores, as it has done since PISA began in 2000. The U.S. shows steady progress on Trends in International Mathematics and Science Study (TIMSS) however, scores are flat on PISA—even declining in mathematics on the last two rounds. Finland on the other hand, scored among the top countries on PISA in the early 2000s, making it a popular destination for American "edutour-ists," eager to learn from Finland's schools. However, since 2006, Finland's PISA scores have declined dramatically. On TIMSS, fourth grade math scores for Finland (535) and the U.S. (539) are statistically indistinguishable, as seen in Loveless (2017). Finnish educator, Pasi Sahlberg is a leading figure in education policy and the author of the best-selling book, "Finnish Lessons 2.0 What can the world learn from educational change in Finland." In an interview by The Washington Post concerning the decline in test scores she identified three trends affecting the Finnish education system at the time. The first was the weakened educational performance of Finnish schoolboys' during the past decade. This troublesome phenomenon is stronger in Finland than in any other OECD country. The second is the aggressive emergence of mobile gadgets such as smartphones among school-aged children. Pasi mentioned emerging research on how the Internet affects the brain — and thereby learning — and suggests three principal consequences: shallower information processing, increased distractibility, and altered self-control mechanisms. These alone can inform concentration on complex conceptual math and science problems can become more difficult for children at this stage. The third was the serious economic downturn that Finland has faced since 2008. This has greatly affected education more than any other public sector. Around 300+ of Finland's municipalities were forced to cut spending, merge schools, increase class sizes, and limit access to professional development and school improvement. But the most harmful consequence of these fiscal constraints is the loss of support staff, classroom assistants, and special education personnel (Heim, 2016). Loveless (2017) accurately portrays this claim by adding, "This is why comparing U.S. test scores with other countries must be done with caution."

Any effective implementation of education reform requires a thorough understanding of the existing system (its strengths, opportunities, and stakeholders and the way they currently affect one another). Healthy economies consist of individuals who have good ideas for new businesses and the ability to grow them and create employment. In 2008, IBM published a survey named, "The Enterprise of the Future" focusing on which characteristics organization leaders need most in their staff. They spoke with fifteen hundred leaders in eighty countries. The two priorities were a*daptability to change and creativity in generating new ideas.* Leaders found that highly qualified graduates were lacking in these very same qualities. Few, if any of the abilities that entrepreneurs need in today's workforce are actually facilitated by our current education model. This leads to a discussion on a vital component of long term happiness— and specifically intrinsic motivation.

The Impact of Intrinsic Motivation

Literature on intrinsic motivation proposes two notions that relate to the impact of rewards on people's lives. The first is a sense of competence and the second is a positive sense of well-being (Csikszentmihalyi, Graef & Gianinno, 2014). In flow, intrinsic motivation is its means of sustainability. Deci and Ryan's (2000) study on intrinsic motivation explains how social context strongly boosts or obstructs a person's social integration in terms of exercising values and responsibilities, "Contexts supportive of autonomy, competence, and relatedness were found to foster greater internalization and integration than contexts that thwart the satisfaction of these needs," (pp.76) reconfirming the fundamental need for social integration within intrinsic motivation.

Among different life activities, a study of the experience of freedom in daily life found sports and games to be highly desirable activities. In both US and Italian teenage groups, students felt the happiest in structured leisure activities like "sports and games" and "art and hobbies," which are both flow-inducing activities (Csikszentmihalyi, Wong 1991). Since structured leisure has also been observed to induce the greatest amount of flow, it is safe to support the claim of Csikszentmihalyi and Graef and Gianinno (2014) that, "If one's daily experiences are more often perceived to be intrinsically rewarding, one ought to feel more happy, confident and self-fulfilled" (pp. 115).

Consider research on East and West coast elementary and junior-high school students, where they have been interviewed about their perceptions of common school learning activities (Block, H. 1984. p. 66). These interviews reveal that students perceive their current assignments, tests, and homework as being work-like and as undermining their emerging sense of self-social competence and self-social determination (Block, H. 1984. p. 66). Such activities suggest that students are incapable of choosing the right substance or form for their work; it must be chosen for them as seen in, "They do not understand their own productive motives; they must be made to engage in work whether they want to or not. And they cannot set and enforce their own standards of learning excellence; these must be set for them (Block, H. 1984. p. 66)." This shows the detrimental effects of an education system that punishes failure instead of celebrating its role in building resilience and informing one's intrinsic motivation.

CONCLUSION

The pursuit of happiness and the experience of flow serve as tools, embodied examples of the innate ability to hone in on quality experience. Csikszentmihalyi (1990) states that one must make a concerted or committed effort to manifest happiness. At the very core of this chapter, the authors believe that anything sustainably worthwhile demands qualities like effort, self-determination, perseverance and discipline.

Flow speaks to the human potential of building perseverance within an engaged activity that merges challenge and skill with enjoyment. This state also allows for the practice of attending to the present moment, a skill critical in today's hyper-stimulated world. Flow creates space for mindful experiences that counterbalance the effects of mindless consumption, boredom, self-absorption, chaos and uncertainty.

The rigid and systematic education system speaks to our potential courage to challenge generational norms based on power dynamics. A creative life is fueled by a willingness to revel in the intricacies or simplicities of life and experience greater purpose. It is vital to nurture this curiosity and playful exploration in children so as to not leave them vulnerable to a mundane life.

This chapter highlights how people are largely responsible for their own happiness, for stress management and engagement in flow and creativity. These interrelated concepts should empower individuals to harness their inner capacity to cultivate flow and happiness in a life they create, not simply to conform to their current life. In fact, empowering individuals with the responsibility to harness their own happiness generates a positive feedback loop that allows happiness to coexist with the realities of everyday challenges.

Children love to soak in wonder and excitement and although it may seem that they are natural born experts in the field of creativity, parents and society at large play a facilitating role in sustaining a child's exploration of the world. By providing them with ways to challenge and inspire existing and new beliefs, we can equip them and ourselves with the right conditions for a meaningful life.

Happiness depends upon ourselves. — Aristotle

REFERENCES

Block, H. (1984). *School Learning Activities More Playlike: Flow and Mastery Learning*. The University of Chicago Press.

Breath, J. (2016). *The Importance of Meditation Breaks for Kids*. Retrieved from https://www.healthychildren.org/English/healthy-living/emotional-wellness/Pages/Just-Breathe-The-Importance-of-Meditation-Breaks-for-Kids.aspx

Butner, D. (2017, November). The World's Happiest Places. *National Geographic: The Search For Happiness*, *232*(5), 30–59.

Carey, B. (2014). *How we learn*. Random House.

Chilcott, L., Birtel, M., & Guggenheim, D. (2010). *Waiting for "Superman"*. Paramount Studios.

Csikszentmihaly, M. (1996). *Creativity Flow and The Psychology of Discovery and Invention*. New York, NY: Harper Collins.

Csikszentmihalyi, M. (1990). *Flow: The psychology of optimal experience*. New York: Harper & Row.

Csikszentmihalyi, M. (2014). *Flow and the foundations of positive psychology* (1st ed.). doi:10.1007/978-94-017-9088-8

Csikszentmihalyi, M., & Csikszentmihalyi, I. (1988). *Optimal Experience: Psychological Studies of Flow in Consciousness*. Cambridge University Press. doi:10.1017/CBO9780511621956

Csikszentmihalyi, M., & Graef, R. (2014). The Experience of Freedom in Daily Life. In *Flow and the Foundations of Positive Psychology*. Dordrecht: Springer. doi:10.1007/978-94-017-9088-8_4

Csikszentmihalyi, M., Montijo, M. N., & Mouton, A. R. (2018). Flow theory: Optimizing elite performance in the creative realm. In S. I. Pfeiffer, E. Shaunessy-Dedrick, M. Foley-Nicpon, & S. I. Pfeiffer (Eds.), *APA Handbook of Giftedness and Talent* (pp. 215–229). Washington, DC: American Psychological Association. doi:10.1037/0000038-014

Csikszentmihalyi, M., & Rathunde, K. (1993). The measurement of flow in everyday life. *Nebraska Symposium on Motivation*, *40*, 57–97. PMID:1340523

Csikszentmihalyi, M., & Wong, M. M.-H. (1991). The situational and personal correlates of happiness: A cross-national comparison. In F. Strack, M. Argyle, & N. Schwarz (Eds.), International series in experimental social psychology, Vol. 21. Subjective well-being: An interdisciplinary perspective (pp. 193-212). Elmsford, NY, US: Pergamon Press.

Deci, E., & Ryan, R. (2000). Self-determination theory and the facilitation of intrinsic motivation, social development, and well-being. *American Psychological Association. Inc.*, *55*(1), 68–67.

Delle Fave, A. (2009). Optimal Experience and Meaning: Which Relationship? *Psihologijske Teme*, 18.

Diener, E., Lucas, R. E., & Scollon, C. N. (2006). Beyond the hedonic treadmill: Revising the adaptation theory of well-being. *The American Psychologist*, *61*(4), 305–314. doi:10.1037/0003-066X.61.4.305 PMID:16719675

Diener, E., & Oishi, S. (2005). *The nonobvious social psychology of happiness.* Taylor Francis.

Evans, S., Ling, M., Hill, B., Rinehart, N., Austin, D., & Sciberras, E. (2007). Systematic review of meditation-based intervention for children with ADHD. *European Child Adolescent Psychiatry, 27*, 9-27.

Galantino, M. L., & Quinn, L. (2008). Therapeutic effects of yoga for children: A systematic review of the literature. *Pediatric Physical Therapy*, *20*(1), 66–80. doi:10.1097/PEP.0b013e31815f1208 PMID:18300936

Gruber, J., Mauss, I., & Tamir, M. (2011). A dark side of happiness? How, when and why happi ness is not always good. *Sage (Atlanta, Ga.)*, *6*(3), 222–233. doi:10.1177/1745691611406927 PMID:26168514

Heim, J. (2016). *Finland's schools were once the envy of the world. Now, they're slipping*. Retrieved from https://www.washingtonpost.com/local/education/finlands-schools-were-once-the-envy-of-the-world-now-theyre-slipping/2016/12/08/dcfd0f56-bd60-11e6-91ee-1adddfe36cbe_story.html

Kahn, D. (2003). Montessori and optimal experience research: Toward building a comprehensive education reform. *The NAMTA Journal*, *28*, 1–9.

Kesebir, P., & Diener, E. (2008). *In pursuit of happiness: Empirical answers to philosophical questions.* Sage Publications, Inc.

Kids & Tech: Tips for Parents in the Digital Age. (2018). Retrieved from https://www.healthychildren.org/English/family-life/Media/Pages/Tips-for-Parents-Digital-Age.aspx

Langer, E. J. (2000). *Mindful learning*. Sage Publications, Inc.

Larsen, J. T., & McKibban, A. R. (2008). *Is happiness having what you want, wanting what you have, or both?* Association for Psychological Science.

Laurent, V., Nidich, S., Wendt, S., Jamie, G., & Nidich, R. (2019). Effect of Meditation on Social- emotional Learning in Middle School Students. *Project Innovation, 139*(3), 111-119.

Lenoir, F. (2015). *Happiness: A Philosopher's Guide*. Brooklyn, NY: Melville House.

Lopez, S., & Snyder, C. (2009). *The oxford handbook of positive psychology* (2nd ed.). Oxford, UK: Oxford University Press.

Lopez, S., & Snyder, C. (2009). *The oxford handbook of positive psychology* (2nd ed.). Oxford, UK: Oxford University Press. doi:10.1093/oxfordhb/9780195187243.001.0001

Loveless, T. (2017). *The 2017 Brown Center Report on American Education: How Well Are American Students Learning?* Brown Center on Education Policy at Brookings. Retrieved from https://www.brookings.edu/wp-content/uploads/2017/03/2017-brown-center-report-on-american-education.pdf

Lyubomirsky, S. (2008). *The how of happiness: A scientific approach to getting the life you want*. New York: Penguin Press.

Lyubomirsky, S., King, L. A., & Diener, E. (2005). The benefits of frequent positive affect: Does happiness lead to success? *Psychological Bulletin*, *131*(6), 803–855. doi:10.1037/0033-2909.131.6.803 PMID:16351326

Lyubomirsky, S., Sheldon, K. M., & Schkade, D. (2005). Pursuing happiness: The architecture of sustainable change. *Review of General Psychology*, *9*(2), 111–113. doi:10.1037/1089-2680.9.2.111

McLeod, M. (2018). *The ultimate happiness: An exclusive interview with the Dalai Lama* (2nd ed.). Lions Roar Foundation.

Meadows, H. D. (2008). *Thinking in Systems: A Primer*. White River Junction, VT: Chelsea Green Publishing Company.

Nakumara, J., & Csikszentmihaly, M. (2009). The concept of flow. In C. R. Snyder & S. J. Lopez (Eds.), *Oxford handbook of positive psychology* (pp. 89–105). Oxford University Press.

Parks, A., Della Porta, M. D., Pierce, R. S., Zilca, R., & Lyubomirsky, S. (2012). Pursuing happiness in everyday life: The characteristics and behaviors of online happiness seekers. *Emotion (Washington, D.C.)*, *12*(6), 1222–1234. doi:10.1037/a0028587 PMID:22642345

Polanczyk, G. V., Willcutt, E. G., Salum, G. A., Kieling, C., & Rohde, L. A. (2014). ADHD prevalence estimates across three decades: An updated systematic review and meta-regression analysis. *International Journal of Epidemiology*, *43*(2), 434–442. doi:10.1093/ije/dyt261 PMID:24464188

Robinson, K., & Aronica, L. (2015). *Creative Schools: The Grassroots Revolution That's Transforming Education*. New York, NY: Viking Penguin.

Seligman, M. E. P., & Csikszentmihalyi, M. (2000). Positive psychology: An introduction. *The American Psychologist*, *55*(1), 5–14. doi:10.1037/0003-066X.55.1.5 PMID:11392865

Shelley, T. (2008). *Health psychology* (7th ed.). New York, NY: McGraw Hill.

Springer Netherlands Csikszentmihalyi, M., Graef, R., & Gianinno, S. M. (2014). Measuring Intrinsic Motivation in Everyday Life. In *Flow and the Foundations of Positive Psychology* (pp. 113–125). Dordrecht: Springer.

The Enterprise of the Future. (n.d.). *IBM 2008 Global CEO Study*. Retrieved from http://globalforum.items-int.com/gf/gf-content/uploads/2014/04/ceostudy2008_fullrep.pdf

Vallerand, R. (2000). Deci and Ryan's Self-Determination Theory: A View from the Hierarchical Model of Intrinsic and Extrinsic Motivation. *Psychological Inquiry*, *11*(4), 312–318. Retrieved from http://www.jstor.org/stable/1449629

Van Ness, P.H. (1999). *Yoga as spiritual but not religious: A pragmatic perspective.* University of Illinois Press.

Zhao, Y. (2012, June 6). *Test Scores vs. Entrepreneurship: PISA, TIMSS, and Confidence*. Retrieved from http://zhaolearning.com/2012/06/06/test-scores-vs-entrepreneurship-pisa-timss-and- confidence/

Zhao, Y. (2017). *What works may hurt: Side effects in Education.* Springer.

KEY TERMS AND DEFINITIONS

Autotelic Personality: Characteristics in personality that enable one to engage in flow activities for the mere enjoyment of the experience; personality traits such as perseverance, curiosity, and low self-absorption.

Creativity: The exploration of generating original ideas and perspectives, which can be implemented into daily living; a willingness to think outside of the box; the ability to create.

Eudemonia: A term originated by the Ancient Greeks as a condition of living well; prosperity.

Feedback Loop: Is a closed chain pattern of cause and effect reaction connections from a stock, activated by decisions, rules, physical laws, or actions.

Flow: A state of consciousness where a person is completely immersed in the present moment while doing something that he/she loves; this state merges optimal experience with a challenge-skill balance and provides multiple benefits to well-being and personal development.

General Self-Efficacy: A personal judgment on how much one believes that he/she can accomplish something.

Happiness: Refers to a subjective experience that can be heightened and sustained through practices that merge pleasure, challenge and purpose (as seen in flow and creativity); a popular term across a variety of realms for its positive influence (seen in culture, government, health, and success).

Hedonic Treadmill: The observed tendency that people return to their average happiness set-point relatively soon after an event takes place, regardless of whether it is a negative or positive situation.

Intrinsic Motivation: A motivation that arises from internal rewards; engaging in a behavior that is naturally pleasurable or satisfying to do.

Mindfulness: The quality of being present in the moment; observing and accepting one's thoughts, feelings, and bodily sensations; a calming and therapeutic technique.

Optimal Experience: An experience that stimulates complex, psychological processes such as motivation and positive emotions.

Perceived Stress: A self-formed awareness on how much stress one is experiencing at any given moment in time; Thoughts and feelings inform perception.

Programme for International Student Assessment (PISA): Every three years, it tests 15-year-old students from all over the world in reading, mathematics and science. The tests are meant to assess how well the students master key subjects. The impact of these international standardized assessments in the field of educational policy has been significant, in terms of the creation of developing new practices, reform in assessment policy, and external influence over national educational policy.

Resilience: The capacity to rapidly recover from a state of difficulty and stress.

System: A group of elements or parts that are organized and interrelated in a pattern of structures that design a specific set of behaviors, often classified as its "function" or "purpose."

Systems Theory: Is an interdisciplinary study of systems that takes a holistic approach to analysis that focuses on the elements within a system, how they interrelate, how they work over time and within the context of larger systems (e.g., natural or man-made).

Trends in International Mathematics and Science Study (TIMSS): Is a series of international assessments of 4th and 8th grade student mathematics and science knowledge. TIMSS Advanced assesses students in the final year of secondary school in advanced mathematics and physics.

APPENDIX

Table 1. Zero-Order Correlations of Age, Total Perceived Stress, General Self-Efficacy and Flow in Diverse Athletes

Measure	1	2	3	4
1. Age	-	-3.07**	.011	.391**
2. Total PSS		-	-.446**	-.246*
3. GSE Total			-	.144
4. Flow Total				-

** Significant at the .01 level

* Significant at the .05 level

Figure 1. Perceived Stress Means and Gender

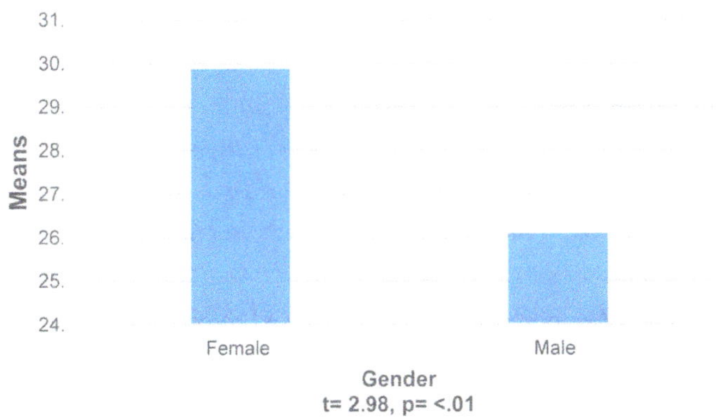

Chapter 2
In the Pursuit of Happiness:
Developing and Sustaining Happiness in Children

Jaclyn Terese Kell
Marymount Manhattan College, USA

ABSTRACT

How can we foster happiness in a child and what happens if it is not done properly? Newborns have to rely on their parents and others to teach them this emotion from the beginning, and there are some that fail to do so. This chapter discusses the theories and methods used in fostering happiness in children from a young age as well as understanding other challenges. Positive psychology, discovered by Martin Seligman, is currently a new industrialized way of catalyzing a more focused view on infusing life with positive qualities. Other topics concerning happiness stem from positive psychology. It is imperative to understand them and consider them throughout a child's life. Children's minds are constantly developing to understand new things around them. Children aren't going to be happy at all times, and there will be moments when they throw tantrums or have other issues. When these moments occur, it is important for parents, teachers, and other adults to handle them the right way.

INTRODUCTION

Understanding Happiness

The idea of happiness and being happy can range from good health, enjoying time with family, or maintaining a prosperous career. The concept of happiness over the

DOI: 10.4018/978-1-7998-2940-9.ch002

past decade has received a lot of attention among researchers (Aaker, Kamvar, and Mogilner, 2012). Psychologists and other scholars have worked to establish the best way to increase, measure, and understand why happiness is so important (Aaker et al., 2012). Happiness is an important individual goal for most, and it's interesting to think that our understanding of how to pursue this happiness, for the most part, has stemmed from media, parents, and peers (O'Brien, 2008). The meaning of this term has a variety of definitions depending on the individual. For individuals who are much older, the concept of happiness has most likely already been accessed and implemented in different ways throughout their lives.

From a very young age, children progress and learn from parental figures in their life and from those around them. Happiness during infancy and childhood may be just as critical as happiness during adulthood for predicting future success and well-being (Coffey, 2019). First however, it is important to consider how to foster this kind of positive emotion in children. When asking a child the meaning of happiness, a child may offer a diverse set of responses compared to an already developed adult. There are psychological determinants that can play a role. Research suggests that childhood happiness is associated with strong social capabilities and healthy behaviors. Those who struggle to achieve happiness experience greater difficulty contending with stress and forging relationships (Batcho, 2019). Fostering happiness in children at a young age can result in various positive outcomes, while failing to nurture happiness, can result in negative consequences. Happiness today is an ongoing subject and is judged by what we experience every day. This emotion sustains life and is not only a consequence of success, but also a cause of it (Perez-Alvarez, 2016). What is it about happiness that is so critical from the beginning, and how does it affect one's future?

Subjective Happiness and Choices

The meaning of happiness is personal for each individual, and researchers suggest that there are many definitions for this emotion. There are two emotional-based subjects that when felt can be recognized as happiness. *High arousal positive affect qualities* include exhilaration, elation, and eagerness. *Low arousal positive affect qualities* include tranquility, peacefulness, and serenity. These are all affirmative emotions, and they can manifest differently depending on the individual. Age is a factor that has been influential in determining if individuals prefer high or low arousals of happiness. From a blog-based data examination, there tends to be a steady shift in happiness wherein individuals transform from excited to peaceful happiness as they age. *Temporal focus* can be used as a more basic psychological factor when discussing age and happiness. Temporal focus refers to how an individual views and thinks about the past, present and future. Younger individuals have a broad future ahead of them, and as they age, their view of what's ahead of them becomes less vast. This concept is defined as a temporal focus, wherein an individual's attention is set more on current events and on what's happening now and so other than age, one's understanding of happiness may expand from this principal of temporal focus. Age is a useful signal of someone's temporal focus, and could regulate whether happiness is supplementary with high or low arousal based on future or present moments. An individual's temporal focus likely aligns with whether the emotion will be experienced as happiness that manifests as excitement or as a sense of calm. The foundation of building on these meanings of happiness allows researchers to investigate a temporal focus and to determine how these forms of pleasure influence the choices of others (Aaker et al., 2012).

Research has shown that an individual's cognitive processing can be affected by positive moods and can therefore influence decision-making. When individuals are in a positive state of mind, they tend to think more creatively when solving a problem and are more optimistic, as well. Positively-minded individuals also tend to make choices that are less risky and tend to provide more options when making more direct decisions. Individuals, who are happier, also tend to make healthier choices in their private lives. The choices one makes are affected by one's definition of happiness and so defining happiness as exciting motivates someone to choose an exciting option over a calm one. Those who are older tend to be influenced by emotional interactions and tend to be persuaded by more meaningful views. Compared to those who are younger, those who are older crave more novel interactions that are modern, fresh, and new. From this information, it is hypothesized that an individual, who is more focused on the future rather than on the present, will regulate which type of happiness is accepted (Aaker et al., 2012)

Positive Psychology

Martin Seligman, born in 1942, is known as the pioneer of Positive Psychology because of how he was able to use specific scientific approaches to investigate how happiness and other positive qualities are cultivated (Pursuit of Happiness, 2019). This approach can be defined as an existential and substantiated way of thinking in an area of research and training (Carr, 2012). This is also a way of examining constructive character personalities and affirmative emotions (Seligman and Steen et al., 2005). The field of psychology has predominantly focused on suffering since World War II. Psychologists now measure concepts such as depression and schizophrenia with reasonable accuracy. Positive Psychology, however, diverges from traditional aspects of psychology such as mental health disorders, trauma, and anger (Seligman 2004). The purpose of research in positive psychology is to create a balance and to garner a more overall comprehensive understanding of the human experience, of disorders, and feebleness (Seligman and Steen et al., 2005). In Seligman's scientific study of Positive Psychology, he evaluates and expands on three different happy lives that relate to three desires (Seligman, 2004). Each of these realms is measurable, can be taught, and is skill-based (Seligman, Ernst, Gillham, Reivich, Linkins, 2009). These realms are called *The Pleasant Life*, *The Good Life*, and *The Meaningful Life* (Seligman, 2004).

Three Realms

The Pleasant Life encompasses positive emotions such as affection, delight, and pleasure in which one's life involves as many wholesome things as conceivable (Seligman & Ernst et al., 2009). Next, *The Good Life* exemplifies affirmative qualities such as strength, but also other aspects like vigor and knowledge (Seligman, 2004). The Good Life involves a state of flow, which is very similar to what Aristotle pursued in his works (Seligman and Ernst et al., 2009). This flow is something that facilitates learning and occurs when an individual is able to utilize strength and intelligence to conquer any challenge that is encountered (Seligman and Ernst et al., 2009). Finally, *The Meaningful Life* relates to positive intuition; including elements like family and democracy (Seligman, 2004). The individuals others are surrounded by, connections with individuals, and future generations are what increase meaning in an individual's life (Seligman and Ernst et al. 2009). These three different concepts all allow psychologists to glean a better understanding of these positive emotions throughout life.

While Martin Seligman focused on Positive Psychology at all different ages, another researcher, Dr. Tal Ben-Shahar, a professor at Harvard University, explains how Positive Psychology can also be useful to aid individuals at younger ages. Often psychology's approach has been simply to ask what is initially wrong with a child and then to analyze the problem and find an efficient answer. Positive Psychology offers a different approach in which more in-depth questions are presented to examine the conditions that allow children to thrive. This method is beneficial in order to encourage children to prosper rather than to focus on more problematic areas. The purpose of Positive Psychology is to allow individuals to perceive situations in life from both positive and negative perspectives. Often negative emotions tend to shut people down, but positive feelings help to create more of a successful and determined life style. Dr. Tal Ben-Shahar shares that "Positive emotions don't make us blind to life's hardship. They are the fuel which enables us to go out and do good in the world (Greenville- Cleave, 2014)." Happiness is critical since it offers significant results and encourages individuals to give the most in life to receive the most positive outcomes (Greenville- Cleave, 2014).

Negatives of Positive Psychology

Those who support Positive Psychology argue that traditional psychology, in general, mainly focuses on the negative characteristics of life. As a result, there tends to be a lack of focus on theories of human understanding that pertain to joy and success. However, Richard Lazarus, a well-known psychologist, has voiced opinions on procedural matters that have plagued Positive Psychology. He states that the Positive Psychology Movement has depicted a miserable image of what it means to be human by grossly exaggerating tragic components of life and failing to include them. He contends that Positive Psychology ironically disregards the productive expansions that could increase pain and loss for humans and that there is not enough attention given to the parts of human life like trauma and death, which are important factors in a person's existence. He suggests that someone must first experience profound anguish in order to understand more meaningful human emotions. Lazarus is implying that suffering major loss allows the most positive aspects of human existence to materialize. He believes that Positive Psychology stresses positive emotions so excessively that other factors like grief and loss are dismissed. Aligned with this critique of Positive Psychology, it is shown that solely implementing positive emotions isn't enough for a human to experience true happiness. Damage and grief act as stimulants to growth and teach others how to give back from experiencing these negative feelings. It can be challenging to balance the existing focus on the positive and negative elements of life (Harvey and Pauwels, 2003).

Benefits of Happiness

Positive emotion counters the out-group homogeneousness effect and allows others to have a more affirmative outlook. Having an increased optimistic feeling pushes one toward enhanced affiliation and social outcomes. Additionally, individuals are able to shift their attention to novel stimuli by enabling intellectual flexibility, and as a result their attentiveness is directed toward more rewarding thought processes. Evidence suggests that increased positive emotion improves one's physical and mental health. One study in particular showed that enhanced happiness improved psychological health and decreased depressive symptoms. Experiencing reduced negative emotions and more positive emotions yields lower risks of psychological disorders like schizophrenia and anxiety. Reducing these negative emotions also help an individual decrease diagnoses of severe heart disease and other major health conditions (Gruber and Mauss et al. 2003).

Positive Emotion

When individuals are aware of a situation, they evaluate it in relation to their desires and values, and then proceed to respond to that situation using certain emotions (Quoidbach, Mikolajczak, & Gross, 2015). Within the framework of positive psychology, positive emotion plays an important role. Joy, happiness, and serenity are some examples of positive emotions that signal action and cognitive suppleness (Bai, Repetti, and Sperling, 2015). Positive emotion is thought to be extremely beneficial in achieving success with mental health and psychological growth, as well. Studies have shown that individuals who engage more in family activities are goal-oriented and pursue more interests to increase their positive emotions and happiness (Quoidbach, Mikolajczak, & Gross, 2015). In 1998, a woman named Barbara Fredrickson introduced *The Broaden-and-Build Theory.* This theory introduced the notion that positive emotions help individuals attain long-term social and substantial resources that are imperative for subsistence (Simon-Thomas and Keltner, et al 2017). Given this theory, unlike negative emotions, which narrow a person's thoughts making it hard to adapt, positive emotions are able to expand individuals' actions in a healthier way (Quoidbach, Mikolajczak, & Gross, 2015).

Fostering these happy and positive feelings within children at a young age promotes success. During infancy, happiness is measured by investigating positive and negative frequencies. These independent concepts are adaptive resolutions rather than falling on one cohesive range. Often within younger children, positive and negative emotions can occur simultaneously (Coffey, 2019). For instance, children might be upset when their parents leave them with a babysitter, but are then happy again when they return. Using the Broaden-and-Build Theory, which links happiness to success, experiencing these positive reactions allows individuals to construct resources to use later in life. Focusing principally on the stages of infancy and childhood, these positive effects have indicated higher rates of social, problem solving, and creative skills (Coffey, 2019). The regulation of positive emotions is often shaped by the environment of the child. Within the earliest stages of childhood, family upbringing plays an important role in fostering these emotions. Parents can promote these positive arousals in their children by being receptive to their needs, helping them problem solve, and by creating a validating and constructive atmosphere (Tan & Smith, 2018).

Self and Emotional Regulation

Researchers have considered a conceptual model based on the transmission of self and emotional regulation from parents to child (Tan & Smith, 2018). This kind of emotional regulation is when individuals are able to influence their feelings based on when they have them and how they can be expressed. Many of the studies on regulating positive emotions have focused on how increasing these emotions can be used to repair negative emotions (Quoidbach, Mikolajczak, & Gross, 2015). Other research has shown that creating positive situations and using humor are able to alleviate negative moods. Being able to increase these regulatory emotions has recently been successful at improving happiness. In a 2012 study, Jose et al. found that these positive regulation approaches, when facilitated and controlled, had positive effects on fostering a cheerful disposition. Using these strategies has not only regulated happiness but has contributed to higher self-esteem and life satisfaction (Quoidbach et al., 2015).

Mothers, in particular, are responsible for modeling emotional expressions and socialization with their children. A study conducted by Bridgett et al. (2015) focuses on how a mother's regulated emotions connect to a child's. Children often use something called *effortful control*, which is how they are able to prevent certain responses and perceive errors. Effortful control is described as the capability to refrain from a central, dominant reaction to perform a subdominant response. Relevant to this concept, children are more likely to exhibit a higher level of positive emotion when mothers are able to do the same. During a computerized distress task geared toward maternal emotional regulation, a mother's capability to tolerate grief was associated with how her young daughter reacted to the same situation. From these results, mothers who contributed more emotion had children who exhibited a similar emotional response. This establishes a correlation between maternal and child emotion regulation. Implementing these positive features within a child's life at an early age is imperative, especially when employing strategies like reappraisal. Reappraisal can be defined as a way of altering the route of a certain emotional reaction before an emotional incentive can be triggered. This is essential since it fosters more positive emotions, rather than negative. For instance, when children receive a good grade on a test, a parent might buy them ice cream in order to connect a good grade with something positive and enjoyable, like sweets (Tan & Smith, 2018).

Overall, a positive emotional climate within families is a powerful mechanism in order to promote happy feelings within children (Tan & Smith, 2018). It's critical to understand how certain family dynamics are able to foster positive expressions. Communicating among adults and sharing pleasantries with one another has been expressed as an interactive strategy that can further extend positive emotions (Bai et al., 2015). Denham et al. (1997) discovered that children of parents, who use more positive reactions rather than negative, were happier with other peers at two to six years of age. This suggests that in terms of emotional regulation, children were more responsive to parents who displayed a greater number of positive emotions over negative emotions (Tan & Smith, 2018).

Introducing Physical Happiness

The sense of touch is able to trigger positive and happy feelings among children. Affection such as hugs, kisses, and cuddling are just a few examples of how physical affection can be practiced. This social performance corresponds to positive forms of emotions from parent to child. Studies have shown that supportive physical contact with a parent or other paternal figures regulates bodily reactivity to acute sensors in children. As a child grows older from infancy to early childhood, there can be significant changes in how the parent displays this affection. As an example, parents might refrain from kissing their older children in public to avoid embarrassing them (Bai et al., 2015).

Conducting leisurely activities can also promote these constructive reactions. Mothers, who pursue interactions like peek-a-boo and face-to-face play with their infants, stimulate and prolong their infants' sense of happiness. Among younger and older children in school, in particular, these displays of affirmative emotions increase with active peer involvement in activities At home, family members can assume the role of a peer or playmate by conducting face-to-face interactions such as coloring with children or teaching them how to ride a bike. From these events, parents are able to engage with their child and to manifest enjoyment (Bai et al. 2015). These actions and behaviors that are rife with positive emotions are likely to be repeated with children as a way to encourage them to be more social within their environment (Akinin, Hamlin, and Dunn 2012). This may include moments such as comforting another child in order to make him/her feel happier or to help a peer reach a specific goal.

Facial Cues

Something as simple as smiling is a reaction and behavior that is closely linked with happiness. When someone smiles, he/she is using almost ten different facial muscles, and this is a complex expression that many humans use to interact with one another, especially parents to children. It is hypothesized that when children smile, that facial signal reduces stress and promotes positive behavior. According to biosocial models, this exchange of happiness between child and parent helps develop a stronger affirmative bond. The importance of fostering these happy cues in children through these positive levels of expression can also function as cues for healthy development. Furthermore, children who are happier tend to be met with a higher level of care and playfulness from their parents, such as playing catch or painting (Franklin & Volk, 2017).

Accurately decoding these facial expressions is critical since parental empathy is linked to the emotional well-being of children. A child's non-verbal behavior is an important emotional cue. For younger children whose negative emotions and verbal abilities are not yet developedm this non-verbal behavior is a principal channel for socialization. Studies have examined children's ability to decode distinctive facial cues. In Bucks (1975) experiment with role-playing theory, children were better at decoding the emotions of happiness than more negative emotions like fear and anger. Focusing on the encoding aspect of non-verbal communication, all age groups improved their ability to decode anger at ten and eleven, while their ability to decode happiness stayed constant. Parents interact more with their children using social skills theory and learning theory compared to those who don't have children. These theories would suggest that the accuracy of decoding these facial cues is different between parents and non-parents (Feinman & Feldman, 2019).

In the development and preservation of social competence, the regulation of one's emotions plays an important role, including the capability to retain applicable parenting conduct. Interpersonal conflict and aggression are thought to be associated with an emotional regulation shortage, which also includes problems in parental actions. When child abuse is present, parents experience emotional recognition deficits when it comes to viewing children's facial emotions. Research has shown that emotional recognition, aggression, and social competence are complex. Emotion recognition accuracy has been linked to the development of social competence in children and other emotional acknowledgment variances have been related to aggression. From this information, it is understood that children who are aggressive are likely to be angrier and because of this general emotion recognition accuracy, they will likely display aggressive behavior. In relation to parental behavior, parents, who have issues with emotional recognition accuracy will relay verbal and physical abuse toward children. According to the model of child physical abuse known as social information processing, parents who are physically abusive, compared to non-abusive parents, are less attentive to their children's conduct. This can then lead to issues in decoding the child's emotional well-being. This lack of identification can result in neglect and can damage a child's overall happiness in the future (Wagner and Milner, 2014).

Children and Stages

According to Alice Honig, Susan Miller, and Ellen Church (2019), authors of the article entitled *Happiness Along,* adults can recognize and reciprocate actions that make children happy. The first stage is "peek-a- boo" starting from birth to age two. A child at 7 months, raises a blanket up and down in front of his/her face and a parent or teacher might respond by saying "peek-a-boo." This warm, high- pitched response is called "parentese" or "motherese," which conveys joy and happiness towards the child even though the child may not have understood the words the parent is conveying. It's also important for parents and other adults to be aware and notice when a baby is performing a new task so that they can reinforce it with happy feelings. Rocking and stroking a child's back is also a source of reinforcement since children love the kinesthetic stimulation from physical touch (Honig et al., 2019).

At ages three and four, toddlers find a different source of satisfaction through playing with other children. They also however, still crave the additional affection of being held by a parent or simply experiencing the extra reassurance. Boosting independence is also a way to make children feel happy. If babies signal that they want to try and feed themselves, it is recommended that parents provide them with the opportunity to do so. This provides additional validation for the child and encourages him/her to try new skills. When children feel that they are being loved and that their parents are attuned to their needs- a child feels happy. It's often the smallest things that trigger a child's joyful emotions, such as receiving small treats after accomplishing a task or having an opportunity to play games (Honig et al., 2019).

Children enjoy creating social relationships with teachers, parents, and peers since their self-esteem is boosted when they feel valued by others. For instance, preschoolers have a desire to please their teachers, so they feel happy being "little helpers" and doing things such as cleaning things up in the classroom. By accomplishing these tasks, children begin to develop a sense of independence and content gratification. There will be moments when children experience frustration and temperament issues, and managing these situations effectively is critical. Taking time to discuss the issue and help children ease their way back into that comforting and happy mindset may not always be easy, but it's the effort and persistence that counts and pays off (Honig et al., 2019).

Kindergarteners, aged five to six, have the amazing ability to express their own thoughts and opinions to others. This is probably one of most stimulating developmental changes that occurs because of how extensive their language capabilities have become. A new toy may be great for toddlers, but for children who are a little older, their happiness originates from forging relationships and from other achievements. They crave interaction and love from those around them as a source of comfort, as well. Research has shown that when a child is able to communicate thoughts and feelings in relationships that they have developed at home and at school, they are able to have more success in the educational environment. Creating these friendships is important in order for children to feel comfortable enough to express themselves in a safe environment (Honig et al., 2019).

Happiness and Education

Fundamentally, an educational environment is perceived by many as a place where children are able to feel safe and a place for them to gain support and assistance from teachers when needed. Jennifer Pepe is a child psychologist at Mary Durand

Elementary School in Vineland, New Jersey. She has observed and seen the effects of how happiness can affect a child within different environments. Durand Elementary is home to many students that come from lower income settings (J. Pepe, personal communication, May 28, 2019). The parents of these children are often separated or raised by other relatives. This can make for a very unstable environment in which emotional, physical, and verbal abuse can occur (J. Pepe, personal communication, May 28 2019). In other situations, the parent of a child is currently in jail or abusing drugs. For most students, their family life doesn't seem to affect their overall emotions at all, and for others it has a significant consequence. Students who often start fights or bully others perceive it as a way for them to alleviate the anger and fear they experience at home (Jennifer Pepe, personal communication, May 28, 2019).

Fostering happiness in children can make or break them as they grow up and can also impact those around them (Jennifer Pepe, personal communication, May 8, 2019). Pepe has dealt with many cases in which a child lives in an abusive household. These students often have trouble staying focused in the classroom or tend to cause problems with other peers (Jennifer Pepe, personal communication, May 28, 2019). Pepe also explained how some students have been victimized by sexual abuse by family members, as well. This trauma has a great effect on a child's view of the world in terms of not being able to trust other adults (Jennifer Pepe, personal communication, May 28, 2019). Certain physical and sexual abuse like this can also cause a child to sometimes defend his/her abuser, especially if it is a parent (Jennifer Pepe, personal communication, May 28, 2019). The child feels attached and a sense of loyalty towards the abuser regardless of what he/she has been through (Jennifer Pepe, personal communication, May 28, 2019). Pepe observed that children, who don't receive these positive affirmations, find happiness in other areas. At school, a child became very possessive of a coloring book and when the teacher tried to take it away, this student became aggressive (Jennifer Pepe, personal communication, May 28, 2019). The child had developed this association to happiness with an object, and when this object was taken away, so was his/her happiness (Jennifer Pepe, personal communication, May 28, 2019).

A variety of research studies have looked at the relationship between infant happiness in relation to childhood IQ and educational attainment. These happiness levels in children have been related to cognitive abilities associated with success. A variety of studies have suggested that there is an association with the positive and negative affect of environmental factors. Significant circumstantial improvements within a child's environment, such as moving from an orphanage to a stable home, have been related to higher levels of educational attainment and a higher IQ. This research also proposes that it is critical to understand the roles of positive and negative affect from analysts of scholastic accomplishment. Factors such as a parent's socioeconomic status, occupation, and marital status are important because they can affect a child's success. Parents, who are from a higher socioeconomic status, are able to provide their children with better resources such as tutoring and private schooling compared to parents from a lower socioeconomic status. Those who have a higher educational attainment might benefit from more positive success and from a happier well-being (Coffey, 2019).

Child's Well-Being

Positive moods and a happier sense of wellbeing among children appear synergistic with enhanced education. Studies have revealed that there have been increases in depression and a lower development of happiness over time, which is why exposing these constructive emotions is so critical. Well-being, overall, promotes more creative and analytical thinking, as opposed to negative moods which can narrow one's attention. Within an educational environment, teaching happiness provides students with the opportunity to reach life satisfaction and to enhance their well-being on a broader scale. Children and young adults spend much of their time at school, which offers a number of well-being initiatives. Statistically in the Unites States, children from ages 6-17, spend around 30-35 hours per week in school. Having these everyday positive interactions among teachers, students, and other staff members, is important for assuring a child's well-being. Enforcing this positive well-being at home and at school allows children to improve their behavior, and overall to engage more extensively in learning (Seligman & Ernst, 2019).

Sustainable Happiness and Education

As discussed previously, Positive Psychology and happiness research have uncovered many additional findings throughout the years: happiness also contributes tremendously towards sustainability. This development has prompted the idea that social, environmental, and economic factors are symbiotic. The concept of sustainable happiness proposes that happiness has a local, global, and positive impact on individuals in the present and future. For individuals, the most challenging aspect is to recognize how to pursue this happiness throughout their lives. Every definition of happiness is relevant to sustainable happiness. On a daily basis. people make choices that affect their happiness and the happiness of others, as well. For instance, if parents, who are alcoholics, show up to their jobs late and intoxicated, which results in their getting fired, this might cause them to get angry and to potentially take their anger out on their children (O'Brien, 2008).

Our understanding of what happiness is originates from everything around us such as family, friends, books, and media. Nodding says that, "Happiness should be an aim of education, and a good education should contribute significantly to a personal and collective happiness" (O'Brien, 2008). At Cape Breton University, Catherin O'Brien teaches a course in which her students are challenged to identify which barriers exists when they leave a legacy of sustainable happiness. Having this type of knowledge is important, especially for young adults, where the goal is to create happiness literacy through which students can better appreciate certain values. Individuals are able to use the concept of sustainable happiness to direct their everyday actions. When fostering happiness in children, introducing sustainable happiness is a concept that is able to guide certain decisions that are being made. This also allows them to consider indicators like social and environmental well-being so that there is stability between happiness and community. When higher levels of satisfaction are being supported by guidelines and behavior, sustainable happiness seems to be consistent and reinforces this relationship (O' Brien 2008).

CONCLUSION

In conclusion, the meaning of happiness is personal for each individual, and there are many versions of this emotion, as well (Aaker et al., 2012). Younger individuals have a broad future ahead of them and as they get older their outlook becomes less extensive. This means that their attention is more set on current events and on understanding more about their own well-being (Aaker et al., 2012). From a very young age, children progress and learn through parental figures in their life and from others around them. Happiness during infancy and childhood is just as important as happiness during adulthood for indicating the potential for future success and well-being (Coffey, 2019). From aforementioned topics, fostering happiness in children can be accomplished through various methods. Understanding Positive Psychology and positive emotions is beneficial in order to ensure that children thrive rather than to focus on the areas in which they struggle. Often negative emotions tend to shut children down, but positive feelings help to create more of a successful and determined life style (Greenville- Cleave 2014). Parents, in particular, play an important role in fostering happiness in children. Being attentive to a child and making sure that he/she feels loved and appreciated, creates a strong foundation. Also offering physical affection like hugs and kisses, as well as positive facial cues, model positive engagement for the child

Within an educational environment, it's important for children to enjoy learning and to feel safe. Many children who come from challenging home environments have a hard time displaying positive emotions. Not many teachers have an opportunity to see or understand what it's like for children who don't receive the proper care they deserve. A lack of happiness within a child can have many adverse outcomes such as lashing out at other students or not being able to trust adults. This is why it's important for teachers to take the time to understand each child and to do what they can to help promote more happiness in their students' lives. Furthermore, informative research on happiness has discussed the association between happiness and childhood IQ and educational attainment. Aligned with these findings, happiness levels have been associated with cognitive abilities associated with success. Significant circumstantial improvements within a child's environment such as moving from an orphanage to a stable home have yielded high levels of educational improvement and higher IQ (Coffey, 2019). As explained, fostering happiness has a plethora of benefits and it is important to always foster happiness throughout a child's life. That is why introducing sustainable happiness is a concept that is able to guide certain decisions that can affect one's life in the present and future. This also allows children to consider indicators like social and environmental well-being so that there is stability between happiness and community (O'Brien 2008). Happiness expands far beyond an emotional level. There are so many physical and cognitive aspects of happiness that help a child along in developing this emotion the right way and, in the process, passing that same joy on to others in the process.

REFERENCES

Akinin, L. B., Hamlin, J. K., & Dunn, E. W. (2012). Giving Leads to Happiness in Young Children. *PLoS One*, *7*(6), e39211. doi:10.1371/journal.pone.0039211 PMID:22720078

Alan, C. (2012). Psychiatric Rehabilitation Journal. *Trustees of Boston University.*, *35*(4), 335–358. doi:10.2975/35.42012.355.358

Bai, S., Repetti, R. L., & Sperling, J. B. (2016). Children's expressions of positive emotion are sustained by smiling, touching, and playing with parents and siblings: A naturalistic observational study of family life. *Developmental Psychology*, *52*(1), 88–101. doi:10.1037/a0039854 PMID:26524382

Coffey, J. K. (2019). *Cascades of infant happiness: Infant positive affect predicts childhood IQ and adult educational attainment. Emotion.* Retrieved from https://slb.mmm.edu:2208/10.1037/emo0000640

Feinman, J., & Feldman, R. (1982). Decoding Children's Expressions of Affect. *Child Development*, *53*(3), 710–716. doi:10.2307/1129384

Franklin, P., & Volk, A. A. (2018). A review of infants' and children's facial cues' influence on adults' perceptions and behaviors. *Evolutionary Behavioral Sciences*, *12*(4), 296–321. doi:10.1037/ebs0000108

Gruber, J., Mauss, I., & Tamir, M. (2011). A Dark Side of Happiness? How, When, and Why Happiness Is Not Always Good. *Perspectives on Psychological Science*, *6*(3), 222–233. doi:10.1177/1745691611406927 PMID:26168514

Happiness, C. (n.d.). *More Than Just Child's Play*. Retrieved from https://www.psychologytoday.com/us/blog/longing-nostalgia/201201/childhood-happiness-more-just-childs-play

Harvey, J., & Pauwels, B. (2003). The Ironies of Positive Psychology. *Psychological Inquiry*, *14*(2), 125–128. Retrieved from http://www.jstor.org/stable/1449818

Honig, Miller, & Church. (2019). *Ages & Stages: Helping Happiness Along*. Retrieved from https://www.scholastic.com/teachers/articles/teaching-content/ages-stages-helping-happiness-along/

Lazarus, R. (2003). Does the Positive Psychology Movement Have Legs? *Psychological Inquiry*, *14*(2), 93–109. doi:10.1207/S15327965PLI1402_02

Mogilner, C., Aaker, J., & Kamvar, S. (2012). How Happiness Affects Choice. *The Journal of Consumer Research*, *39*(2), 429–443. doi:10.1086/663774

O'Brien, C. (2008). Sustainable happiness: How happiness studies can contribute to a more sustainable future. *Canadian Psychology*, *49*(4), 289–295. doi:10.1037/a0013235

Pérez-Álvarez, M. (2016). The science of happiness: As felicitous as it is fallacious. *Journal of Theoretical and Philosophical Psychology*, *36*(1), 1–19. doi:10.1037/teo0000030

Quoidbach, J., Mikolajczak, M., & Gross, J. J. (2015). Positive interventions: An emotion regulation perspective. *Psychological Bulletin*, *141*(3), 655–693. doi:10.1037/a0038648 PMID:25621978

Seligman, M. (2004). Can Happiness Be Taught? *Daedalus*, *133*(2), 80–87. doi:10.1162/001152604323049424

SeligmanM. (n.d.). Retrieved from https://www.pursuit-of-happiness.org/history-of-happiness/martin-seligman-psychology/

Seligman, M., Ernst, R., Gillham, J., Reivich, K., & Linkins, M. (2009). Positive education: Positive psychology and classroom interventions. *Oxford Review of Education*, *35*(3), 293–311. doi:10.1080/03054980902934563

Seligman, M. E. P., Steen, T. A., Park, N., & Peterson, C. (2005). Positive Psychology Progress: Empirical Validation of Interventions. *The American Psychologist*, *60*(5), 410–421. doi:10.1037/0003-066X.60.5.410 PMID:16045394

Shiota, M. N., Campos, B., Oveis, C., Hertenstein, M. J., Simon-Thomas, E., & Keltner, D. (2017). Beyond happiness: Building a science of discrete positive emotions. *The American Psychologist*, *72*(7), 617–643. doi:10.1037/a0040456 PMID:29016167

Tan, L., & Smith, C. L. (2018). *Intergenerational transmission of maternal emotion regulation to child emotion regulation: Moderated mediation of maternal positive and negative emotions. Emotion*. Retrieved from https://slb.mmm.edu:2208/10.1037/emo0000523

Temperament: Temperamental Effortful Control (Self-Regulation). (n.d.). Retrieved from http://www.child-encyclopedia.com/temperament/according-experts/temperamental-effortful-control-self-regulation

The Science of a Meaningful Life. (n.d.). Retrieved from https://greatergood.berkeley.edu/

The Science of Happiness – Tal Ben-Shahar. (n.d.). Retrieved from https://positivepsychologynews.com/news/bridget-grenville-cleave/2014080629622

Wagner, M. F., Milner, J. S., McCarthy, R. J., Crouch, J. L., McCanne, T. R., & Skowronski, J. J. (2015). Facial emotion recognition accuracy and child physical abuse: An experiment and a meta-analysis. *Psychology of Violence*, *5*(2), 154–162. Retrieved from https://slb.mmm.edu:2208/10.1037/a0036014

KEY TERMS AND DEFINITIONS

Cognitive Processing: The function of mental activity, thinking, remembering, and acting.

Emotional Regulation: A response to certain experiences in a sufficient manner using a variety of emotions.

Foster: To encourage and nurture, develop.

Framework: Format or structure that supports a theory.

Parentese: "Baby talk," parents expressing high pitched and repetitive words to gain a reaction from a child.

Physical Affection: Developmental or nurturing actions exchanged between people such as hugging, kissing, and cuddling.

Positive Emotion: Lacking negative feeling and having a sense of joy, happiness, and serenity.

Positive Psychology: An existential and substantiated way of thinking in an area of research, studying constructive personalities, and affirmative emotion.

Stimulants: An element or something that raises levels of bodily or psychological activity.

Sustainable Happiness: Happiness that extends further towards the environment, community, and future individuals.

Temporal Focus: How an individual views and thinks about the past, present and future.

Wellbeing: Positive feelings, happiness, gaining a sense of personal growth, and having purpose in life.

Chapter 3
How Children Fail:
Exploring Parent and Family Factors That Foster Grit

Emily Hotez
UCLA Center for Healthier Children, Families, and Communities, USA

ABSTRACT

In recent years, there has been widespread interest across both the research and public sectors in understanding how to promote children's lifelong success in a range of domains. While a focus on promoting success in children remains salient, equally salient in the research is how children fail—specifically, how children prevail in the face of failure, adversity, and other challenges over time. The chapter explores parenting and family factors that predict grit. This chapter investigates a range of parenting and family factors, including demographic characteristics, parenting behaviors and styles, and family cultural and environmental factors. Based on this research, the chapter provides overarching recommendations to researchers seeking to understand grit in a family context.

INTRODUCTION

In 2012, Dr. Paul Tough published the renowned book, "How Children Succeed: Grit, Curiosity, and the Hidden Power of Character," contributing to widespread interest in why "some children succeed, while others fail" across the research and public sectors. In this book, Tough synthesized research that emphasizes the critical role of "character" in child development, which catalyzed efforts among families, practitioners, and researchers to explore the mechanisms underlying character

DOI: 10.4018/978-1-7998-2940-9.ch003

development and how children succeed more broadly. While Dr. Tough's focus on promoting success in children remains salient, equally salient is how children *fail*—specifically, how children prevail in the face of failure, adversity, and other challenges over time.

The purpose of this chapter is to explore parenting and family factors that predict a key element of character— grit, i.e., "perseverance and passion for long-term goals" (Duckworth, Peterson, Matthews, & Kelly, 2007), a construct that has been substantially developed and explored by Dr. Angela Duckworth. This chapter will provide a rationale for the importance of grit; review research on parenting practices and aspects of families' environment that may promote grit in children; and synthesize findings to provide overarching recommendations to families, professionals, and researchers. Specifically, this chapter will address the following objectives:

- Review the research on grit across developmental contexts to underscore its significance in the empirical research and highlight the rationale for exploring predictors of grit;
- Investigate the role of specific parenting characteristics in predicting children's grit, including demographic characteristics and parenting behaviors and styles;
- Explore the impact of broader family factors in promoting grit, including cultural, socioeconomic, and environmental factors; and
- Provide overarching recommendations to researchers interested in understanding and cultivating grit in the family context.

BACKGROUND

Rationale for Investigating Grit

The last decade has witnessed an emergence of numerous research studies on grit, defined as "perseverance and passion for long-term goals" (Duckworth, Peterson, Matthews, & Kelly, 2007). Grit has garnered widespread attention, largely due to the finding that it accounts for an average of four percent of the variance in lifetime success outcomes and has been found to be more predictive of success than traditional measures of IQ. Moreover, research has found that outcomes associated with grit are wide-ranging and diverse. Grit has been found to be predictive of numerous educational outcomes, including educational attainment in adults, grade point average among Ivy League undergraduates, and ranking in the National Spelling Bee (Duckworth, Peterson, Matthews, & Kelly, 2007). In addition, grit has been identified as an important predictor of professional success due to its role in predicting retention in

United States Military Academy West Point cadets, success among entrepreneurs, and overall career decision self-efficacy (Duckworth, Peterson, Matthews, & Kelly, 2007; Mooradian, Matzler, Uzelac, & Bauer, 2016; Vela, Sparrow, Whittenberg, & Rodriguez, 2018).

Further, the implications of grit extend far beyond educational or professional success, predicting a range of non-cognitive skills including the Big Five conscientiousness component, forgiveness, and positive well-being (Arya & Lal, 2018; Duckworth, Peterson, Matthews, & Kelly, 2007; Walker, 2017). In fact, Eskreis-Winkler, Duckworth, Shulman, & Beal (2014) investigated "the grit effect" by exploring grit in four contexts: the military, the workplace, high school, and marriage. This study found that grit was a more effective predictor of retention in these contexts than more traditional predictors of retention, including intelligence, physical aptitude, the Big Five personality traits, and job tenure.

Measuring Grit and Related Constructs

As context, grit is primarily assessed through Angela Duckworth's twelve-item (Grit-O) and eight-item (Grit-S) self-report scales and these are the primary measures of grit applied across the majority of research studies on grit. Factor analysis procedures with these measures have identified that grit is comprised of two components, or factors (Duckworth et al., 2007). The Grit-S (i.e., the Short Grit Scale) retains this two-factor structure with four fewer items and improved psychometric properties (Duckworth & Quinn, 2009).

The first factor, *consistency of interests*, has been defined in the literature as goal- and action-oriented long-term behavior—this is distinct from an individual or situational interest (Muenks et al., 2017). Consistency of interests is assessed via six items on the Grit-O, each measured using a five-point Likert scale: 1) I often set a goal, but later choose to pursue a different one; 2) New ideas and new projects sometimes distract me from previous ones; 3) I become interested in new pursuits every few months; 4) My interests change from year to year; 5) I have been obsessed with a certain idea or project for a short time but later lost interest; and 6) I have difficulty maintaining my focus on projects that take more than a few months to complete.

The second factor, *perseverance of effort,* is conceptualized as the tendency to continue working toward a particular goal (Muenks et al., 2017). Perseverance of effort is also assessed via six items on the Grit-O, each measured using a five-point Likert scale: 1) I have achieved a goal that took years of work; 2) I have overcome setbacks to conquer an important challenge; 3) I finish whatever I begin; 4) Setbacks don't discourage me; 5) I am a hard worker; and 6) I am diligent.

While the majority of the research on grit presented in this chapter will focus on grit as measured on the Grit-O and Grit-S, research that investigates similar or related constructs to grit (e.g., resilience, determination, persistence) utilizing different data collection instruments will also be considered. The purpose of applying a broader lens is to ensure that this chapter does not negate important findings in the literature that relate to grit. For example, *resilience* has been defined as a"positive adaptation despite experience of significant adversity or trauma" (Luthar, 2015, p. 742). According to scholars of resilience and grit, "grit is not just having resilience in the face of failure, but also having deep commitments that you remain loyal to over many years" (Perkins-Gough, 2013). In addition, *perseverance* has been conceptualized as the capacity to remain focused and committed to both short- and long-term goals in the face of adversity (Constantin, Holman, & Hojbotă, 2011). Thus, perseverance reflects the perseverance of effort component of grit, but does not necessarily address consistency of interests. Although constructs related to grit may have slight deviations in their operational definitions, they may provide important insight into relevant relationships within the current body of literature. Researchers have sought to disentangle grit from conceptually similar constructs and their findings provide support for investigating grit along with these related constructs. For example, Credé, Tynan, & Harms (2017) conducted a full meta-analysis to disentangle grit from other constructs, including conscientiousness, self-control, mental toughness, and cognitive ability. This research identified that grit is highly correlated with conscientiousness. In addition, this research identified that several of these related constructs were also strongly associated with academic performance. Thus, while grit research will be prioritized in the current chapter, research supports that there may be utility in exploring related constructs to grit.

In addition to investigating related terms, the current chapter will also investigate research pertaining to various *mindsets*, i.e., "beliefs about the capacity to grow one's abilities" (Haimovitz & Dweck, 2016). A key aspect of grit is a *growth mindset*, i.e., the perception that abilities are "malleable" rather than fixed characteristics that do not change (Hochanadel & Finamore, 2015, p.48). According to Duckworth (2013), embracing a growth mindset is an important component of grit. In fact, the field of social cognitive and affective neuroscience has utilized functional magnetic resonance imaging techniques to identify commonalities in neural networks between grit and growth mindset (Myers, Wang, Black, Bugescu, & Hoeft, 2016). In addition to a growth mindset, a *failure mindset* (i.e., the belief that failure is "enhancing" rather than "debilitating") is a key component of grit. While success across educational, professional, and interpersonal domains remains a critical goal for families, educators, researchers, and practitioners, examining how children fail may be a vital consideration to this line of inquiry (Haimovitz & Dweck, 2016, p. 860).

Rationale for Synthesizing Parenting and Family Predictors of Grit

The vast majority of grit research has been conducted among adult samples, with a particular focus on college students. This research has found that grit and/or its components are associated with a range of important traditional educational measures, e.g., academic adjustment, college grade point average, college satisfaction, sense of belonging, faculty-student interactions, and intent to persist (Bowman, Hill, Denson, & Bronkema, 2015). Findings on grit in college students have also extended beyond traditional educational success measures, including subjective and mental well-being, resilience, self-control, and a growth-oriented mindset (Akbag & Ummet, 2017; Kannangara et al., 2018).

Although there is a large body of research on grit in college students, there is also a burgeoning body of research on grit earlier on in life. This research demonstrates the role of grit in contributing to academic motivation, academic locus of control, and positive thinking in adolescence (Celik & Saricam, 2018; Pina-Watson, Lopez, Ojeda, & Rodriguez, 2015). Among youth samples, grit has also been suggested to serve as a potential protective factor against adversity. For example, Guerrero, Dudovitz, Chung, Dosanjh, & Wong (2016) analyzed survey data with a sample comprised of mostly Latino ninth-graders from low-income neighborhoods in Los Angeles. Those with higher levels of grit had significantly lower odds of alcohol and marijuana use and getting into fights in the last 30 days compared with those with lower levels of grit. The authors suggested that grit might serve as a buffer against risk behavior involvement.

The multi-faceted outcomes associated with grit across educational, professional, and interpersonal contexts for a range of developmental stages and diverse samples underscores the utility of investigating whether various social or cultural contexts can *foster* or *enhance* grit. Indeed, research investigating change in grit over time is currently emerging. As an example of extant research in this area, Park, Baelen, Tsukayama, & Duckworth (2018) conducted a year-long prospective, longitudinal study investigating how perceptions of school culture influence the development of grit in middle school students. The authors explored whether students perceived their school to be mastery goal oriented (i.e., the school focuses on enhancing skills "for their own sake," p. 121) versus, performance goal oriented (i.e., the school focuses on students' capacity to demonstrate ability in relation to other students). Longitudinal findings demonstrated that changes in the extent to which students perceived their schools as more mastery goal oriented predicted changes in grit over the school year. The authors interpreted this finding to indicate that school environments that emphasize the value of learning "for learning's sake" are particularly fruitful environments for fostering grit.

However, Datu (2017) aptly notes that the majority of studies on grit emphasize "person-related correlates of grittiness," yet do not adequately pay heed to "social factors" that may be important for fostering grit (p. 135). As research on grit across the lifespan continues to emerge, there is a need to identify parenting- and family-specific factors that are associated with grit so that parents and families can potentially be more effectively equipped to foster grit in their children.

MAIN FOCUS OF THE CHAPTER

Parenting and Family Predictors of Grit

Parent and Family Demographic Factors

Research has begun to identify particular parental characteristics that may predict children's development of grit. Jiang et al. (2019) conducted a study on grit and academic achievement among Chinese primary school students. Findings demonstrated that grit predicted later academic achievement, even after controlling for a range of demographic factors, including family socioeconomic status. Thus, parental demographic factors did not play a role in the relationship between grit and academic achievement. Indeed, this finding has been further supported in additional research studies. For example, Park, Kwak, & Kim (2018) investigated antecedents of grit among Korean adolescents in South Korea. This research did not identify parental education as a predictor of grit.

An exception to these findings pertains to immigrant status (i.e., citizen versus non-citizen). O'Neal et al. (2016) conducted a mixed methods study with Latino college students and although they did not find citizens versus non-citizens to have significantly different levels of grit, they found that immigrant status moderated the relationship between grit and depression. Specifically, grit was associated with depression in the full sample, however there was a stronger association between grit and depression for non-citizens than for citizens, with depression higher at lower levels of grit for non-citizens. Taken together with a qualitative analysis, the authors interpreted this research to suggesting that non-citizen students may need to utilize grit to combat stress and adversity that they may experience in higher education as non-citizens. This research contributes important nuance into the question of demographics and grit, although this study is limited to college students and thus cannot provide insight into the role of family immigrant status on grit over the course of children's lifespans.

Research exploring parent and family demographic predictors of grit inevitably must address the critique in the literature and in public spheres that grit and related constructs minimize the influence of structural inequalities in society that impede an individual's ability to attain success (Scelfo, April 8, 2016). Relatedly, limited research has been conducted to address whether grit is, in part, a byproduct of broader socioeconomic factors. As an example of research in this area, Akos & Kretchmar (2017) statistically controlled for gender, race, and first-generation college student status in their analysis of grit. Although they found no differences in total grit scores between racial minorities and non-minorities, they found that racial minorities rated themselves lower on the perseverance of effort scale relative to non-minorities. The finding that minorities may rate themselves lower on grit should be further investigated in additional research studies, particularly in light of the self-report nature of the Grit-O and Grit-S. In a recent interview, Duckworth responds to some critiques of grit by noting, "That's not the message...It's not that poverty or racism doesn't matter, it's just that hard work does matter" (Scelfo, April 8, 2016). In other words, although grit is an important factor to investigate, it should not be analyzed without consideration of broader contextual factors.

In general, additional research is required to determine the relationship between parent and family demographic characteristics and grit—the small body of extant research suggests that grit may develop independently of socioeconomic circumstances; in contrast, various socioeconomic challenges may present a greater need for children to develop grit to succeed.

Parental Cognitions

Previous research demonstrates that parenting-related schemas and perceptions, reflective functioning abilities, and emotional experiences (i.e., *parental cognitions*) may play a role in children's development of grit. For example, Haimovitz & Dweck (2016) investigated parents' *failure mindsets* (i.e., the belief that failure is either "enhancing" or "debilitating," p. 860) in relation to "intelligence mindsets" (i.e., "beliefs about whether intelligence is fixed or malleable," which is in direct opposition to the notion of growth mindsets p. 860). The researchers conducted a series of three studies with parent-child dyads to investigate the role of failure mindsets and found that parents who viewed failure as "debilitating" had children with fixed intelligence mindsets, suggesting that a growth mindset may actually be fostered in children based on how parents exhibit their beliefs surrounding failure.

Importantly, the authors emphasized that children's non-cognitive characteristics will not simply be "transmitted" via any qualities that parents exhibit—rather, parents are responsible for "creating conditions" in the learning environment at home that are particularly conducive to the growth mindset (p. 1855). In addition, parents have other beliefs, e.g., "their theories of how to motivate children" that often drive their behaviors, which may not align with parents' growth mindsets (Haimovitz &

Dweck, 2016, p. 1851). Examples of theories of motivation may include whether they believe failure is motivating or discouraging. Thus, research suggests that the way in which parents convey their beliefs surrounding growth and failure may foster a growth mindset (and, theoretically, grit) in children, although a range of other parental cognitions should be examined in conjunction with mindsets. Future research should investigate this interplay of factors to further disentangle processes that encourage grit in the home.

Parenting Style and Behaviors

Carol Dweck, a leading researcher in the mindset arena, emphasizes that parenting behaviors, such as how parents offer praise, can be important for cultivating a growth or failure-positive mindset. For example, praising children's intelligence encourages a fixed mindset, because intelligence is often thought to be an immutable characteristic that does not increase or change. Instead, Dweck emphasizes that encouraging children's effort is more conducive to a growth mindset (Dweck, 2009). In addition, highlighting that challenges and obstacles are typical aspects of the learning process may be beneficial in fostering growth mindsets (Haimovitz & Dweck, 2016). Importantly, Haimovitz & Dweck (2016) emphasize that although praise and other parental behaviors likely contribute to the development of children's mindsets, these factors should be investigated in the context of the broader constellation of parental cognitions which also are likely to play a role.

Other existing research also supports the role of a specific parenting style for promoting children's grit. As an example of research that investigates parenting style and grit, Howard, Nicholson, & Chesnut (2019) investigated the influence of a range of parenting factors, including "overparenting" and components of authoritative parenting (e.g., parental acceptance and involvement) on college students' academic success. Parenting factors were determined via participants' recollections of parenting behaviors, via the Helicopter Parenting Index (Odenwaller, Booth-Butterfield, & Weber, 2014) and the Parenting Style Index (Steinberg, Lamborn, Dornbusch, & Darling, 1992). Overparenting and parental acceptance were significantly associated with grit such that overparenting was associated with lower levels of grit and parental acceptance was associated with higher levels of grit. The authors also found that grit mediated the relationship between overparenting and academic success, such that parenting behaviors influence grit, which in turn has an impact on academic success. This finding demonstrates the important role of parenting style in predicting grit, as well as the broader implications of parenting style on academic success.

Although these findings represent compelling evidence that parenting behaviors and parenting style may predict grit, the results are somewhat limited by the self-report and retrospective nature of the available research. There is limited prospective research on parenting style and grit, although previous research with grit proxies (e.g., persistence) suggests that prospective studies may yield similar results. For example, Padilla-Walker, Day, Dyer, & Black (2013) investigated two-parent families with a child between the ages of 11 and 14. This study utilized three waves of data from the Flourishing Families Project and found that authoritative fathering at time two was positively associated with adolescent persistence at time three, and adolescent persistence was positively associated with school engagement and negatively associated with delinquency at time four. Taken together, findings further underscore that parenting style and behaviors may indeed have important implications for promoting grit and growth mindsets, although the research is somewhat limited in this area, making it difficult to draw robust conclusions. Further complicating the process is that little is known about how children's behaviors may influence parenting behaviors that may cultivate grit, mindsets, or related constructs, which suggests that future research should investigate bi-directional relationships among these variables (Haimovitz & Dweck, 2016).

Parent-Child Relationships

In addition to investigating specific parenting behaviors and styles, researchers have also investigated the bi-directional parent-child relationship and any relational factors that may predict grit. Levy & Steele (2011) was the first study to investigate grit in relation to attachment. This study investigated self-reported attachment styles to parents in childhood and to romantic partners during adulthood utilizing a range of attachment-related assessments. For example, this study measured subjectively perceived past parental care and protection, current self-reported anxiety and avoidance patterns, and current self-reported security, avoidance, and anxiety/ambivalence (using the Adult Attachment Scale [Collins & Read, 1990]). Findings revealed that grit was significantly associated with both current and past attachment. Given that this research focused on retrospective analyses of child-parent attachment, it would be highly beneficial for future research to conduct prospective longitudinal analyses to investigate the role of attachment and grit.

Research has not consistently supported the link between parent-child relationships and grit. For example, Argyros & Johnson (2018) investigated a range of predictors of resilience. The findings of this study identified numerous individual characteristics (e.g., self-esteem and personality) that were significant predictors. The authors also investigated the role of perceived social support and found that along with other external or contextual factors, social support was not predictive of resilience. The authors interpreted the findings to suggest that psychological resilience is better predicted by individual characteristics rather than external characteristics. Taken together, findings suggest that parent-child relationships may be important environments for cultivating grit in children—however, it is necessary to evaluate both individual and contextual factors to gain a more nuanced perspective into the role of parent-child relationships.

Familial Culture Factors

Researchers have further expanded the lens on grit to investigate the role of familial cultural factors on grit. Several studies have sought to expand the extant research (which primarily focuses on Western samples) to investigate grit in collectivist contexts. For example, Datu (2017) investigated Filipino high school students' "relatedness" to parents, teachers, and friends and whether there were associations between relatedness and grit, for the purposes of drawing broader conclusions about collectivist cultures. Findings revealed that relatedness to parents was associated with greater consistency and overall grit, suggesting that parental relatedness with children may be a contributor to children's grit in families with more collectivist orientations.

This finding has been further supported in additional research studies. Lin & Chang (2017) investigated family context in a sample of Taiwanese high school students. Specifically, they investigated the degree to which an individual perceives that his or her family influences him or her as well as the degree to which an individual perceives that his or her family adopts a democratic parenting style. Findings revealed that family influence, but not democratic parenting style, predicted children's levels of grit. Thus, the perception of a strong family influence, which may include perception of a combination of robust social support as well as high pressure and expectations in regards to an individual's goals and ambitions, may be particularly conducive to the development of grit for children in collectivist cultures. These findings underscore the need for research to continue to investigate parenting style across cultures to assess the role of parenting styles and grit in context.

Research on predictors of grit in Latino families has yielded somewhat inconsistent results. Vela, Lu, Lenz, & Hinojosa (2015) investigated "familismo" (i.e., "loyalty and solidarity to the family unit") among families of Latino college students and found that familismo did not predict grit (Vela, Lu, Lenz, & Hinojosa, 2015, p. 290). This is in contrast to other studies with Latino students that found family support to be associated with academic resilience (Cavazos et al., 2010). Vela, Lu, Lenz, & Hinojosa (2015) interpreted these findings to suggest that although familismo may be an important predictor of grit in Latino factors, other factors may be equally or more important in predicting grit among this sample. This finding speaks to the broader notion that researchers should be cautious in drawing broad generalizations about specific cultures or ethnic groups, since these groups are by no means homogenous.

Future research should explore a comprehensive set of predictors of grit in diverse samples to build on this line of research.

While these studies provide important insight into the role of familial culture and grit, the most comprehensive study investigating the relationship between grit and familial culture was conducted by Disabato, Goodman, & Kashdan (2018). This study utilized online survey methodology to investigate an international sample of over 7,000 participants spanning seven continents. Regions with individualist-oriented cultures showed similar grit score reliability to the total sample. However, the reliability of grit total scores for Latin America and East and South Asia were lower than other world regions. The authors interpreted these findings as indicating that grit may be more robustly supported in individualist-oriented countries, as opposed to collectivist-oriented countries (i.e., those in Latin America and Asia). Indeed, the inconclusive findings on diverse samples underscore the need for additional research on the role of familial culture in predicting grit.

Parental and Family Factors for Predicting Grit in at-risk Youth

An important component of the literature on the associations among parents, families, and grit is research that supports grit as a potential protective factor for risk behaviors. It is particularly salient to investigate grit in samples of risk, given that an important component of grit is the ability to persist, often in contexts of adversity. Research generally supports the notion that parent-child relationship factors are particularly important for children's grit in at-risk samples.

For example, a cross-sectional study by O'Gara, Calzada, & Kim (2010) investigated resilience as a proxy for grit, defined conceptually in this study as "overcoming serious threats to healthy development and experiencing positive outcomes despite exposure to such threats" (p. 2). The researchers applied structural equation modeling techniques to investigate relationships among parent-child alienation, parental displays of warmth and hostility, and adolescent resilience and delinquency in Mexican American families. Parent-child alienation was assessed based on adolescents' self-reported sense of alienation from their parents on items including "I have to rely on myself when I have a problem to solve" and "I don't get much attention from my parents." Findings from this research suggested that lower adolescent perceived alienation from parents predicted both higher resilience and lower delinquency. The authors interpreted these findings to suggest that strong parent-child relationships can potentially promote resilience in adolescents—these results provide support for the aforementioned association between parent-child relationships, and suggest that these findings also hold true for at-risk samples.

Additional research underscores the role of parenting factors in predicting grit among at-risk youth and also identifies individual variation within these relationships.

Suizzo et al. (2017) conducted structural equation modeling analyses to investigate the pathways through which fathers' warmth influences adolescents' grades, with a focus on academic determination and self-efficacy (which can serve as theoretical proxies for grit). In this research, academic determination was based on a questionnaire assessing students' self-reported "level of determination and persistence when engaging in challenging school tasks." This questionnaire includes items such as "I continue working on difficult tasks despite the frustrations I encounter" and "When I start a project, I make up my mind to see it through," which are somewhat akin to the items assessed in measures of grit. Measures of academic self-efficacy assessed self-efficacy specific to language arts and math.

Findings from this research revealed gender differences—for male adolescents, the association between fathers' warmth and English language art grades were mediated by academic self-efficacy and determination to persist on challenging schoolwork. For female adolescents' associations between fathers' warmth and math grades were mediated by optimism and determination. The authors interpreted these findings to suggest that fathers' warmth uniquely contributes to boys' and girls' school performance and, importantly, to the non-cognitive factors found to be predictive of school performance (e.g., self-efficacy, determination to persist, etc.). These findings underscore the need to further investigate interactions between individual and social factors, particularly among high-risk samples. In addition, this research supports the utility of investigating individual variation between parents and children based on characteristics such as gender.

Findings with higher risk youth suggest that although parenting factors and parent-child relationships appear to play an important role in children's grit, broader family and contextual factors may also be important for further understanding this relationship. For example, Tiet, Huizinga, & Bynes (2010) conducted a longitudinal study of youth living in high-risk neighborhoods with a specific eye towards identifying predictors of resilience. Results revealed that over time, resilience was predicted by bonding to family and teachers, involvement in extracurricular activities, lower levels of parental discord, fewer adverse life events, and being less involved with delinquent peers. Particularly notable was the fact that resilience predicted future resilience, thus creating a positive feedback loop that continuously strengthened resilience.

Along these lines, researchers of at-risk youth have also specifically examined the extent to which families encourage or permit children to engage in a wide range of extracurricular activities, and whether participation in these activities, in turn, promotes grit. Peck, Roeser, Zarrett, & Eccles (2008) conducted a longitudinal study to examine the role of extracurricular activity involvement in contributing to "educational resilience" (i.e., "the unexpectedly positive academic achievement and educational attainments among youth whose lives are characterized by multiple personal and social risks," p. 137). This study specifically examined "educationally vulnerable youth" (i.e., adolescents who are "at risk for dropping completely out of formal education systems," p. 136). Findings suggested that positive extracurricular involvement may promote educational resilience among vulnerable youth. Specifically, educationally vulnerable adolescents who were engaged in both sports and school clubs were significantly more likely to enroll in college compared to vulnerable youth who were not involved in extracurricular activities.

Considerations for the Role of Parents and Families in Children's Grit

The aforementioned findings on parenting and family factors that promote children's grit should be understood in the context of several important caveats, particularly as they apply to vulnerable populations. One consideration pertains to the critical importance of understanding the ways in which "individual characteristics" interact with "structural context," rather than investigating these factors in isolation (Anderson, Turner, Heath, & Payne, 2016, p. 198). Indeed, the extant body of literature has largely established the role of grit in predicting individual outcomes, as well as concurrent associations among grit and other individual characteristics. As a result, the research on parenting and family predictors of grit is fairly limited. Therefore, the research reviewed in the current chapter consistently underscores the need to broaden the research lens to investigate the interplay among the wide range of factors that likely contribute to the development of grit.

Another important consideration relates to the utility of the construct of grit itself. Credé, Tynan, & Harms (2017) conducted a meta-analytic review of grit that suggested that the two grit components (perseverance of effort and consistency of interests) may not equally contribute to the myriad of positive outcomes associated with grit. Rather, perseverance of effort was found to be a stronger predictor of performance, suggesting that this factor should be investigated separately in relation to performance. Moreover, this research also identified grit as highly correlated with related constructs, including conscientiousness and self-control. Given these findings, when seeking to identify family predictors of grit, researchers may want to consider evaluating grit components separately, as well as testing a range of related constructs so that it may be possible to disentangle any identified associations. Indeed, research is beginning to move in this direction. Tang, Wang, Guo, & Salmela-Aro (2019) investigated longitudinal relationships among growth mindset, goal commitment, grit, academic achievement and school engagement among sixth through ninth graders in Finland. The authors also included several constructs conceptually related to grit as covariates, including conscientiousness and academic persistence. Consistent with findings from the aforementioned meta-analysis, this study also found that the perseverance of effort component (but not the consistency of interests component) uniquely contributed to academic outcomes and engagement. Moving forward, research exploring the distinct contributions of each grit component should include familial and parental antecedents of each component as well as investigate related constructs.

RECOMMENDATIONS AND FUTURE RESEARCH DIRECTIONS

The current chapter explored parenting and family factors that predict a key element of character— grit, i.e., "perseverance and passion for long-term goals" (Duckworth, Peterson, Matthews, & Kelly, 2007). The research points to a range of overarching recommendations to researchers interested in understanding ways in which to potentially cultivate grit in the family context. There is a strong rationale for exploring grit— the last decade has witnessed an emergence of research studies on grit and grit has been found to be associated with outcomes in multiple domains, including educational, professional, and interpersonal measures of success.

Given these important findings, the current chapter explored research on parenting characteristics, practices, and behaviors that may promote these characteristics in children. First, the current research does not support that any particular family demographic characteristics promote grit in children. However, there appears to be utility in investigating grit within particular demographics contexts—it may be the case that certain socioeconomic challenges require individuals to harness grit as a means to overcome stress and adversity. In addition, due to the self-report nature of the Grit-O and Grit-S, it is important for researchers to continue to investigate potential self-report bias in their research, particularly for minority groups who may exhibit different reporting patterns relative to non-minority groups. More broadly, it is necessary to investigate and interpret grit within the broader socioeconomic context of the research.

In terms of the role of other parent or family characteristics— previous research demonstrates that parental cognitions may play a role in children's development of grit. It is not simply the case that gritty parents produce gritty children—rather, parents have the potential to foster learning environments at home that may be particularly conducive to children's growth mindset and grit by demonstrating failure as an opportunity for growth and praising children's efforts rather than intelligence or other fixed characteristics. The research on parenting style suggests that the extent to which parents demonstrate acceptance and authoritative parenting is also predictive of grit. Additionally, the quality of the parent-child relationship appears to also be an important predictor of grit, including in at-risk samples. However, the research in these areas is limited and often relies on retrospective design and self-report. Additional research should further explore these important areas by employing prospective designs and observational measures of parenting style and parent-child relationships. Moreover, research suggests that certain individual characteristics, e.g., self-esteem and personality, and gender, may influence the relationship between parent-child relationships and grit, suggesting that researchers need to include a wide range of measurement strategies to capture the complexities of these associations.

This chapter also reviewed the impact of broader familial factors in promoting grit, including cultural beliefs. The current research suggests that the utility of grit may vary by cultural context or region. Specifically, research suggests that parent-child relatedness may be an important predictor of children's grit in collectivist cultures, although research is not consistent with respect to this finding. Research examining broader contexts in relation to grit has also pointed out a range of environmental factors that are necessary to consider, including children's relationships with teachers and peers and extracurricular activities. Additional research should assess the role of cultural beliefs, region, and other broader contextual factors to more effectively understand the role of grit in diverse samples.

CONCLUSION

The current chapter explored parenting and family factors that may predict children's development of grit throughout the lifespan. This chapter: 1) reviewed findings on grit across developmental contexts to underscore its significance in the research and highlight the rationale for exploring predictors of grit; 2) investigated the role of specific parenting characteristics in predicting children's grit, including demographic characteristics and parenting behaviors and styles; 3) explored the broader impact of contextual factors in promoting grit, including cultural, socioeconomic, and other environmental factors; and 4) provided overarching recommendations to researchers seeking to understand grit in the family context. Although the last decade has witnessed a burgeoning body of research highlighting the utility of grit and the relationships between grit and other individual constructs, there remains limited research on parent and family predictors of grit. This dearth of research makes it challenging to draw robust conclusions regarding these relationships and underscores the need for future research on grit to include prospective, longitudinal studies with diverse samples.

REFERENCES

Akbag, M., & Ümmet, D. (2017). Predictive Role of Grit and Basic Psychological Needs Satisfaction on Subjective Well-Being for Young Adults. *Online Submission*, *8*(26), 127–135.

Akos, P., & Kretchmar, J. (2017). Investigating grit at a non-cognitive predictor of college success. *The Review of Higher Education*, *40*(2), 163–186. doi:10.1353/rhe.2017.0000

Anderson, C., Turner, A. C., Heath, R. D., & Payne, C. M. (2016). On the meaning of grit... and hope... and fate control... and alienation... and locus of control... and... self-efficacy... and... effort optimism... and.... *The Urban Review*, *48*(2), 198–219. doi:10.100711256-016-0351-3

Argyros, G., & Johnson, C. (2018). *Psychological Resilience in Higher Education Students: A Systematic Investigation of Predictive Factors*. Academic Press.

Arya, B., & Lal, D. S. (2018). Grit and sense of coherence as predictors of well-being. *Indian Journal of Positive Psychology*, *9*(1), 169–172. doi:10.15614/ijpp.v9i01.11766

Bowman, N. A., Hill, P. L., Denson, N., & Bronkema, R. (2015). Keep on truckin'or stay the course? Exploring grit dimensions as differential predictors of educational achievement, satisfaction, and intentions. *Social Psychological & Personality Science*, *6*(6), 639–645. doi:10.1177/1948550615574300

Cavazos, J. Jr, Johnson, M. B., Fielding, C., Cavazos, A. G., Castro, V., & Vela, L. (2010). A qualitative study of resilient Latina/o college students. *Journal of Latinos and Education*, *9*(3), 172–188. doi:10.1080/15348431003761166

Çelik, İ., & Sariçam, H. (2018). The Relationships between Positive Thinking Skills, Academic Locus of Control and Grit in Adolescents. *Universal Journal of Educational Research*, *6*(3), 392–398. doi:10.13189/ujer.2018.060305

Collins, N. L., & Read, S. J. (1990). Adult attachment, working models, and relationship quality in dating couples. *Journal of Personality and Social Psychology*, *58*(4), 64. doi:10.1037/0022-3514.58.4.644 PMID:14570079

Constantin, T., Holman, A., & Hojbotă, M. A. (2011). Development and validation of a motivational persistence scale. *Psihologija (Beograd)*, *45*(2), 99–120. doi:10.2298/PSI1202099C

Credé, M., Tynan, M. C., & Harms, P. D. (2017). Much ado about grit: A meta-analytic synthesis of the grit literature. *Journal of Personality and Social Psychology, 113*(3), 492–511. doi:10.1037/pspp0000102 PMID:27845531

Datu, J. A. D. (2017). Sense of relatedness is linked to higher grit in a collectivist setting. *Personality and Individual Differences, 105*, 135–138. Retrieved from org.proxy.wexler.hunter.cuny.edu/10.1016/j.paid.2016.09.039

Disabato, D. J., Goodman, F. R., & Kashdan, T. B. (2019). Is grit relevant to well-being and strengths? Evidence across the globe for separating perseverance of effort and consistency of interests. *Journal of Personality, 87*(2), 194–211. doi:10.1111/jopy.12382 PMID:29573415

Duckworth, A. L., & Eskreis-Winkler, L. (2013). True grit. *APS Observer, 26*(4).

Duckworth, A. L., Peterson, C., Matthews, M. D., & Kelly, D. R. (2007). Grit: Perseverance and passion for long-term goals. *Journal of Personality and Social Psychology, 92*(6), 1087–1101. doi:10.1037/0022-3514.92.6.1087 PMID:17547490

Duckworth, A. L., & Quinn, P. D. (2009). Development and validation of the Short Grit Scale (GRIT–S). *Journal of Personality Assessment, 91*(2), 166–174. doi:10.1080/00223890802634290 PMID:19205937

Dweck, C. S. (2009). Developing Talent Through a Growth Mindset. *Olympic Coach, 21*(1).

Eskreis-Winkler, L., Duckworth, A. L., Shulman, E. P., & Beal, S. (2014). The grit effect: Predicting retention in the military, the workplace, school and marriage. *Frontiers in Psychology, 5*, 36. doi:10.3389/fpsyg.2014.00036 PMID:24550863

Guerrero, L. R., Dudovitz, R., Chung, P. J., Dosanjh, K. K., & Wong, M. D. (2016). Grit: A potential protective factor against substance use and other risk behaviors among Latino adolescents. *Academic Pediatrics, 16*(3), 275–281. doi:10.1016/j.acap.2015.12.016 PMID:26796576

Haimovitz, K., & Dweck, C. S. (2016). What predicts children's fixed and growth intelligence mind-sets? Not their parents' views of intelligence but their parents' views of failure. *Psychological Science, 27*(6), 859–869. doi:10.1177/0956797616639727 PMID:27113733

Hochanadel, A., & Finamore, D. (2015). Fixed and growth mindset in education and how grit helps students persist in the face of adversity. *Journal of International Education Research, 11*(1), 47–50.

Howard, J. M., Nicholson, B. C., & Chesnut, S. R. (2019). Relationships Between Positive Parenting, Overparenting, Grit, and Academic Success. *Journal of College Student Development*, *60*(2), 189–202. doi:10.1353/csd.2019.0018

Jiang, W., Xiao, Z., Liu, Y., Guo, K., Jiang, J., & Du, X. (2019). Reciprocal relations between grit and academic achievement: A longitudinal study. *Learning and Individual Differences*, *71*, 13–22. doi:10.1016/j.lindif.2019.02.004

Kannangara, C. S., Allen, R. E., Waugh, G., Nahar, N., Khan, S. Z. N., Rogerson, S., & Carson, J. (2018). All that glitters is not grit: Three studies of grit in university students. *Frontiers in Psychology*, 9. PMID:30210389

Levy, J. M., & Steele, H. (2011). Attachment and grit: Exploring possible contributions of attachment styles (from past and present life) to the adult personality construct of grit. *Journal of Social and Psychological Sciences*, *4*(2), 16–49.

Lin, C. L. S., & Chang, C. Y. (2017). Personality and Family Context in Explaining Grit of Taiwanese High School Students. *Eurasia Journal of Mathematics. Science and Technology Education*, *13*(6), 2197–2213.

Luthar, S. S. (2015). Resilience in development: A synthesis of research across five decades. Developmental Psychopathology: Volume Three: Risk, Disorder, and Adaptation, 739-795

Mooradian, T., Matzler, K., Uzelac, B., & Bauer, F. (2016). Perspiration and inspiration: Grit and innovativeness as antecedents of entrepreneurial success. *Journal of Economic Psychology*, *56*, 232–243. doi:10.1016/j.joep.2016.08.001

Muenks, K., Wigfield, A., Yang, J. S., & O'Neal, C. R. (2017). How true is grit? Assessing its relations to high school and college students' personality characteristics, self-regulation, engagement, and achievement. *Journal of Educational Psychology*, *109*(5), 599–620. doi:10.1037/edu0000153

Myers, C. A., Wang, C., Black, J. M., Bugescu, N., & Hoeft, F. (2016). The matter of motivation: Striatal resting-state connectivity is dissociable between grit and growth mindset. *Social Cognitive and Affective Neuroscience*, *11*(10), 1521–1527. doi:10.1093can/nsw065 PMID:27217105

O'Gara, J. L., Calzada, E. J., & Kim, S. Y. (2019). The father's role in risk and resilience among Mexican-American adolescents. *The American Journal of Orthopsychiatry*. PMID:30628806

O'Neal, C. R., Espino, M. M., Goldthrite, A., Morin, M. F., Weston, L., Hernandez, P., & Fuhrmann, A. (2016). Grit under duress: Stress, strengths, and academic success among non-citizen and citizen Latina/o first-generation college students. *Hispanic Journal of Behavioral Sciences, 38*(4), 446–466. Retrieved from org.proxy.wexler.hunter.cuny.edu/10.1177/0739986316660775

Odenweller, K. G., Booth-Butterfield, M., & Weber, K. (2014). Investigating helicopter parenting, family environments, and relational outcomes for millennials. *Communication Studies*, *65*(4), 407–425. doi:10.1080/10510974.2013.811434

Padilla-Walker, L. M., Day, R. D., Dyer, W. J., & Black, B. C. (2013). "Keep on Keeping On, Even When It's Hard!" Predictors and Outcomes of Adolescent Persistence. *The Journal of Early Adolescence*, *33*(4), 433–457. doi:10.1177/0272431612449387

Park, D., Yu, A., Baelen, R. N., Tsukayama, E., & Duckworth, A. L. (2018). Fostering grit: Perceived school goal-structure predicts growth in grit and grades. *Contemporary Educational Psychology*, *55*, 120–128. doi:10.1016/j.cedpsych.2018.09.007

Park, S., Kwak, K., & Kim, Y. (2018). Psychological variables related to grit among adolescents in South Korea: A longitudinal study from age 4 to 14. *Current Psychology,* 1–6.

Peck, S. C., Roeser, R. W., Zarrett, N., & Eccles, J. S. (2008). Exploring the roles of extracurricular activity quantity and quality in the educational resilience of vulnerable adolescents: Variable-and pattern-centered approaches. *The Journal of Social Issues*, *64*(1), 135–156. doi:10.1111/j.1540-4560.2008.00552.x PMID:19543445

Perkins-Gough, D. (2013). The significance of grit: A conversation with Angela Lee Duckworth. *Educational Leadership*, *71*(1), 14–20.

Piña-Watson, B., López, B., Ojeda, L., & Rodriguez, K. M. (2015). Cultural and cognitive predictors of academic motivation among Mexican American adolescents: Caution against discounting the impact of cultural processes. *Journal of Multicultural Counseling and Development*, *43*(2), 109–121. doi:10.1002/j.2161-1912.2015.00068.x

Scelfo, J. (2016, Apr. 8). Angela Duckworth on Passion, Grit and Success. *The New York Times*. Retrieved from: https://www.nytimes.com/2016/04/10/education/edlife/passion-grit- success.html

Steinberg, L., Lamborn, S. D., Dornbusch, S. M., & Darling, N. (1992). Impact of parenting practices on adolescent achievement: Authoritative parenting, school involvement, and encouragement to succeed. *Child Development*, *63*(5), 1266–1281. doi:10.2307/1131532 PMID:1446552

Suizzo, M. A., Rackley, K. R., Robbins, P. A., Jackson, K. M., Rarick, J. R., & McClain, S. (2017). The unique effects of fathers' warmth on adolescents' positive beliefs and behaviors: Pathways to resilience in low-income families. *Sex Roles*, *77*(1-2), 46–58. doi:10.100711199-016-0696-9

Tang, X., Wang, M. T., Guo, J., & Salmela-Aro, K. (2019). Building grit: The longitudinal pathways between mindset, commitment, grit, and academic outcomes. *Journal of Youth and Adolescence*, *48*(5), 850–863. doi:10.100710964-019-00998-0 PMID:30788767

Tiet, Q. Q., Huizinga, D., & Byrnes, H. F. (2010). Predictors of resilience among inner city youths. *Journal of Child and Family Studies*, *19*(3), 360–378. doi:10.100710826-009-9307-5

Tough, P. (2012). *How children succeed: Grit, curiosity, and the hidden power of character*. Houghton Mifflin Harcourt.

Vela, J. C., Lu, M.-T. P., Lenz, A. S., & Hinojosa, K. (2015). Positive psychology and familial factors as predictors of Latina/o students' psychological grit. *Hispanic Journal of Behavioral Sciences, 37*(3), 287–303. Retrieved from org.proxy.wexler.hunter.cuny.edu/10.1177/0739986315588917

Vela, J. C., Sparrow, G. S., Whittenberg, J. F., & Rodriguez, B. (2018). The Role of Character Strengths and Importance of Family on Mexican American College Students' Career Decision Self-Efficacy. *Journal of Employment Counseling*, *55*(1), 16–26. doi:10.1002/joec.12070

Walker, C. O. (2017). Exploring the contributions of grit and personality in the prediction of self-and other-forgiveness. *Journal of Individual Differences*, *38*(3), 196–202. doi:10.1027/1614-0001/a000236

KEY TERMS AND DEFINITIONS

Consistency of Interests: The first factor measured in the Grit-O, *consistency of interests*, has been defined in the literature as goal- and action-oriented long-term behavior. This is distinct from an individual or situational interest (Muenks et al., 2017). Consistency of interests is assessed via six items on the Grit-O, each measured using a five-point Likert scale: 1) I often set a goal, but later choose to pursue a different one; 2) New ideas and new projects sometimes distract me from previous ones; 3) I become interested in new pursuits every few months; 4) My interests change from year to year; 5) I have been obsessed with a certain idea or project for a short time but later lost interest; and 6) I have difficulty maintaining my focus on projects that take more than a few months to complete.

Failure Mindset: Failure mindset is the belief that failure is "enhancing" rather than debilitating"). Failure mindset is considered a key component of grit--while success across educational, professional, and interpersonal domains remains a critical goal for families, educators, researchers, and practitioners, examining how children fail may be a vital consideration to this line of inquiry (Haimovitz & Dweck, 2016, p. 860).

Grit: Defined as "perseverance and passion for long-term goals" (Duckworth, Peterson, Matthews, & Kelly, 2007). According to the scholars of resilience and grit, "grit is not just having resilience in the face of failure, but also having deep commitments that you remain loyal to over many years" (Perkins-Gough, 2013).

Growth Mindset: Conceptualized as the perception that abilities are "malleable" rather than fixed characteristics that do not change (Hochanadel & Finamore, 2015, p.48). According to Duckworth & Eskreis-Winkler (2013), embracing a growth mindset is an important component of grit.

Mindset: Defined as "beliefs about the capacity to grow one's abilities" (Haimovitz & Dweck, 2016). Examples include growth and failure mindset.

Parental Cognitions: Previous research demonstrates that parenting-related schemas and perceptions, reflective functioning abilities, and emotional experiences (i.e., *parental cognitions*) may play a role in children's development of grit.

Perseverance of Effort: The second factor measured in the Grit-O, *perseverance of effort* is conceptualized as the tendency to continue working toward a particular goal (Muenks et al., 2017). Perseverance of effort is also assessed via six items on the Grit-O, each measured using a five-point Likert scale: 1) I have achieved a goal that took years of work; 2) I have overcome setbacks to conquer an important challenge; 3) I finish whatever I begin; 4) Setbacks don't discourage me; 5) I am a hard worker; and 6) I am diligent.

Resilience: Resilience has been defined as "positive adaptation despite experience of significant adversity or trauma" (Luthar, 2015, p. 742). According to scholars of resilience and grit, "grit is not just having resilience in the face of failure, but also having deep commitments that you remain loyal to over many years" (Perkins-Gough, 2013).

Chapter 4
Grit, Goal Setting, and Social Support as It Pertains to Family Dynamics and Romantic Relationships

Valerie Lynn Blanchard-McGehee
University of Louisiana at Lafayette, USA

ABSTRACT

This chapter explores interpersonal relationships in family dynamics and romantic relationships as they pertain to grit, goal setting, and social support. Individuals in various types of relationships will be explored, such as married and non-married couples, couples with children, and couples without children. In addition, this chapter will examine the influence that partners and family members have on one another and the several outcomes that result in different kinds of family and relational supports. The chapter will also explore the importance of using all three methods (grit, goal setting, social support) in conjunction with one another, since the three are vital to long-term success in interpersonal relationships and positive family dynamics, regardless of environmental or socio-economic differences in each case. Examples with evidentiary and anecdotal support will be used to explain the benefits or detriments of having or not having these traits in interpersonal relationships and family dynamics. These examples were selected to be inclusive and to relate to family, parental, and spousal relationship structures.

DOI: 10.4018/978-1-7998-2940-9.ch004

INTRODUCTION

Achieving a goal as complex and subjective as having a successful long-term relationship or being a good parent can be difficult, regardless of previous successes or financial tools available. However, in analyzing cases in which success in these areas is prevalent, certain ingredients have consistently revealed themselves as being vital, if used in combination, towards ultimate success. Among these ingredients are the character trait of grit (growth mindset), the tools of setting goals, and utilizing social support to aid in successful relationships or in obtaining positive family dynamics. When used in conjunction, grit, goal setting, and social support will lead to positive family dynamics and successful long-term romantic relationships regardless of race, social class, ethnicity, gender, or other distinctions. The three concepts will be explored throughout this chapter in relation to family dynamics and romantic partnerships, as evidenced through cited research as well as anecdotal evidence.

GRIT

Grit is a word that can be defined in many ways. Martin Seligman (2014), a lead expert in the field of Positive Psychology, describes grit as, "the combination of high persistence and high passion towards the fulfillment of an objective." Angela Duckworth, a psychologist who coined the term grit, defines it as "the tendency to sustain interest in and effort toward long-term goals" (Duckworth et al., 2007). Malcolm Gladwell, author of *Outliers*, describes individuals with true grit to have dedicated a minimum of 10,000 hours of practice, or about twenty hours a week for ten years, to their practice.

What does grit look like? Grit is the high school student from a low income, high crime neighborhood who has a 4.0 grade point average, perfect school attendance, attends his after school job for four hours, then comes home and makes dinner for his family as a co-parent to his younger siblings because his single mother must attend work at her night job. Grit is a single mother who raises three children while working the night shift in order to pay for private school, because public schools in her district are not the best option for their future. Grit is also the couple who just celebrated their fiftieth wedding anniversary, who despite their good and bad years, they stayed married because they knew they were stronger together than apart and could rely on each other through the hard times. Grit is the couple that creates goals for themselves and achieves those goals when their partner supports them and holds them accountable. With enough grit, parents of children with severe illnesses can sustain long hours driving to a specialty hospital to endure numerous surgeries and hospital stays, persevere through financial hardships from the ensuing medical bills, and tough it out together. Despite their long days of worry and stress, they know they can rely on each other to get through the hard times and overcome adversity together as long as they choose to never to give up.

When a relationship is perceived by both parties as being a great success despite times of adversity, the reason for the success is never a singular one. Both parties have given great effort, time, and energy towards the maintenance of the relationship. The two individuals made sacrifices when necessary, and developed resilience when faced with turbulence. Success in a marriage or long-term partnership of any type cannot be gauged through numerical processes, but there are consistent measurables seen in every successful partnership regardless of the individuals' differences.

Achieving difficult goals and leading a rewarding life of success can be seen as a sign of talent, intelligence, or even luck. Although these character traits are nice to have, they are much less important than the ability to overcome great adversity and persevere towards completing a goal. Some people are inherently tenacious, while others have developed fortitude and grit as the byproduct of failure or experience. These same principals can be applied to every facet of one's life: financial freedom, enduring long-term meaningful relationships, or being a great parent.

Angela Duckworth has researched and developed numerous findings on grit and its effect on success. This "Guru of Grit," as she is known in the research world, created the grit survey in 2007 which helps individuals understand their level of grit based on a scale of 1-5 (5 being very gritty and 1 being not gritty at all). Research suggests that grit may be as essential as high levels of intelligence and more essential to high achievement and success in life (Chang, 2014). "Grit has been shown to be predictive of several aspects of success ranging from retention in the West Point cadet-training program, higher GPAs amongst undergraduates, higher education attainment among adults, and further progress in the Scripps Spelling Bee" (Duckworth et al., 2007, p.1095).

In a study of doctoral completion (Blanchard, 2018), grittier individuals stood out among those who completed their doctorate and took longer to finish. The very gritty doctoral graduates endured a rollercoaster of success and upsets throughout their doctoral program and managed to complete their studies, even if it took a lot longer to complete than they had planned. Students in the traditional PhD program planned on completing four years of coursework and one year of dissertation research. This group of students, on average, took an extra two years to complete their doctorate. Ironically, the students who scored higher on the grit survey took, on average, an additional two to three years to complete their doctorate. This group of students experienced adversity in their lives, as well as personal and professional distractions (i.e. divorce, career change, pregnancy, personal illness, became a caretaker for a loved one), while in their doctoral program. Most of the doctoral graduates in the non-traditional EdD cohort completed their doctorate within the two to three year time frame set by the doctoral program. Similar to the traditional PhD graduates, the graduates that took longer to complete their dissertation scored higher on the grit survey. The EdD graduates who took longer to complete their doctorate, on average, took an extra year, but these individuals also experienced adversity in their lives and endured personal and professional distractions while attending their doctoral program. “On average, individuals who are gritty are more self-controlled, but the correlation between these two traits is not perfect: Some individuals are paragons of grit but not self-control, and some exceptionally well-regulated individuals are not especially gritty” (Duckworth et al., 2014, p.1).

Gritty Relationships

As grit pertains to relationships, it takes sacrifice, patience, and perseverance to sustain the ups and downs of any relationship over many years. The perfect relationship does not exist. However, those who persevere through the inevitable adversities that arise will manage to maintain a long-term meaningful relationship with their significant other. This takes grit at a high emotional level, from both partners, or the relationship will struggle or become stagnant. (It is important to note that staying in unhealthy relationships, such as abusive ones, are not considered signs of grit). Non-abusive relationships require work, patience, dedication, and grit. According to Angela Duckworth, “People who can set long-term goals and stick to them have a leg up on success in school and life” (as cited in Perkins-Gough, 2013). Duckworth continued, “Grit is related to resilience because part of what it means to be gritty is to be resilient in the face of failure or adversity” (p.14).

People display various levels of grit in different areas of their life. For example, individuals can have a high level of grit (4 or 5) as it relates to his or her career. He or she can put in many hours at work, make personal sacrifices, learn from his or her setbacks and move on, and strive to work his or her way up in the organization. However, this person may not be gritty when it comes to his or her relationship. His or her relationship grit may be a 3 or 4 and tend to not be willing to commit to a relationship for long-term or he or she does not put much effort into his/her relationships and finds him/herself back to being single often. Other people who are work gritty and not relationship gritty may be in a committed relationship but may struggle with his or her marriage. This person does not want to put the time or effort in to work on his or her relationship because they lack the grit and desire for a successful marriage.

Narrative on Relationship Grit

To understand this concept further, let us examine Bill and Debbie's relationship dynamic. Bill and Debbie were high school sweethearts and married after Bill completed four years in the Navy. They had two children, a boy and a girl, that were five years apart. Bill and Debbie struggled with their relationship for many reasons. One reason was because Bill was very much inclined to move up in his career because he felt the need to financially support his family to prove his personal success. Debbie worked part-time in real estate but was mostly at home to raise the children and was content at being a stay-at-home mom. Debbie viewed their relationship and family as a high priority, and although Bill loved his family, he often put his work demands as a priority over his family. "While some can balance their various roles as spouse, worker, and home maintainer, many find themselves unable to switch off these roles and relax enough to get absorbed in their personal interests. The result is to make their personal time more fragmented, stressful, and much less enjoyable," according to psychologists Pascale and Primavera (2017). This difference led to daily arguments, falling out of love, and eventually the dissolution of their marriage. Since Debbie and Bill lacked the communication necessary to understand each other's goals and needs, the marriage ended in divorce. According to Debbie, Bill lacked relationship grit and according to Bill, Debbie lacked work grit. The viewpoints they had for each other were opinion, but both may be partially true. Bill and Debbie both lacked the grit to work on their relationship together, in the good times and bad times, and to persevere no matter what. They did not discuss seeking professional marriage counseling nor were they able to seek to understand each other, rather than to be understood themselves. Many marriage-saving tools they could have utilized were overlooked, and instead they chose not to make the effort. They simply did not have the passion and perseverance to weather the storm.

Now let us look at James and Virginia's marriage dynamics. Both James and Virginia were college graduates, but after college, Virginia decided to be a stay-at-home mom and to raise their five children. James went to work and was promoted frequently in his organization. James found balance between work and family. Virginia found balance between being a wife, a mother, and taking the time to socialize with friends. When times were rough financially, Virginia would pick up a part-time job for a few months to help support the family. She never criticized James for not being a provider, even though she would come home exhausted. James realized the effort that Virginia had put in to support the family and took on the household chores, such as doing the laundry and cooking dinner, to help alleviate the tasks that Virginia normally did. James and Virginia had grit in their approach to the hard work it took to maintain a long-lasting marriage. They made each other a priority, worked on themselves to be better for each other, and assisted the other when needed. James believed that a husband and wife's responsibilities in a good marriage were not fifty-fifty, because that balance is almost impossible to achieve. Instead, he believed that if both he and his wife gave 75%, the combined result would always be more than 100% of what their family life needed. They stuck it out, persevered, and were gritty about their marriage. Virginia and James experienced the highs and lows of a relationship for the sixty plus years they were married, until their deaths, which were six months apart from one another.

Jachimowicza et al. (2018) suggest that, "Passion is essential for perseverance to unfold its beneficial effects because it combines with perseverance to increase immersion in an activity, evidenced by increased focus and pursuit of activities related to their passionate endeavor. That is, the increased immersion produced by the combination of perseverance and passion leads individuals to devote greater cognitive effort and investment to their goals, as evidenced in more intense concentration. This heightened immersion, in turn, provides the energy and dedication that makes it more likely that individuals attain their goals."

Marriage is full of many dynamics. It comes down to how much effort the individuals in it want to make it work, and how gritty the partners are to withstand the tides of a long-term commitment. Communication with a partner and self-care are important practices to exercise daily. "Neuroscientific discoveries have shown that we can increase our neural growth by the actions we take, such as using good strategies, asking questions, practicing, and following good nutrition and sleep habits" (Mindset Works, 2015). This finding led researchers to understand the link between mindsets and achievement.

Gritty Parenting

Gritty parenting is another important dynamic. Although the amount of available research on this topic is not substantial, evidence shows that when parents are loving, respectful, and demanding, children admire them (Duckworth 2016). Duckworth's research on raising gritty parents who are gritty themselves and model their passion and perseverance for their children, will more likely raise children who have higher levels of grit than those parents who do not model grit. Authoritative and loving parents hold high expectations of their children and provide support to their children. Children tend to emulate their gritty, authoritative (not authoritarian) parents, which can result in gritty children. In Duckworth's (2016) book on Grit, she states, "If you want to bring forth grit in your child, first ask how much passion and perseverance you have for your own life goals. Then ask yourself how likely it is that your approach to parenting encourages your child to emulate you. If the answer to the first question is "a great deal," and your answer to the second is "very likely," you're already parenting for grit." Duckworth (2016) suggests that extra-curricular activities is a great way for children to develop grit because they can be interesting and challenging. Her rule is that children should choose an activity that they are very interested in and encourage children to complete the activity to its natural end (i.e. the end of a season, the end of the year). Parents should also choose an extra-curricular activity and see it through to the end (i.e. train for a 5K, plant a garden). When parents can stick to a hobby or an extracurricular activity, they become gritty role models for their children.

Narrative on Gritty Parenting

Victoria works for a very influential organization as a sales manager for a large territory in the northeast. When she began her position as a sales representative, she did not know much about sales or selling products, but she was an ambitious person who dove head first into the sales world. Victoria grew up emulating her stepmother, who was kind and caring to her stepdaughter, as well as ambitious and proactive in her own life. As a little girl, Victoria marveled at the accomplishments that her stepmother achieved, and was impressed with her stepmother's talent to be able to do anything. Victoria learned as she got older that her stepmother did not always know how to do "everything," but her stepmother learned from her failures and figured things out. Victoria's stepmother was a great role model for her growing up because she had the opportunity to see firsthand what it meant to have grit and a growth mindset. Psychologist Carol Dweck states, "Having a growth mindset is the belief that your abilities can be developed," (as cited by France, 2016). When it came time for Victoria to decide whether she should move on in her career, she weighed her decisions and decided to take a chance by leaving her comfortable career to start over in an industry that she was passionate about, even though she did not yet have experience in it. By witnessing her stepmother's growth mindset throughout her young life, she had the confidence to take a risk, knowing she could achieve success in her new career by learning from her mistakes.

Raising a child with grit can reflect parenting skills. But how do individuals turn into gritty adults when they do not have gritty parents? In research conducted with doctoral graduates (Blanchard 2018), individuals who were not raised by gritty parents felt the need to overcome their adversity and prove their self-worth by taking their education seriously and by pursuing a doctoral degree. Through financial burdens, hours studying, and overall surviving a doctoral program, these individuals persevered and stuck to their goals. Unlike Victoria's stepmom, who was a positive influence on her growth mindset, individuals with parents who are lazy, uninvolved, or unmotivated to set goals can become gritty adults because they see the negative impact of this lack of grit on their parents' lives. Oftentimes, people who grow up in an environment of adversity and are surrounded by adults with a fixed mindset can become very gritty and driven to succeed in a very powerful way despite the negative influence of their upbringing. Furthermore, parents do not necessarily need to be the sole role model in a child's life and are allowed to make mistakes like anyone else. Siblings, grandparents, teachers, and friends can all have their hand in raising a child with grit and a growth mindset.

A growth mindset is a wonderful character trait to have or to learn. Any time a person fails, he can choose one of two outcomes: He will either experience this failure as an opportunity to learn and grow, or as a reason to quit and stop trying. The person who fails and learns from his mistakes becomes smarter, gains experience, and becomes more capable of positive change. His ceiling for being able to handle adversity has been raised considerably. This is what makes a person grittier. Grit is associated with an "optimistic explanatory style (Duckworth, Quinn, & Seligman, 2009) and with growth mindset (Galla et al., 2013) cognitive dispositions that incline individuals to look for changeable causes for their current problems" (p.9).

Interventions and studies have proven that a person's mindset can change from fixed to growth, and when it does, it leads to increased motivation and achievement (Mindset Works, 2015). A partner willing to actively improve after making a mistake in a relationship is practicing a growth mindset. It can be a learned behavior for those honest, self-aware, and most importantly for those willing enough to take direction from those who are more knowledgeable. These skills are helpful in maintaining a relationship, keeping a steady job, or making personal changes in one's life. It also requires a cosmic shift in perceiving success and failure: Failure becomes an opportunity for growth instead of a reason to stop trying. Only those with grit realize that failing is a byproduct of the long path to success and achievement. "Perseverance without passion isn't grit, but merely a grind," (Jachimowicza et. al., 2018)

Goal Setting

The term *goal* is defined by goal setting theorists as the object or aim of an action (Locke & Latham, 1990). According to Locke and Latham (2002), a goal is defined simply as what the individual is consciously trying to do. Goals direct attention and action, and challenging goals mobilize energy, lead to higher effort, and increase persistent effort. Goals motivate people to develop strategies that will enable him or her to perform at the required goal levels. Accomplishing the goal can lead to satisfaction and further motivation, or frustration and lower motivation if the goal is not accomplished (p.705).

In Blanchard's research of doctoral completion (2018), she discovered that participants in her study changed their fixed mindset to a growth mindset once they figured out their workable strategy to finish their research and writing. They no longer felt that doctoral degree attainment was impossible (after they created succinct goals with the end in mind). For example, one participant's strategy was to reward herself for the small wins that led up to her big win. The participant said, "My goal was to look up five articles on Sunday and read an article a day during the week. This to me was manageable." To reward herself, she would take Saturdays off from doing any doctoral work whatsoever. She continued, "I had to create a system, reward myself by taking a day off, and those were the things that got me motivated. Before I knew it, I had almost finished chapter two and didn't even realize it."

Another goal-setting strategy that participants used to finish their doctoral program was to create timelines and due dates for themselves. More specifically, during the dissertation phase, the participants committed themselves to submit portions of their dissertation to their adviser in a timely manner. To keep themselves on track, some participants created schedules, timelines, and calendars to post in their office. Although doctoral completion was a top priority to the participants in this study, they still needed to manage their personal life and career. A popular technique used by participants was to create a schedule, but to communicate it with their family and friends to reinforce the timeline and to hold themselves accountable. A goal-setting technique that another participant tried was to make his dissertation work part of his daily routine and always uphold the date and time for his thesis work as he would with every item on his schedule. Creating the specific task of dissertation work during a specific time frame instead of a broad one made it easier for him to dedicate a structured amount of time for his goal to be completed.

All participants in Blanchard's Study (2018) set goals to complete their doctorate, executed their plan, and received the results when they successfully defended their dissertations. Creating what Locke and Latham (1990) referred to as accuracy goals, the doctoral graduates were able to "carefully plan and identify the best paths to achieve their goals with minimal deviation" to achieve their doctorate. "Having a clear, compelling goal mobilizes your focus toward actionable behavior," (Boss, 2017, para.3) and achieving goals builds self-efficacy. Furthermore, goal-setting was intrinsic to doctoral completion for the participants in Blanchard's (2018) study.

Goal Setting in Relationships

Many family goals are financial in nature, such as saving money to purchase a new car or saving to pay off student loans to be debt free. Talking about financial goals may be a sensitive topic but avoiding the conversation can lead to disastrous outcomes. Couples benefit when managing money together. "While it doesn't make discussing a sensitive topic any easier, know that working hard to get on the same page financially with your spouse is worth it in the long run," (Jaggernath, 2019). It is important for couples to set small, realistic goals that are important to each person. Once a couple can attain the small financial goals together, then they should plan to reach long term goals as a pair.

Other common goals may include a couple deciding to get into a fitness and nutrition routine together. Creating a healthy lifestyle are great goals to embark on for a couple. The commitment and hard work to make this lifestyle change together results in strengthening the relationship, especially when the pair start to see the positive results of their hard work. A study from the journal, JAMA Internal Medicine, found that, "Men and women were more likely to stop smoking, exercise more or lose weight if their partner joined them in becoming healthier….For example, a smoker was more likely to quit if their partner also stopped smoking than if their partner had never smoked," (LiveScience, 2015). Partners can become a great role model for their spouse when attempting to reach a goal. The data in the same study (Jackson, Steptoe, Wardle, 2015), discovered, "When one person changed an unhealthy behavior, having a mate who was also making efforts to become healthier in the same area over the same time period had a stronger influence than having a mate who already exhibited that healthy behavior and could serve as a role model," (LiveScience, 2015).

It is also important for couples to reward themselves when they do attain their goals. Celebrating a goal in which the couple achieved together can promote future accomplishments because it is a reward they can both look forward to doing. When two people are working towards a shared goal, it brings them together to form a common bond. The major finding of goal setting, which is based on hundreds of studies, is that individuals who are provided with specific, difficult but attainable goals perform better than those given easy, nonspecific, or no goals at all (Lunenburg, 2011). Coinciding with this finding, the individuals must have ample capability, accept the goals, and accept feedback related to performance (Latham, 2003). According to Latham and Locke (2002):

The 1990 theory of goal setting developed from studies involving close to 40,000 participants in eight countries performing 88 different tasks in laboratory and field settings, using experimental and correlational designs, over a time span of one minute to three years where the goal was assigned, self-set, or set participatory with an individual or group is this: (1) a specific, high goal leads to a higher performance than no goal, or an abstract goal such as do your best, (2) there is a linear relationship between the difficulty level of the goal and job performance, (3) performance feedback, participation in decision making, and competition only affect performance to the extent that they lead to the setting of a specific, high goal (p.705)

Goal Setting for Families

When couples and families set goals, it is important that the goals are agreed upon. The family should ask, "Is this goal feasible, and if so, what are the parameters by which we consider the goal to be completed?" In asking these questions, the family is not only making the goal's "completeness" more clearly defined, they are setting reasonable expectations for the amount of work and time it will take to complete the project. According to Stephen Covey (1989), to begin with the end in mind, "Is the ability to envision in your mind what you cannot at present see with your eyes. It is based on the principle that all things are created twice. There is a mental (first) creation, and a physical (second) creation. The physical creation follows the mental, just as a building follows a blueprint. If you don't make a conscious effort to visualize who you are and what you want in life, then you empower other people and circumstances to shape you and your life by default. It's about connecting again with your own uniqueness and then defining the personal, moral, and ethical guidelines within which you can most happily express and fulfill yourself." Dweck's research about mindset is comparable with many of Covey's principles about being proactive (Dweck, 2006). "A review of the supporting literature about each concept reveals that proactivity and a growth mindset require a similar frame of mind that motivates individuals to take greater responsibility for personal progress" (Franklin Covey, 2015, p.2).

The willingness for a family to set specific parameters at the start of the process and stick to them to completion is vital to the family's success. Projects can continue on much longer than they should because the proper parameters for completion have not been clearly mapped out, and this can lead to frustration and confusion within a family unit.

For example, is a home renovation ever really finished unless the family has made clearly defined goals to an ultimate end? Adi Tatarko, co-founder and CEO of Houzz (Pullen, 2017), says, "12% of couples consider divorce when remodeling or renovating their home." It is also important that the goals are attainable and realistic (Pullen, 2017). According to psychotherapist Tina Tessina (2016), "You need to discuss budget, your individual wants for the result of the renovation, your different style preferences and how you're going to manage the disruption of the renovation… You need to be able to talk about your disagreements and resolve them. If you can't do this about everyday things, you won't be able to do it about the special stressful situation of renovation." Family projects are healthy to do in order to create lasting memories, but it is imperative that deadlines are created to match the goals, and this is what Covey refers to as creating an end in mind.

Narrative on Goal Setting in Relationships

Gabe wanted to help Sharon pay off her student loan debt of $110,000. Sharon wanted to pay it off in three years and thought if she lived to the bare minimum then she could do this. Gabe appreciated Sharon's motivation and willingness to make sacrifices so they would not have the burden of the student loan debt, but Gabe did not think this was possible. After explaining to Sharon that the seven percent interest would affect the monthly payments that Sharon estimated, Sharon soon realized that it would take her eight years to pay off her loans if she was aggressive with them. Gabe wanted to help Sharon with the payments so they came up with a plan that would help Sharon not live paycheck to paycheck. After committing to their payoff plan, Gabe and Sharon were able to pay off Sharon's student loans in five years. They decided to take the bonuses they received at work and put it towards the student loans. They also had paid off their car payments and were able to take the extra amount of money they now had and put that towards the student loans as well. Gabe and Sharon worked as a team and accomplished a common goal. They no longer had the burden of the huge monthly payment and celebrated with a Caribbean vacation. Attaining their common goal brought them closer together and relieved the stress that Sharon endured from such a huge loan she thought would never go away.

After a couple agrees to the terms and strategy of goal completion, the result of completing this joint venture should always result in a positive change for both parties. The best way to implement the success of both parties is to set goals that result in a win-win outcome. "Win–win conflict resolution is a cognitive and behavioral skill that can well serve your relationship's happiness," (Grieger, 2014). A true win-win, according to Stephen Covey (1989), occurs when both people develop an idea and together, they expand on the idea to create an even better outcome because they synergized. Covey's win-win philosophy is founded on principles like Mary Parker Follett's early work in conflict resolution. Follett's integrated approach forms the basis of what is now commonly referred to as "win-win" (Tonn, 2003). Follett taught that there are three main ways of dealing with conflict: domination, which creates a win-lose scenario; compromise, where both parties settle; and integrated, where a solution has been found in which both desires have found a place. The first two methods result in a scenario where one party sacrifices something to the benefit of the other. Follett explains that both are unsatisfactory because "conflict will come up again and again in some other form" since "we give up part of our desire" (Graham, 2003, p.5). "If we start from the proposition that there will be differences and disagreements in all relationships, then it follows that how you resolve these disagreements will be critical to on-going success of those relationships… Every disagreement will have a resolution. You want to make sure that the resolution does not leave lingering hurt or resentment in either of you. In resolving differences and disagreements, there are only four possible outcomes," (Grieger, 2014).

One of the variables that moderates the goal-performance relationship is commitment. Locke and Latham (1990, p. 124) stated, "It is virtually axiomatic that a goal that a person is not really trying for is not really a goal and cannot have much effect on subsequent action." Commitment is a broader term than goal acceptance in that it refers to one's attachment to or determination to attain the goal, regardless of its source (Latham & Locke, 2002). The causes of commitment fall into two broad categories: factors that make goal attainment important and factors that make an individual confident that the goal can be attained. Factors that were found to affect an individual's desire to attain a specific, high goal include authority, peers, making the goal public, incentives, internal rewards, punishment, and instrumentality (Latham & Locke, 2002). "Although perseverance helps individuals by remaining committed to their goal pursuit, passion provides individuals with the focus necessary to achieve their goals. Thus, when individuals pursue goals, they are not passionate for, perseverance may not produce increased performance," (Jachimowicza, et. al., 2018).

SOCIAL SUPPORT

Social support is an invaluable emotional tool in goal completion. Having a supportive spouse, friend, or family member leads to alleviating emotionally charged conflicts and aids in growth mindset. "A social support network is comprised of several individuals within one's environment who influence one's perceptions of his or her environment and might include family members, friends, and co-workers" (Kelly, 2005, p.57). Social support can take various forms, including "emotional support (attempts to alleviate negative affects), professional support (mentoring and guidance), and practical support (money or help with task completion)," (Jairam & Kahl, 2012, p.317). One of the most potent types of social support that will be discussed in this section is parental support towards children and the importance of this in goal completion. Other powerful social support constructs are spousal support from one party to the other (singular), or joint spousal support, in which both parties are participating in a shared goal or endeavor.

Social Support for Parenting

Of all relationship types, parenting is one of the hardest and most complicated. "While there are challenges in bringing up a baby, during the first year in particular, some couples grow stronger as they find a new respect for each other as parents and share experiences that bind them together. It can help to deal with any relationship problems you face after having a baby as they happen," (NCT, 2019). Parenting is a job in which singular success is almost always gauged subjectively. It is often difficult for new parents to find balance between working while simultaneously dedicating enough time to contribute to household productivity or provide emotional support for the child and spouse. According to findings by Nelson and Lyubomirsky (2015), "More than half of workers report difficulties balancing the responsibilities of work and family (Parker and Wang, 2013), and parents frequently experience fatigue associated with being 'on call' 24/7 (Feldman and Nash, 1984)." Parents themselves are individually supported through their own networks of friends, colleagues, and family. Some families choose to outsource support for children in the form of nannies, babysitters, or daycare. "Support from friends and family helps new mothers deal better with stress, and this has been proven to help mothers see their children in a more positive light," (Narvaez 2013). As children get older, their daily schedule and activities become progressively more complicated and time consuming, and it can be difficult to keep up with their schedules, especially when parents themselves have work obligations. The value of getting support from likeminded parents is smart and healthy and can result in creating a social network of friends, peers, or other parents to lighten the load. Parents often align other parents to more efficiently manage their time via carpool, for example. Navarez (2013) suggests that, "Mothers who have the help of people they trust feel more self-esteem, confidence as a parent, and struggle less to access information that helps them problem-solve for their bundle of joy."

Parents themselves can also benefit from their own social support apart from their family as a way to maintain a healthy balance and emotional state. According to Charney (2004), having a network of friends that are available to talk to on the phone or to grab a quick bite to eat with can help to "sharpen the saw" as referenced in *Seven Habits of Highly Effect People* (Covey, 1989). Covey describes the renewal of self through mind, body, heart, and spirit. "As you renew yourself in each of the four areas, you create growth and change in your life. You increase your capacity to produce and handle the challenges around you. Without this renewal, the body becomes weak, the mind mechanical, the emotions raw, the spirit insensitive, and the person selfish," (Covey, 1989).

Scheduling personal time away from work and family is an important and healthy way to refocus, regroup, and relax one's mind, especially in times of heavy workload or stress. Sharpening the saw adds much needed variety to those with strict routines and full schedules and is vital to positive mental health and fostering outside relationships. Theoretical models of social support specify the following two important dimensions: (1) a structural dimension, which includes network size and frequency of social interactions, and (2) a functional dimension with emotional (such as receiving love and empathy) and instrumental (practical help such as assistance with child care) components (Covey, 1989, p.208).

Narrative on Family Social Support

When Kelly had her first child, she felt that she was finally in a place in her life, career, and finances, where she would be able to effectively raise a child. Once the baby was born, she was a great mother, but started to neglect the time she spent with her husband. Kelly and her husband, John, lacked the great communication they once had before their son was born, because they did not prioritize time to work on their relationship. Kelly's husband began to express that he was beginning to feel distant from Kelly. Although he considered her a fantastic mother, he needed her to be more mindful of her role as a wife through communication and support. For Kelly's husband, giving their marriage more attention and time would be beneficial to his emotional state, and was much needed to strengthen their relationship after the baby was born. This social support was vital for Kelly herself, although she may not have recognized it until their conversation. Once the couple finally decided to actively block out time for their relationship, they decided to schedule one date night a month, and made a point to prioritize this time in the same way they prioritized time spent on their careers or with the baby. Soon, they discovered their communication with each other improved dramatically, and surprisingly, their ability to parent as a team grew more effective. After a few months, date night became an enjoyable activity, and one in which Kelly and her husband looked forward to each month. Kelly's career and parenting seemed to benefit from her "sharpening the saw." After a few more months, Kelly joined a book club and her husband joined a men's night at their church. These short breaks from their regular routine were a joyous reprieve from their daily stressors and gave Kelly a boost of excitement each month.

Research psychologist, Dr. Rob Pascale, found that (2017), "Marriages also benefit when spouses have time for themselves, either to pursue their own interests or just to relax. Personal time allows us to maintain our individual identities, provides opportunities to do things we like to do, and lets us feel like we have some control over our lives. Alone time can actually help to keep a relationship fresh and less stressful." Kelly and John's relationship improved dramatically once they prioritized their marriage, and the addition of social activities allowed them to receive social support from peers outside of their immediate family. According to family counselor, Daniel White (2017), "Good parents aren't necessarily the ones that sacrifice themselves entirely for their child, but rather the ones that know they can't pour from an empty cup, and as such, work to balance their own needs with that of their child in order to provide the very best for their little one."

Social Support for Relationships

Social support is just as important for couples without children. When one spouse takes issue with the other for spending too much time away from the marriage in favor of outside activities or friends, it results in resentment and emotional imbalance. Although it is healthy for either spouse to have his/her own interests and passions, it is possible for one spouse to feel alienated or detached if the other is spending an overabundance of time outside of the relationship. Communicating this feeling of detachment is important for a healthy marriage to sustain long term. If the injured spouse does not communicate his/her concerns quickly to the other, feelings of resentment will continue to build over time, and the relationship will deteriorate. The spouse who is spending more time apart from his relationship may not be aware of the negative effect his activities are having on his partner. As such, verbalizing these concerns is the responsibility of the injured party in order for the conflict to be resolved. "What's most important is that spouses agree how much time they want together and apart. When handled correctly, each partner feels he/she is getting his/her fair share. Here perceptions are more important than the actual number of hours. Even if couples spend very little time together or very little time apart, the relationship is fine if the proportion is what they both want. If each partner has different perspectives, however, the amount of time together and apart can be a source of conflict. For some partners, too much together time can be suffocating, while for others too little can make them feel insecure and isolated," (Pascale & Primavera, 2017).

Being mindful and empathetic are great traits to have, but ultimately, being solution-based is key in alleviating a lot of the balance in a relationship. For example, creating an agreed upon schedule is an invaluable tool which allows both partners to prioritize date nights as well as social interactions with others. "Balance and compromise are essential when it comes to using time. A mix of time with friends and family, time together as a couple, and separate time for each partner add to marital quality, as does an equal split between our circle and activities and those of our partner. If balance is missing, it's wise to have a straightforward discussion with your partner and work out the necessary negotiations to get to a better place, (Pascale & Primavera, 2017).

Feelings of detachment or alienation can be resolved by scheduling a men's group event on the same night as a girls' night out. Since both partners are enjoying social activities away from the other, this can reduce loneliness and create better balance in the marriage. Nonetheless, it is important to spend time away from the significant other and even more important, to prioritize and enjoy it. According to Dr. Fairbrother (2011), "Social support is the physical and emotional comfort given to us by our family, friends, co-workers and others. It's knowing that we are part of a community of people who love and care for us, and value and think well of us," (p.7).

CONCLUSION

Grit, goal setting and social support are three-character traits that lead towards progressive achievement. When all three traits are implemented, an individual is more likely to succeed than if the three traits were not applied. Relationships in any form require commitment and tenacity, and couples who can commit to work out their problems through patience and open communication will find success. "Solid relationships are built on solid individuals. To bring the best version of ourselves into relationships, we sometimes need to work on ourselves first. Patience builds character," (Palmiotto, 2018). Relationships also require resilience to learn from mistakes and grow as a couple or a family through times of great success or when faced with adversity. "Resilience is one of the keys to life satisfaction. It can help prevent depression and enhance relationships. It helps us deal with sudden and unexpected challenges as well as those we anticipate and cannot avoid. It also safeguards us against long-term difficulties," (Collingwood, 2018). A healthy growth mindset does not look at failures as faults, but rather as learning experiences. This change in perception is palpable for those who aspire to achieve a growth mindset. Failure is an opportunity to grow, rather than a reason to quit. It is not the easiest method to apply when facing great failure at the start, but with enough practice, it is a learned trait. Those who fail in the right direction can still stumble towards great success, if their perception of failure is an opportunity to grow.

Creating a vision for the future in a relationship or as a family leads to setting goals and accomplishments that can be celebrated with one another. These goals can be broad and sweeping, or incremental and detailed. Child and family therapist, Angela Pruess (2018), states, "When we take the time to reflect on how we'd like our family to grow, we invest in our family's success. It's highly likely that if we don't take the time to develop goals for our family, we won't take the steps necessary to move closer to them. When families come together to work toward a common goal, they're more likely to succeed."

Support from spouses, family, and friends is also important to sustain one's mental health. When times are difficult, a loyal support group to help keep our head above water and stay the course is an invaluable tool, especially when coupled with having grit and setting goals. "Psychologists and other mental health professionals often talk about the importance of having a strong social support network. When trying to reach our goals or deal with a crisis, experts frequently implore people to lean on their friends and family for support. Research has also demonstrated the link between social relationships and many different aspects of health and wellness," (Cherry, 2019). Having these support networks helps the individual weather the inevitable ups and downs any family or relationship will endure. A phone call, email, or supportive text message from a supportive person can aid in getting through the day's troubles or a motivating reason to keep striving towards a goal.

Sustaining any type of relationship over a period of time is not always easy. In romantic relationships for example, couples put their best self forward initially. Over time, character flaws tend to reveal themselves. Just like the courting stages of a romantic relationship are bound by bliss, so are the prenatal stages of becoming pregnant and anticipating the bundle of joy that will complete the family. No one can foresee the challenges of raising a child and the impact it will have on their relationship before it actually happens. "If we fail to effectively meet these inevitable differences when they eventually arise, they can become ordeals or even deal-breakers. Dealing with personality differences, spending habits, child-rearing philosophies, household responsibilities, sexual issues, or any of the many concerns that couples routinely find themselves addressing, can challenge even the most dedicated lovers," (Bloom, 2014). No amount of preparatory book reading about parenting can prepare a young parent for the stressors that come with having a baby, just as one cannot know what it is like to be married until he/she has experienced it firsthand.

In conclusion, grit, goal setting and social support can be individually utilized in a relationship of any type. However, when the three character traits are combined, the outcome leads to advanced accomplishment. Stephen Covey's Seven Habits of Highly Effective People teaches us that, "knowledge, skill, and desire are all within our control. We can work on any one [area] to improve the balance of the three" (Covey, 1989, p.89). This concept is especially important for couples and families to communicate and grow as a unit. Understanding that each family member must stay within his/her circle of influence will keep families bonded. Being proactive in a relationship or as a parent means taking initiative, setting goals, and pushing through no matter the circumstances. Healthy relationships are important because they bring out the best in each person. No relationship is perfect, but it is worth the effort to be a better spouse or to be a more effective parent.

REFERENCES

Blanchard, V. (2018). *Doctoral Program Completion: Grit, Goal setting, Social Support.* Seton Hall University Dissertations and Theses (ETDs). 2552.

Bloom, C., & Bloom, L. (2014). *Got Grit?* Retrieved from https://www.psychologytoday.com/us/blog/stronger-the-broken-places/201410/got-grit

Borresen, K. (2019). *How to prevent a home renovation from wrecking your relationship.* Retrieved from https://www.huffpost.com/entry/home-renovation-relationship-marriage_1_5cae1371e4b03ab9f24f4604

Chang, W. (2014). *Grit and Academic Performance: Is Being Grittier Better?* Retrieved from https://scholarlyrepository.miami.edu/oa_dissertations/1306

Charney, D. (2004). *Psychobiological mechanism of resilience and vulnerability: Implications for successful adaptation to extreme stress*. Retrieved from doi:10.1176/appi.ajp.161.2.195

Cherry, K. (2019). *How Social Support Contributes to Psychological Health*. Retrieved from https://www.verywellmind.com/social-support-for-psychological-health-4119970

Collingwood, J. (2018). *Building resilience*. Retrieved from https://psychcentral.com/lib/building-resilience/

Covey, S. R. (1989). *The seven habits of highly effective people*. New York: Free Press.

Covey, F. (2015). *Using Stephen R. Covey's The 7 Habits of Highly Effective People in Education*. Retrieved from https://www.theleaderinme.org/uploads/Documents/results/7_Habits_Lit_Review_for_Ed ucation.pdf

Duckworth, A. (2016). *Grit: The power of passion and perseverance*. New York: Scribner.

Duckworth, A., Gendler, T., & Gross, J. (2014). Self-control in school-age children. *Educational Psychologist, 49*(3), 199–217. doi:10.1080/00461520.2014.926225

Duckworth, A., Peterson, C., Matthews, M., & Kelly, D. (2007). Grit: Perseverance and passion for long-term goals. *Journal of Personality and Social Psychology, 92*(6), 1087–1101. doi:10.1037/0022-3514.92.6.1087 PMID:17547490

Duckworth, A., Quinn, P., & Seligman, M. (2009). Positive predictors of teacher effectiveness. *The Journal of Positive Psychology*, *4*(6), 540–547. doi:10.1080/17439760903157232

Fairbrother, N. (2011). *Social support*. Retrieved from http://www.heretohelp.bc.ca/sites/default/files/images/visions-ss.pdf

Feldman, S., & Nash, S. (1984). The transition from expectancy to parenthood: Impact of the firstborn children on men and women. *Sex Roles*, *11*(1–2), 61–78. doi:10.1007/BF00287441

France, S. (2016). *The Fixed Mindset vs. The Growth Mindset*. Retrieved from http://executivesecretary.com/the-fixed-mindset-vs-the-growth-mindset/

Galla, B., & Duckworth, A. (2013). More than resisting temptation: Habits mediate the association between self-control and positive life outcomes. *Journal of Personality and Social Psychology, 109*(3), 508–525. doi:10.1037/pspp0000026 PMID:25643222

Graham, P. (2003). *Mark Parker Follett: Prohpet of Management*. Washington, DC: Beard Books.

Grieger, R. (2014). *Happiness with Others: Practice Win–Win*. Retrieved from https://www.psychologytoday.com/us/blog/happiness-purpose/201407/happiness-others-practice-win-win

Jachimowicza, J., Wihlerb, A., Baileya, E., & Galinskya, A. (2018). Why grit requires perseverance and passion to positively predict performance. *Proceedings of the National Academy of Sciences of the United States of America Journal*, 115(40). 10.1073/pnas.1803561115

Jackson, S., Steptoe, A., & Wardle, J. (2015). The Influence of Partner's Behavior on Health Behavior Change The English Longitudinal Study of Ageing. *JAMA Internal Medicine*, *175*(3), 385–392. doi:10.1001/jamainternmed.2014.7554 PMID:25599511

Jaggernath, J. (2019). *How to Talk to Your Spouse About Setting Financial Goals-Money & Relationships*. Retrieved from https://www.mymoneycoach.ca/blog/communicate-about-money-with-spouse-set-financial-goals.html

Jairam, D., & Kahl, D. (2012). Navigating the doctoral experience: The role of social support in the successful degree completion. *International Journal of Doctoral Studies*, *7*. doi:10.28945/1700

Kelly, M. (2005). Psychological adaptation to graduate school: How to smell the roses while burning the midnight oil. *Behavior Therapist*, *28*, 57–59.

Latham, G. P. (2003). Goal setting: A five-step approach to behavior change. *Organizational Dynamics*, *32*(3), 309–318. doi:10.1016/S0090-2616(03)00028-7

LiveScience. (2015). *Couples who set health goals together have more success, study suggests*. Retrieved from https://www.foxnews.com/health/couples-who-set-health-goals-together-have-more-success-study-suggests

Locke, E. A., & Latham, G. P. (1990). *A theory of goal setting and task performance*. Academic Press.

Locke, E. A., & Latham, G. P. (2002). Building a practically useful theory of goal setting and task motivation. *The American Psychologist*, *57*(9), 705–717. doi:10.1037/0003-066X.57.9.705 PMID:12237980

Lunenburg, F. (2011). Goal-setting theory of motivation. *International Journal of Management, Business, and Administration*, *15*(1), 5.

Mindset Works. (2015). *Dr. Dweck's discovery of fixed and growth mindsets have shaped our understanding of learning*. Retrieved from https://www.mindsetworks.com/science/

Narvaez, D. (2013). *New Moms Need Social Support.* Retrieved from https://www.psychologytoday.com/us/blog/moral-landscapes/201301/new-moms-need-social-support

Narvaez, D., Panksepp, J., Schore, A., & Gleason, T. (Eds.). (2013). *Evolution, Early Experience and Human Development: From Research to Practice and Policy*. New York: Oxford University Press.

National Childbirth Trust (NCT). (2019). *Changes in your relationships after having a baby*. Retrieved from https://www.nct.org.uk/life-parent/your-relationship-couple/relationship-changes/changes-your-relationships-after-having-baby

Nelson, S., Kushlev, K., & Lyubomirsky, S. (2014). The pains and pleasures of parenting: When, why, and how is parenthood associated with more or less well-being? *Psychological Bulletin, 140*(3), 846–895. doi:10.1037/a0035444 PMID:24491021

Palmitotto, J. (2018). *Patience and Your Relationships*. Retrieved from https://familyguidanceandtherapy.com/patience-and-your-relationships/

Parker, K., & Wang, W. (2013). *Modern parenthood: Roles of moms and dads converge as they balance work and family*. Retrieved from http://www.pewsocialtrends.org/2013/03/14/ modern-parenthood-roles-of-moms-and-dads-converge-as-they-balance-workand-family/

Pascale, R., & Primavera, L. (2017). *Time Together and Time Apart*. Retrieved from https://www.psychologytoday.com/us/blog/so-happy-together/201702/time-together-and-time-apart

Perkins-Gough, D. (2013). The Significance of Grit: A Conversation with Angela Lee Duckworth. *Resilience and Learning, 71*, 14-20.

Pruess, A. (2018). *The Importance of Setting Family Goals and How to Do It.* Retrieved from https://www.mother.ly/parenting/the-importance-of-setting-family-goals-and-how-to-do-it

Pruess, A. (2019). *The Importance of Setting Family Goals – and How to Do It.* Academic Press.

Pullen, J. (2017). *Renovating a house can be such a nightmare that it leads over 10% of couples to consider divorce.* Retrieved from https://www.businessinsider.com/12-of-couples-consider-divorce-when-they-are-remodeling-their-home-2017-11

Seligman, A. (2014). *Flow and the foundations of positive psychology*. New York: Springer Publishing.

Tessina, T., Smith, R. (2016). *How to Be Happy Partners: Working it out Together.* CreateSpace Independent Publishing Platform.

Tonn, J. C. (2003). *Mary P. Follett: Creating Democracy, Transforming Management*. New Haven, CT: Yale University Press. doi:10.12987/yale/9780300096217.001.0001

White, D. (2017). *How to Overcome Relationship Problems After Having a Baby*. Retrieved from https://www.bergencounselingcenter.com/articles/relationship-problems-after-baby/

KEY TERMS AND DEFINITIONS

Empathic: Showing an ability to understand and share the feelings of another (Lexico, 2019).

Fixed Mindset: When people believe their basic qualities, like their intelligence or talent, are simply fixed traits. They spend their time documenting their intelligence or talent instead of developing them. They also believe that talent alone creates success, without the effort (Dweck, 2015).

Goal-Setting Theory: To the process of identifying something that you want to accomplish and establishing measurable goals and time frames (Locke & Latham, 2002).

Grit: The tendency to sustain interest in and effort toward very long-term goals (Duckworth et al., 2007).

Growth Mindset: When people believe that their most basic abilities can be developed through dedication and hard work. This view creates a love of learning and a resilience that is essential for great accomplishment (Dweck, 2015).

Resilience: How well a person can adapt to the events in his/her life when a person is faced with a tragedy, natural disaster, health concern, relationship, work, or school problem. A person with good resilience has the ability to bounce back more quickly and with less stress than someone whose resilience is less developed (Cohen, 2018).

Social Support: The degree to which a person's basic social needs are fulfilled by interacting with others. Social support systems can be composed of individuals and/or groups. Social support systems may provide affection, sympathy, acceptance, esteem from others, advice, information, and help with work responsibilities (Kaplan, Cassel, and Gore [1977]; Thoits [1982]).

Social Support Network: A network of several individuals within one's environment who influence one's perceptions of his or her environment and might include family members, friends, and co-workers (Kelly, 2005).

Chapter 5
Key Ingredients for Fostering Emotional Intelligence in Children

Nava R. Silton
Marymount Manhattan College, USA

Amanda Anzovino
Marymount Manhattan College, USA

ABSTRACT

This chapter delves into the history of emotional intelligence, from early allusions in the 1920s to contemporary times. It describes the various facets and components of emotional intelligence, discusses how it can be measured, and will discriminate between the emotional quotient (EQ) and the intelligence quotient (IQ) in terms of predicting future life success. The chapter then delineates key ingredients for becoming an emotionally intelligent parent and for promoting emotionally intelligent strategies in the home. Finally, the chapter concludes with comprehensive sections of how to foster emotional intelligence in the workplace and in the school system. The benefits of infusing emotional intelligence in the home, the school, and the workplace are emphasized and discussed.

DOI: 10.4018/978-1-7998-2940-9.ch005

INTRODUCTION, BACKGROUND AND HISTORY

History

While the publication of Daniel Goleman's best-selling book, *Emotional Intelligence* in 1995 strongly popularized the construct of emotional intelligence, intelligence has been an evolving concept with multiple definitions and different subtypes. Thorndike (1920) identified three categorizations of intelligence: abstract, mechanical, and social. Abstract intelligence is related to one's verbal abilities, mechanical intelligence is related to one's visual and spatial abilities, and social intelligence is related to one's ability to interact with others. Thorndike (1937) continued to build on the concept of social intelligence and further defined it as the ability to understand your own mental state, motives, and behaviors and the ability to use that understanding as a basis for decision-making. Additionally, social intelligence also includes the ability to understand and manage relationships with other individuals. In the 1940s, David Wechsler, of the renowned Wechsler Intelligence Tests, suggested that affective or emotional components of intelligence may be critical to success in life. In the 1950s, Humanistic Psychologists, like Abraham Maslow, who proposed the famous Hierarchy of Needs, discussed how individuals can build their own emotional strength. In 1975, Howard Gardner introduced the concept of Multiple Intelligence Theory in his text, *The Shattered Mind,* which introduced Intrapersonal (self-awareness) and Interpersonal (social relationship) skills." In 1981, Sternberg, Conway, Ketron, and Bernstein conducted a study wherein participants were asked to describe an intelligent person. Many of the responses included characteristics related to social abilities such as being able to admit to mistakes, to accept others, and to display interest in the world. Research continued on the topic of social intelligence and the theory continued to develop into what we refer to today as emotional intelligence. In 1985, Wayne Payne introduced the term "emotional intelligence" in his doctoral dissertation entitled, "A Study of Emotion: Developing Emotional Intelligence; Self-integration; Relating to Fear, Pain, and Desire." In 1987, Keith Beasley & Reuven Bar-On utilized the term "emotional quotient (EQ)." Beasley discussed the term in an issue of Mensa Magazine while Bar-On mentioned the term in the unpublished version of his graduate thesis. In 1990, Yale researchers, Peter Salovey and John Mayer published their landmark article, "Emotional Intelligence" in the Journal, *Imagination, Cognition, and Personality.* As aforementioned, in 1995 Daniel Goleman wrote his best-selling *Emotional Intelligence* text and described why Emotional Intelligence (EI) can matter more than one's Intelligence Quotient (IQ) in predicting future life success. Finally, in 1996, The Consortium for Research on Emotional Intelligence in Organizations conducted research to identify emotional and social factors that are integral to later job success (Cory, 2019).

Emotions and Moods

In order to comprehend the construct of emotional intelligence, it is important to understand the basics of the theory: emotions and moods. Morris (1989) and Forgas (1992) define emotions as intense feelings that are triggered by internal and/or external stimuli. Emotions are demanding of attention and cause an interruption in cognition and behavior. Since emotions are so high in intensity, they are more fleeting than moods- however- emotions may persist over time in a less intense manner. Plutchik (2001) categorized human feelings into eight basic emotions: fear, anger, joy, sadness, acceptance, disgust, anticipation, and surprise. These eight emotions act as messages that aid in the decision-making process. When a stimulus invokes the emotion of *fear*, the message is that a change needs to occur. When a stimulus invokes the emotion of *anger*, the message is that one needs to fight against the issues caused by the stimulus. When a stimulus invokes the emotion of *joy*, the message is an indication of what is important in our life. When a stimulus invokes the emotion of *sadness*, the message implies that we need to reconnect with loved ones. When a stimulus invokes the emotion of *acceptance*, the message is to be open-minded. When a stimulus invokes the emotion of *disgust*, the message serves as a warning to reject the stimulus. When a stimulus invokes the emotion of *anticipation*, the message is an indication to start planning for the future. Lastly, when a stimulus invokes the emotion of *surprise*, the message serves to turn our attention to new situations and events. Salovey & Mayer (1990) further explain that emotions are adaptive and can ignite the transformation of personal and social interactions into experiences that are enriching for the individuals involved.

Whereas emotions are high in intensity, short-lasting, and interruptive - moods are the opposite. Morris (1989) defines moods as being general states of feelings that are not rooted in the original stimuli that caused the mood. Moods are low intensity and pervasive. Furthermore, moods have been found to have an effect on cognition. Both positive and negative moods are functionally beneficial. Forgas, Bower, and Moylan (1990) discovered that positive moods can increase perceptions of one's own self-efficacy and success. Moreover, George (2000) found that positive moods can increase creativity, inductive reasoning, and integrative thinking. Negative moods on the other hand, have been found to increase diligent information processing, attention to detail, and the detection of error (Isen, Daubman, & Nowicki, 1987; Salvoey, Hsee, & Mayer, 1993).

Emotional Intelligence

Leading researchers in the field, Salovey and Mayer (1990), define four components of emotional intelligence, 1) understanding and expressing one's own emotions, 2) the ability to perceive emotions in others, 3) regulating affect, and 4) using moods and emotions to influence one's own behavior. Emotional intelligence is viewed as a skill-set that can be cultivated and developed over time. Further research has identified two types of emotional intelligence: trait and ability, as well as four major aspects of emotional intelligence: 1) appraisal and expression of emotion, 2) use of emotion to enhance cognitive processes and decision making, 3) knowledge of emotions, and 4) managing emotions. Emotional intelligence is a critical construct because of its positive connection to increased functioning, developmental outcomes, healthy relationships, and achievement (Salovey & Mayer, 1990; Goleman, 1995).

Types of Emotional Intelligence

Trait Emotional Intelligence

Petrides and Furnham (2003) define trait emotional intelligence as a personality trait rooted in self-perceived emotional capabilities and dispositions measured by self-reported surveys. Characteristics of trait emotional intelligence reported in surveys include social awareness, adaptability, empathy, assertiveness, self-motivation, emotion perception, expression, management, and regulation (Petrides, 2011).

Ability Emotional Intelligence

Ability emotional intelligence is more connected with the Salovey and Mayer (1990) definition which views emotional intelligence as a skill that can be developed. Moreover, Petrides and Furnham (2003) add that ability emotional intelligence is measured through ability tests and is connected to information processes within the brain.

FOUR MAJOR ASPECTS OF EMOTIONAL INTELLIGENCE

Appraisal and Expression of Emotion

Salovey and Mayer (1990) separate appraisal and expression of emotion into two categories: verbal and non-verbal. The key element of verbal appraisal and expression is using language to clearly speak about one's own or others' emotions, whereas non-verbal appraisal and expression use body language and other silent cues.

A major aspect of the appraisal and expression of emotion is empathy. *Empathy* is defined as the ability of an individual to understand another person' emotions and then experience those same emotions him/herself (Salovey & Mayer, 1990). Further empathic skills include the accurate identification of another's emotions (Buck, 1984), understanding others' point of views (Dymond, 1949), experiencing the same or a different appropriate emotion as a response to another person (Mehrabian & Epstein, 1972), and communicating or acting on the responsive emotion (Krebs, 1975). Being able to empathize with another individual is linked to the finding of Kessler, Price, and Wortman (1985) that positive and healthy relationships with other individuals lead to lower levels of stress and to increased life satisfaction. Additional findings by Salovey and Mayer (1990) state that having more friends, who are emotionally intelligent, leads to having a more supportive and empathic social structure.

Using Emotions to Enhance Cognition and Decision Making

Emotions can be used in functional ways to enhance cognition such as acting as a signal to direct one's attention to specific stimuli (Frigda, 1988) or aiding in the decision- making process (Damasio, 1994). For instance, Damasio (1994) found that being able to predict how others' will emotionally react to an event, a trait of emotional intelligence, can help in the decision-making process by providing multiple options. Moreover, Salovey and Mayer (1990) discovered that emotional shifts can be beneficial to flexible planning, since it leads to wider perspective-taking and helps generate a multitude of ideas.

Knowledge About Emotions

Knowledge about emotions relates to understanding both the determinants and consequences of moods and emotions and how they evolve and change over time (George, 2000)

Managing Emotions

The management of emotions is critical to emotional intelligence since it involves the distinct abilities individuals possess in terms of how to regulate their own and others' emotions and moods (George, 2000). Wasielewski (1985) found that the ability to manage emotions, such as inciting excitement or caution in others, is an advantageous skill in social influence. The ability to successfully manage moods and emotions relies on knowledge and on the consideration of determinants, appropriateness, and malleability of moods and emotions (George, 2000). Moreover, it is a reflective process involving a meta-regulation of mood (Mayer & Salovey, 1997).

COMPONENTS OF EMOTIONAL INTELLIGENCE

In his renowned Emotional Intelligence text (1995), Goleman delineates five key components of emotional intelligence and then separates these five realms into four quadrants. Goleman's five realms include, 1) *Self-Awareness* (knowing and understanding your own emotions), 2) *Self-Regulation* (controlling inner states and managing yourself), 3) *Motivation* (a general willingness to do something), 4) *Empathy* (sharing and recognizing other people's emotions), and 5) *Social skills* (managing and maintaining relationships with others). These five realms are then separated into *Personal Competence* and *Social Competence*. *Personal Competence* involves two key ingredients, 1) Self-Awareness, understanding your own emotions as they occur, and 2) Self-Management, using an awareness of your emotions to positively direct your behavior. *Social competence*, on the other hand, encompasses, 1) Social-Awareness, the ability to understand and recognize emotions in others, and 2) Relationship Management, using knowledge of your emotions and the emotions of others to successfully manage your social interactions (Riopel, 2019).

MEASURING EMOTIONAL INTELLIEGENCE

The BarOn Emotional Quotient Inventory, also known as BarOn EQ-I, is used to measure emotional intelligence. The EQ-I asks individuals to read a multitude of statements and to rank how much each statement describes them. There are five rank options on the test: 1) Very seldom or not true of me, 2) Seldom true of me, 3) Sometimes true of me, 4) Often true of me, and 5) Very often true of me. Examples of statements on the EQ-i include: "I know how to deal with upsetting problems," "I'm unable to show affection," "I feel sure of myself in most situations," and "It's fairly easy for me to express my feelings (BarOn, 1997)."

Emotional Intelligence (EI) vs. Intelligence Quotient (IQ)

Two major types of intelligence include the Emotional Quotient (EQ) and the Intelligence Quotient (IQ). Wechsler (1958) defines intelligence as an individual's capacity to think rationally, to effectively manage his/her environment, and to act with intent. More simply, Bradberry (2014) defines intelligence as one's ability to learn. Intelligence is perceived as being stable over time. For example, your IQ can be the same at age 18 as it is at age 60. Therefore, a key difference between the emotional quotient (EQ) and intelligence quotient (IQ) is that one's emotional quotient is malleable and can change and evolve over time. Furthermore, the intelligence quotient is related more to technical skills, whereas emotional intelligence is related to social skills. As an article in *Time Magazine* stated, "IQ gets you hired, but EQ gets you promoted (Gibbs, 2001)."

Emotional Intelligence and Effective Leadership in the Workplace

Enhancing one's emotional intelligence (EI) is critical for enhancing a variety of skill-sets in the workplace. In fact, Bradberry (2014) reveals how EI can predict work performance. He suggests that 90% of top performers in the workplace have high EI, while only 20% of bottom performers have high EI. Moreover, individuals with high EI earn $29,000 more per year than those with low EI and one additional point of EI could result in a $1,300 increase in salary per EI point. This strong relationship between EI and success in the workplace may relate closely to the following findings, increased emotional intelligence has been related to better communication and listening, stronger decision-making, more positive interactions among colleagues in the workplace, more positive work attitudes, and more positive work outcomes. Moreover, it is has been related to more altruistic behavior, higher employee engagement, stronger group dynamics and better relationships, lower burnout and turnover, less anger and stress and higher overall productivity in the workplace (Bradberry, 2014).

When emotional intelligence was tested alongside thirty-three other important workplace skills, emotional intelligence was identified as the strongest predictor of performance, accounting for a full 58% of success in all types of jobs (Bradberry, 2014). Emotional intelligence was also considered to be the strongest driver of leadership and personal excellence.

More specifically, George (2000) identified five aspects of effective leadership: 1) Create collective goals and objectives, 2) Cultivate an appreciation in others for the importance of work-related activities, 3) Establish and maintain trust, confidence, and optimism in the workplace, 4) Encourage flexible decision-making processes, and 5) Develop an identity for the organization.

The first element of effective leadership is creating collective goals and objectives. According to George (2000), this is connected to emotional intelligence since emotional intelligence contributes to the development of an organization's vision. This connection is also made by Isen, Daubman, & Nowiciki (1987), who found a relationship between positive moods and increased creativity and therefore, leaders with emotional intelligence, who can better regulate their emotions, are more likely to create compelling organizational visions. This is a great example of leaders managing their emotions to enhance cognitive processes and decision-making. Moreover, George (2000) highlights the importance of not only creating an organizational vision, but also of being able to communicate that vision throughout the workplace to ensure employees understand it and see it as a collective or shared idea. Leaders can accomplish this by understanding how their emotions may be perceived, anticipating how others will react, and managing their own reactions.

The second element of effective leadership is cultivating an appreciation in others for the importance of work-related activities. Leaders with high emotional intelligence are able to accomplish this task more efficiently since they can better understand and manage emotions and they possess more self-awareness and social awareness (George, 2000). This skill can be used in subtle ways to influence their employees. For example, Salovey, Hsee, & Mayer (1993) found that leaders with high emotional intelligence are more likely to realize that people react more positively to organizational changes when those changes are framed as improvements over the current condition. Furthermore, the highly emotional intelligent leader will be able to individualize tactics to ensure each employee is positively impacted.

The third element of effective leadership is establishing and maintaining trust, confidence, and optimism in the workplace. George (2000) connected the second and third elements of effective leadership by once again highlighting the importance of leaders having the ability to appraise how their employees feel and being able to influence those emotions.. Emotional intelligence is critical for this element since leaders with high emotional intelligence may be more likely to create a work atmosphere that encourages cooperation and trust through the development of quality relationships with their employees and the use of constructive thinking (George, 2000).

The fourth element of effective leadership is encouraging flexible decision making processes. Decision-making is connected to emotional intelligence in multiple ways. Frigda (1988) noted that emotions can act as signals to redirect one's attention to more pressing matters. Additionally, Schwarz (1990) found that the management of emotions can improve decision-making as well as provides leaders with more details about the challenges they are encountering. Therefore, emotional intelligence can be beneficial to leaders since leaders have the ability to use emotions to make their decision-making more effective and are able to recognize emotions which interfere with decision-making. Regarding flexible thinking, emotional intelligence allows individuals to link more information together and to forge new connections, which increase one's understanding of how issues are related.

The fifth and final element of effective leadership is to develop an identity of the organization. According to Trice & Beyer (1993), an organization's identity is created by the collective culture and shared ideologies of employees such as having similar beliefs, norms, and values. This is related to emotional intelligence because George (2000) defines the management of culture as the management of the organization and its members' emotions. Therefore, effective leaders require a high emotional intelligence since they need to understand their own emotions and their organization's emotions by recognizing all of the shared norms, beliefs, and values. Furthermore, an effective leader should be able to do the above as well as using this understanding to generate even stronger collective feelings amongst all employees. One way to prepare for future emotional intelligence in the workplace is to establish important emotional intelligence strategies early on in development.

Emotional Intelligence and Parenting

Family is the first and most critical context in which early socialization and emotional development take place (Argyriou, Bakoyannis, & Tantaros, 2016). Moreover, diverse parenting styles relate to adaptability, emotion regulation and impulsiveness (Argyriou, Bakoyannis, & Tantaros, 2016). Fortunately, our brains benefits from plasticity, suggesting that it is flexible enough to adapt, grow and compensate in the case of any damage. As new brain cells develop and more connections are made, new skills emerge. In fact, strategies to enhance emotional intelligence (EI) are critical to ensure the emotional parts of the brain (i.e. the amygdala) do not hijack the more rational parts of the brain (i.e. the frontal lobe) when important decisions have to be made. By enhancing the connections between these brain areas, one can transform EI strategies into daily habits. In this manner, EI can evolve and improve the strategies individuals use throughout life. Moreover, parents can model emotional intelligence or can teach emotionally intelligent strategies to their children.

With respect to modeling, parents can model positive emotions and behaviors for children. They can be responsive to their children's emotions and behaviors. Parents can also offer role-playing strategies, vignettes, or "what would you do?" scenarios to encourage their children to practice pursuing emotionally intelligent strategies. To enhance their children's self-awareness, parents can help their children identify and/or recognize their own basic or complex emotions and how best to cope with them. Parents can also introduce games to encourage their children to practice turn-taking, winning and losing, sharing and negotiating. In addition, parents can view TV programs or read books with their children and discuss the storylines with them. This could offer ample opportunities for parents to discuss how characters are acting in the storylines and how the characters could improve their behaviors or reactions to specific situations.

In order for parents to model Emotional Intelligence (EI) for their children, they need to benefit from and to practice strong EI strategies themselves. Researchers suggest that the following ten steps may be critical towards developing one's EI: 1) Manage your emotions, 2) Utilize a careful vocabulary, 3) Practice empathy, 4) Know your stressors, 5) Pause, 6) Benefit from criticism, 7) Praise others and provide positive feedback, 8) Apologize and forgive, 9) Keep commitments, and 10) Feel emotions (Barison, 2018).

With respect to the first EI strategy of *managing emotions*, it is recommended that individuals be knowledgeable about their strengths and weaknesses and consider how their mood may be impacting their daily thoughts and decisions. Individuals are encouraged to stop negative self-talk in its tracks and to reduce negativity by separating out negative thoughts and perceptions from actual facts. Individuals are encouraged to be the masters of their own happiness and to not let others take the wind out of their sails or threaten their happiness (Bariso, 2018).

The second EI strategy involves *selecting a careful vocabulary.* Researchers recommend that individuals transform their vocabulary to utilize more *careful vocabulary,* or specific as opposed to general words to express how they are feeling. Achieving fluency in one's emotional vocabulary wherein you replace the general feeling, "bad" with the specific feelings of "frustration," "anxiety," "disappointment," or "embarrassment," allows the individual to address the emotion or situation more directly. Individuals can better manage their emotions when they know how to more effectively identify them (Bariso, 2018)

The third EI strategy, *practicing empathy* is critical towards developing a strong emotional intelligence. Empathy differs from sympathy, in that empathy requires you to actually place yourself in the shoes of another individual, while sympathy simply relates to pitying or feeling badly when someone is suffering. When an individual places him/herself in the shoes of another individual or wears his/her glasses, he/she can more effectively comprehend the motivations of the other individual and can understand their pain points, what upsets them, frustrates them or inversely, what comforts them. This helps with customer relations and in various other realms of the workplace (Bariso, 2018).

The fourth EI strategy relates to *knowing your stressors and triggers.* Researchers suggest that individuals should conduct a self-check-in, wherein they determine which types of comments or actions set them off. Individuals tend to experience comments or experiences as more negative, once they are already fearful, threatened or frustrated. If individuals can be knowledgeable about these triggers, they can ward off future negative behaviors or can prevent exacerbating an already difficult situation (Bariso, 2018).

The fifth EI strategy of *pausing* reminds individuals to take a step back for a moment. Some clinicians recommend counting from one to three and watching one's breath rise and fall, which helps increase brain circuits for attention and helps reduce stress. In children, one can say, "Breathe in the roses, blow out the candles," so they use visual imagery to help them better breathe or participate in breathing exercises (Bariso, 2018).

The sixth EI strategy involves *benefitting from criticism.* While many individuals struggle to hear or to appreciate criticism, researchers suggest that accepting criticism and being difficult to offend, can be very helpful for knowing how other people think and for helping us to improve.

The seventh EI strategy of *praising others and providing positive feedback* reminds us how important it is to offer affirmation to other individuals. Individuals crave appreciation and accolades. If you can hone in on an individuals' strengths and offer praise to him/her with some specific feedback on what he/she is doing well, it can go a long way in building a trusting and positive relationship with others (Bariso, 2018).

Researchers strongly encourage the eighth EI strategy of *apologizing and forgiving others* since there is a strong correlation between removing these tensions and one's positive, physical and mental health functioning. It is highly beneficial to take responsibility for one's actions and to release grudges and associated stressors (Bariso, 2018).

The ninth EI strategy of *keeping commitments and helping others* assists individuals in building a strong reputation for reliability, trustworthiness and leadership both inside and outside of the workplace. It's important to consider how your actions will affect others and help other individuals even if there is no quid pro quo or help in return (Bariso, 2018).

Finally, the tenth EI strategy relates to *recording your emotions and physically feeling those emotions in your body*. It's important to know that when someone is sad, he/she may feel decreased sensations in his/her heir limbs. When one is angry, he/she might feel increased sensations in his/her upper limbs. When one is feeling a sense of disgust, he/she might experience sensations in his/her throat and digestive system. If one is experiencing surprise or fear, he/she might feel sensations in his/her chest. Moreover, if one is feeling happiness, he/she will likely feel sensations all over his/her body. Being aware of your bodily sensations may help you better decode what basic or complex emotion you may be experiencing at various points in time. Being able to identify these emotions can then help you better manage them. In addition to these child and parent-directed EI strategies, it is important to look at which parenting dimensions may be most closely related to strong socio-emotional outcomes in children (Bariso, 2018).

PARENTING DIMENSIONS

Alegre (2011) categorizes parenting related to emotional intelligence into four dimensions: 1) parental responsiveness, 2) parental positive demandingness, 3) parental negative demandingness, and 4) parental emotion-related coaching. Alegre's (2011) research found that three of the four parenting dimensions (parental responsiveness, parental positive demandingness, and parental emotion-related coaching) correlated with higher emotional intelligence in children.

Parental Responsiveness

With respect to parental responsiveness, researchers operationalize the construct as a combination of parental warmth, nurturance, and support (Alegre, 2011). This combination tends to be associated with positive outcomes in development such as higher child self-regulation and lower externalizing behaviors (Eiden, Edwards, & Leonard, 2007), higher self-esteem (Rohner, 1990), and better psychological adjustment (Khaleque, Rohner, and Riaz, 2007).

Parental Positive Demandingness

Examples of parental positive demandingness strategies include monitoring and supervising children's behavior, allowing children autonomy, reasonable and appropriate discipline, and setting achievable expectations for children to meet (De Clercq, Van Leeuwen, De Fruyt, Van Heil, & Mervielde, 2008; Sanders, 2008). Research has found many beneficial outcomes for children who are raised using parental positive demandingness. The benefits for children include, having higher confidence (Collins & Barber, 2005), higher life satisfaction (Suldo & Huebner, 2004), and higher academic functioning (Wang, Pomerantz & Chen, 2007). Further connections have been made between parental positive demandingness and reduced alcohol consumption (Morgo-Wilson, 2008) and reduced risky sexual behavior (Baptiste, Tolou-Shams, Miller, Mcbride, & Paikoff, 2007).

Parental Negative Demandingness

Examples of parental negative demandingness strategies include controlling children psychologically and punishing children in an inappropriate, harsh, or retaliative manner (Barnett, Deng, Mills-Koonce, Willoughby, & Cox, 2008; Shelton & Harold, 2008). Research has found many adverse developmental outcomes for children raised using parental negative demandingness. For instance, children raised with parental negative demandingness tend to have a lower emotional well-being, fewer prosocial behaviors, and tend to be more prone to learning how to internalize and externalize their problems. The development of cognitive anxiety and personality disorders can also result from children being raised using parental negative demandingness (Alegre, 2011).

EMOTIONAL INTELLIGENCE AT SCHOOL

One of the most optimal places to inculcate healthy EI in children is in the classroom. In school, students with higher EI tend to benefit from more sustainable friendships (Jones, Barnes, Bailey, & Doolittle, 2017), to have greater confidence and self-esteem, to possess greater knowledge of their strengths and limitations, are more versed in conflict resolution, are better at managing stress and anxiety and are better at making decisions and at showing empathy (Bradberry, 2014).

Children who benefit from higher EI in schools, also tend to have better grades and higher standardized test scores, are more likely to initiate positive relationships with teachers, to participate in classroom activities, and to be positively engaged in learning (Jones et al., 2017).

One of Fatum's (2013) essential elements for a healthy classroom environment is creating a space in the classroom where emotional intelligence is encouraged and cultivated in children. Fatum (2013) identifies ten practical suggestions for teachers and parents to help children develop a more robust emotional intelligence: 1) Observe children at home and in the classroom, 2) Create stories to assist with learning, 3) Give choices and encourage connections, 4) Teach the importance of emotions, 5) Create a collaborative atmosphere, 6) Make reflection and journaling a daily habit, 7) Reframe mistakes, 8) Celebrate feelings, 9) Support children's aspirations, and 10) Actively model emotional intelligence skills.

The first suggestion is to observe children in their daily environment such as their home or classroom. During the observation, parents and teachers should take notes about how the children are behaving and how they are relating to other children. For instance, they may hone in on their children's moods, how they communicate with others, and on their personalities. These observations can help provide clues as to the child's ability to manage his/her emotions, his/her learning style, and it can help assess how he/she relates to others.

The second suggestion is to create stories to assist children with learning. Stories help stimulate the integration of multiple senses and story memory is not affected by anxiety, compared to short-term memory which is impacted by stress and anxiety (Cozolino, 2009). Moreover, stories help to foster collectivism amongst individuals and creates the sense of "we" that is rooted in emotional intelligence (Fatum, 2013).

The third suggestion is to give children choices and to encourage connections with others. Fatum (2008) found that the action of making a choice stimulates intrinsic motivation in individuals. Additionally, having a safe environment where choices and consequences can be evaluated provides individuals with the opportunity to learn more about themselves. Therefore, creating safe environments for decision-making within homes and classrooms encourages independence and self-efficacy within children.

The fourth suggestion is to teach the importance of emotions, as well as to emphasize the meaning of different emotions. In most western cultures, the importance of understanding emotions is often overlooked. According to Damasio (1994), the lack of emotion recognition is rooted in the behaviorist belief that emotions are dangerous and should be avoided. However, Fatum (2013) believes that understanding emotions is connected to one's ability to make informed decisions. Therefore, it is important for parents and teachers to validate children's feelings and to help identify the appropriate actions that should be made based on the experienced emotions.

The fifth suggestion is to create a collaborative atmosphere at home and in the classroom. Medina (2008) found that competition amongst peers can create stress which can lead to challenges with learning. In comparison, Vail (1981) found that a calm and relaxed learning environment can lead to increased memory and cognitive processing. Therefore, creating a collaborative home and classroom environment will provide children with an optimal opportunity to learn and grow.

The sixth suggestion is to encourage reflection and daily journaling since both have been found to be beneficial to brain functioning (Medina, 2008). Fatum (2013) suggests that time should be taken to reflect every ninety minutes since it provides our brains with an opportunity to encode new material and to combine it with older memories. Furthermore, practicing these new concepts, through journaling or other means, provides children with the opportunity to actively learn. Journaling can also provide children with the opportunity to actively experience the second suggestion of creating stories, and the fourth suggestion of understanding the meaning of different emotions, on their own.

The seventh suggestion is to reframe mistakes children make to assist them with learning and to maintain a safe environment. Fatum (2013) highlights that providing a safe home or classroom environment to help children reframe their mistakes increases cognitive processing, while also reducing stress. Furthermore, it promotes intrinsic motivation and self-efficacy since children are learning how to develop and correctly use a variety of skills.

The eighth suggestion is to celebrate feelings. This is a critical suggestion since our brains naturally focus on negative elements, and therefore, children need help recognizing and focusing on positive elements to create balance (Fatum, 2013). Moreover, Fatum (2013) identifies celebrating emotions and accomplishments as a way for children to develop realistic optimism and to focus on their strengths while contending with challenges. An example of a child finding balance is acknowledging that he/she may have a weakness in one area, but may have a strength in another (such as struggling with grammar, but being very good at math). This demonstrates a child's ability to recognize his/her own values and balance his/her emotional responses.

The ninth suggestion is to support children's aspirations in a serious manner. Fatum (2013) states that children- who set goals and actively work toward achieving them- develop a lifelong beneficial skill-set that enhances executive functioning. Furthermore, goal setting is linked to increased self-efficacy and self-perceptions of effectiveness. Therefore, it is highly beneficial for parents and teachers to support children and to help them achieve their goals.

The tenth suggestion is to actively model emotional intelligence skills since the emotional intelligence of adults is linked to the emotional intelligence skills of children (Fatum, 2013). Grayson (2012) discovered that parents with high emotional intelligence skills were more likely to manage their emotions, to trust their feelings, and to solve problems. Moreover, modeling emotional intelligence is important because children are able to identify when adults' actions are different then the expectations set by the same adults (Fatum, 2013).

Emotional Intelligence Programs in the Schools

Due to the importance of fostering emotional intelligence in the schools, a variety of robust programs have been developed to both nurture and improve the socio-emotional development of children in and outside of the classroom. Programs tend to break emotional intelligence (EI) into three principal categories: *cognitive regulation, emotional processes, and social/interpersonal skills* (Jones, Barnes, Bailey, & Doolittle, 2017).

Cognitive regulation refers to the basic cognitive skills that are required to direct behavior toward attaining a goal. This construct is related to executive functioning, which involves planning and decision-making and tends to require a certain level of inhibition. Therefore, children tend to use cognitive skills for tasks that require concentration, planning, problem solving, coordination, making conscious choices among alternatives, and inhibiting impulses (Jones et al., 2017).

Emotional processes refer to skills that help children recognize, express, and regulate their own emotions, as well as understand the emotional perspectives of others. These processes are fundamental toward establishing positive social interactions and toward building relationships with peers or adults. Programs related to scaffolding emotional processes tend to target skills like emotion knowledge, vocabulary, and expression (Jones et al., 2017).

Finally, *social and interpersonal skills* relate to accurately interpreting the behaviors of others, effectively navigating social situations, and interacting positively with peers or adults. More specifically, interpersonal skills include the ability to develop friendships, to engage in prosocial and ethical behaviors, and to solve social conflicts. Garnering this emotional knowledge helps individuals effectively solve social problems and collaborate with others (Jones et al., 2017).

Fortunately, many of these school-based programs have shown statistically significant positive effects on socio-emotional outcomes. Immediate outcomes include improvements in the classroom social and instructional environment, as well as in students' socio-emotional skills. Over the long-term, these programs have also shown success at not only enhancing children's social skills, but in boosting their behavioral and academic outcomes, as well. For instance, with respect to behavior, improving EI is expected to produce positive behavioral outcomes such as reducing aggression, depression, and anxiety in children. These programs can positively impact mental processes that underlie behaviors, instead of focusing on directly changing the behaviors (Jones et al., 2017).

In evaluating the efficacy of these programs, it is important to consider that programs usually require a significant time commitment, both with respect to training and implementation. The majority of these programs also focus on skills in the classroom, but children would also benefit from these skills in unstructured environments, like playgrounds, lunchrooms, school hallways, and in out-of-school settings. Programs should also consider further the role of parents and the home environment. It is recommended that these programs also focus more on teachers and classrooms, target skills that reflect developmental growth and age-appropriate outcomes and that measures for the program extend to classrooms, schools, to out-of-school settings and to adult outcomes (Jones et al., 2017).

A number of other programs attempt to teach socio-emotional skills and development to children. The Fast Track PATHS Program (Biernman et al., 2010), The Incredible Year Series (Webster-Stratton & Herman, 2010) and The Strong Kids Social Emotional Learning Program (Alegre, 2011) are just a few of the plethora of programs out there.

The Fast Track PATHS (Promoting Alternative Thinking Strategies) (Biernman et al., 2010) teaches self-control, emotional awareness and understanding, peer-related social skills, and social problem-solving to promote social and emotional competence. Research has shown its efficacy in reducing aggressive behaviors and increasing prosocial behavior, especially in boys (Biernman et al., 2010).

The Incredible Years Series (Webster-Stratton & Herman, 2010) is a set of programs based on social cognitive theory and uses an intervention consisting of sixty socioemotional lessons from kindergarten to second grade. The program has boasted improvements in problem-solving and conflict resolution skills. When the program has been taught by parents and teachers, study results were even stronger and children showed fewer aggressive behaviors and better prosocial skills (Webster-Stratton & Herman, 2010).

The Strong Kids Social Emotional Learning Programs (Alegre, 2011) are programs catered to Kindergarten to eighth-grade students. These programs teach social-emotional skills, with a particular emphasis on enhancing emotional knowledge, self-management strategies, and coping strategies in children (Alegre, 2011).

CONCLUSION

Children with strong emotional intelligence (EI) skills have better mental and physical health as adults, get along better with others, do better in school, and have more successful future careers (Jones et al., 2017). These positive outcomes are just a few of the multitude of positive benefits children and adults can glean from having a strong and healthy emotional intelligence. If parents, employers, school teachers and administrators can tap into emotionally intelligent strategies for use in the home, the workplace, the school and outside of the school, children and adults could benefit immensely from this investment in socio-emotional development.

As aforementioned, programs that aim to enhance children's social skills, are often able to boost children's behavioral and academic outcomes, as well. With respect to behavior, these programs can positively impact mental processes that underlie behaviors, which can help reduce depression, anxiety, aggression and other internalizing or externalizing behaviors in children (Jones et al., 2017).

In terms of academics and/or future life success, as aforementioned, Bradberry (2014) notes that 90% of top performers in the workplace have high EI, while only 20% of bottom performers have high EI. Moreover, individuals with high EI earn $29,000 more per year than those with low EI and one additional point of EI could result in a $1,300 increase in salary per EI point. These impressive statistics likely relate to the fact that employees with higher EI in the workplace, tend to have stronger communication and listening skills, stronger decision-making, more positive interactions with colleagues in the workplace, more positive work attitudes, more positive work outcomes, lower burnout and turnover, less anger and stress and higher overall productivity in the workplace (Bradberry, 2014). This also aligns with the aforementioned research that compared to thirty-three other workplace skills, emotional intelligence was identified as the strongest predictor of performance, accounting for a full 58% of success in all types of jobs. It was also deemed to be the strongest driver of leadership and of personal excellence (Bradberry, 2014).

It is for these reasons that a commitment toward fostering emotional intelligence in the home, in schools and in the workplace has to figure prominently in the minds of parents, teachers, administrators and employers. This investment in human and emotional capital will garner significant benefits over the course of the individual's lifetime and in the success and productivity of the workplace.

REFERENCES

Alegre, A. (2011). Parenting styles and children's emotional intelligence: What do we know? *The Family Journal*, *19*(1), 56–62. doi:10.1177/1066480710387486

Baptiste, D. R., Tolou-Shams, M., Miller, S. R., Mcbride, C. K., & Paikoff, R. L. (2007). Determinants of parental monitoring and preadolescent sexual risk situations among African American families living in urban public housing. *Journal of Child and Family Studies*, *16*(2), 261–274. doi:10.100710826-006-9083-4

Bariso, J. (2018, Feb. 28). 13 Signs of High Emotional Intelligence: Wonder what emotional intelligence looks like in everyday life? *Inc.,* 1-5.

BarOn, R. (1997). *The BarOn Emotional Quotient inventory* (BarOn EQ-i). Author.

Bradberry, T. (2014). Emotional Intelligence. *Forbes*.

Buck, R. (1984). *The Communication of Emotion*. New York: The Guilford Press.

Collins, K., & Barber, H. (2005). Female athletes' perceptions of parental influences. *Journal of Sport Behavior*, *28*(4), 295.

Cory, D. (2019). *EQ-i Certification Course*. The Emotional Intelligence Training Company Inc.

Cozolino, L. (2014). *The neuroscience of human relationships: Attachment and the developing social brain.* WW Norton & Company.

Damasio, A. R. (1994). *Descartes' error: emotion, reason, and the human brain.* New York: GP Putnam's Sons.

De Clercq, B., Van Leeuwen, K., De Fruyt, F., Van Hiel, A., & Mervielde, I. (2008). Maladaptive personality traits and psychopathology in childhood and adolescence: The moderating effect of parenting. *Journal of Personality*, *76*(2), 357–383. doi:10.1111/j.1467-6494.2007.00489.x PMID:18331276

Dymond, R. F. (1949). A scale for the measurement of empathic ability. *Journal of Consulting Psychology*, *13*(2), 127–133. doi:10.1037/h0061728 PMID:18118267

Fatum, B. (2013). Healthy Classrooms, Emotional Intelligence, and Brain Research. *Six seconds: The emotional intelligence network.* Retrieved from http://www.6seconds.org/2013/05/29/healthy-classrooms-emotionalintelligence-and-brain-research

Forgas, J. P. (1992). Affect in social judgments and decisions: A multiprocess model. *Advances in Experimental Social Psychology*, *25*, 227–275. doi:10.1016/S0065-2601(08)60285-3

Forgas, J. P., Bower, G. H., & Moylan, S. J. (1990). Praise or blame? Affective influences on attributions for achievement. *Journal of Personality and Social Psychology*, *59*(4), 809–819. doi:10.1037/0022-3514.59.4.809 PMID:2254856

Frigda, N. H. (1988). The laws of emotion. *The American Psychologist*, *43*(5), 349–358. doi:10.1037/0003-066X.43.5.349 PMID:3389582

Gibbs, N. (2001, June 24). The EQ Factor. *TIME*. Retrieved from http://content.time.com/time/magazine/article/0,9171,133181,00.html

Goleman, D. (1995). *Emotional intelligence*. New York: Academic Press.

Grayson, R. (2012). *Social, developmental, & organizational psychology applied to camp*. Retrieved from www.visionrealization.com

Isen, A. M., Daubman, K. A., & Nowicki, G. P. (1987). Positive affect facilitates creative problem solving. *Journal of Personality and Social Psychology*, *52*(6), 1122–1131. doi:10.1037/0022-3514.52.6.1122 PMID:3598858

Kessler, R. C., Price, R. H., & Wortman, C. B. (1985). Social factors in psychopathology: Stress, social support, and coping processes. *Annual Review of Psychology*, *36*(1), 531–572. doi:10.1146/annurev.ps.36.020185.002531 PMID:3883893

Krebs, D. (1975). Empathy and altruism. *Journal of Personality and Social Psychology*, *32*(6), 1134–1146. doi:10.1037/0022-3514.32.6.1134 PMID:1214217

Medina, J. (2008). *Brain rules*. Seattle, WA: Pear Press.

Mehrabian, A., & Epstein, N. (1972). A measure of emotional empathy 1. *Journal of Personality*, *40*(4), 525–543. doi:10.1111/j.1467-6494.1972.tb00078.x PMID:4642390

Mogro-Wilson, C. (2008). The influence of parental warmth and control on Latino adolescent alcohol use. *Hispanic Journal of Behavioral Sciences*, *30*(1), 89–105. doi:10.1177/0739986307310881

Morris, W. N. (1989). *Mood: The frame of mind*. New York: Springer-Verlag. doi:10.1007/978-1-4612-3648-1

Petrides, K. V. (2011). Ability and trait emotional intelligence. In The Wiley-Blackwell handbook of individual differences, (pp. 656–678). Chichester, UK: Wiley-Blackwell.

Petrides, K. V., & Furnham, A. (2003). Trait emotional intelligence: Behavioural validation in two studies of emotion recognition and reactivity to mood induction. *European Journal of Personality*, *17*(1), 39–57. doi:10.1002/per.466

Riopel, L. (2019). *Emotional Intelligence Frameworks, Charts, Diagrams and Graphs*. Retrieved from www.positivepsychology.com

Salovey, P., Hsee, C. K., & Mayer, J. D. (1993). *Emotional intelligence and the self-regulation of affect. In Handbook of mental control* (pp. 258–277). Englewood Cliffs, NJ: Prentice Hall.

Salovey, P., & Mayer, J. D. (1990). Emotional intelligence. *Imagination, Cognition and Personality*, *9*(3), 185–211. doi:10.2190/DUGG-P24E-52WK-6CDG

Sanders, M. R. (2008). Triple P-Positive Parenting Program as a public health approach to strengthening parenting. *Journal of Family Psychology*, *22*(4), 506–517. doi:10.1037/0893-3200.22.3.506 PMID:18729665

Schwarz, N. (1990). Feelings as information: Informational and motivational functions of affective states. In *Handbook of motivation and cognition: Foundations of social behavior* (Vol. 2, pp. 527–561). New York: Guilford Press.

Sternberg, R. J., Conway, B. E., Ketron, J. L., & Bernstein, M. (1981). People's conceptions of intelligence. *Journal of Personality and Social Psychology*, *41*(1), 37–55. doi:10.1037/0022-3514.41.1.37

Suldo, S. M., & Huebner, E. S. (2004). The role of life satisfaction in the relationship between authoritative parenting dimensions and adolescent problem behavior. *Social Indicators Research*, *66*(1-2), 165–195. doi:10.1023/B:SOCI.0000007498.62080.1e

Thorndike, E. L. (1920). Intelligence and its uses. *Harper's Magazine.*

Thorndike, R. L., & Stein, S. (1937). An evaluation of the attempts to measure social intelligence. *Psychological Bulletin*, *34*(5), 275–285. doi:10.1037/h0053850

Trice, H. M., & Beyer, J. M. (1993). *The cultures of work organizations*. Prentice-Hall, Inc.

Vail, P. (1981). *Emotion: The On Off Switch for learning*. Rosemont, NJ: Modern Learning Press.

Wang, Q., Pomerantz, E. M., & Chen, H. (2007). The role of parents' control in early adolescents' psychological functioning: A longitudinal investigation in the United States and China. *Child Development*, *78*(5), 1592–1610. doi:10.1111/j.1467-8624.2007.01085.x PMID:17883450

Wechsler, D. (1958). *The measurement and appraisal of adult intelligence*. Academic Press.

KEY TERMS AND DEFINITIONS

Ability Emotional Intelligence (Ability EI): Perceives emotional intelligence as a skill that can be developed, can be measured through ability tests and is connected to information processes within the brain.

Emotional Intelligence: The ability to be cognizant of, control, and express one's emotions, and to manage interpersonal relationships judiciously and empathically.

Emotions: Natural instinctive states of mind which derive from one's circumstances, mood, or relationships with others.

Empathy: Stepping into the shoes of another person and perceiving and understanding the emotions that other individuals are experiencing.

Mood: A temporary state of mind or feeling.

Parental Emotion-Related Coaching: Involves recognizing your children's feelings and helping your children learn how emotions work and how to react to feelings in healthy ways.

Parental Negative Demandingness: Children of uninvolved parents tend to experience impairments in attachment, cognition, and social-emotional skills. They also often show poor self-control and low self-esteem

Parental Positive Demandingness: Monitoring and supervision, control, independence granting, setting age appropriate demands and expectations, and applying inductive discipline.

Parental Responsiveness: The degree to which parents are accepting and sensitive to their children's emotional and developmental needs.

Trait Emotional Intelligence (Trait EI): A constellation of emotional self-perceptions located at the lower levels of personality hierarchies that integrates the affective or emotional aspects of personality.

Chapter 6
Kindness Makes a Difference:
Assessing the Efficacy of *Addy & Uno*, an Off-Broadway Musical, and the *Realabilities* Educational Comic Book Series Curriculum in Enhancing Children's Kindness, Empathy, and Interest in Their Peers With Disabilities and Mental Health Disorders

Nava R. Silton
Marymount Manhattan College, USA

Patrick Riley
Marymount Manhattan College, USA

Amanda Anzovino
Marymount Manhattan College, USA

ABSTRACT

High quality interventions, which employ an extended contact model, wherein stories, roleplaying, and other appealing informational media are used to promote more positive intergroup attitudes, tend to be effective at enhancing the attitudes, intentions, and interests of typical children toward their peers with differences. The following four studies assess the efficacy of The Realabilities *comic book series and the* Addy & Uno *off-Broadway musical, which promote kindness, empathy, and a stop-bullying platform while teaching about disabilities and/or mental health disorders. The studies include 1) a qualitative study of 19 fourth grade students from an elementary*

DOI: 10.4018/978-1-7998-2940-9.ch006

school in Paramus, NJ, who viewed the Addy & Uno off-Broadway musical and participated in the full Realabilities educational comic book series intervention; 2) a qualitative study of 20 high school students with diverse disabilities, who participated in the full Realabilities comic book series intervention; 3) a quantitative study of 76 students from a high school in Long Island City, NY, who read the first mental health-based Realabilities comic book; and finally, 4) a quantitative study of 66 students from a high school in Long Island City, NY, who read the first and second mental-health based Realabilities comics. The researchers used a coding system to find principal themes in the qualitative data and used modified versions of the adjective checklist (ACL) and shared activities questionnaire (SAQ), along with a knowledge measure, to assess quantitative changes from pre to post-testing of the comic book series. Study findings help support the efficacy of an extended contact model and suggest that programs like these may serve as useful antidotes to counter negative attitudes of children and adolescents towards disabilities and mental health disorders, respectively.

INTRODUCTION

According to the Centers for Disease Control and Prevention (CDC) (Okoro, Hollis, Cyrus, & Griffin-Blake, 2018), 1 in 4 adults in the United States is currently living with a disability. Despite the fact that twenty-five percent of American adults have a disability, disabilities are rarely showcased favorably on TV and in the media. Unfortunately, when individuals with disabilities are depicted in the media, they are often being portrayed in an odd, pathetic or poor fashion. It is critical to change the landscape and to focus less on a deficit-based model of disability and more on the refined and unique abilities and strengths individuals with disabilities possess, since they are continuously seeking creative solutions and "work-arounds" to succeed in life (Respectability, 2018).

Children and Disabilities

Recent statistics suggest that from 2013-2014, 95% of all children and youth between the ages of 6 and 21, who were accommodated by IDEA, were enrolled in typical schools (National Center for Education Statistics, 2016). Moreover, the number of students who spent the lion's share of their school day (80% or more time) in regular education classrooms increased from 33% from 1990-1991 to 62% from 2013-2014 (NCES, 2016). This significant rise in just over a decade, suggests that regular education schools will need to be increasingly well-equipped to accommodate students with disabilities in the typical classroom. Research suggests that simply including children with disabilities in the classroom does not ensure that typical children will increase their interest, positive attitudes, intentions and socialization with individuals with disabilities. In contrast, high quality interventions that effectively educate typical children about disabilities and encourage children to befriend individuals with disabilities are critical towards fostering attitudes, intentions and promoting the socialization of typical children toward their peers with disabilities (Silton, 2015; Vignes et al., 2009). Moreover, if programs are not created to promote acceptance and social integration, then children with disabilities will be less accepted by their typically developing peers in the classroom (Favazza, Phillepson, & Kumar, 2000). Research consistently reveals that students with disabilities are not only more vulnerable to negative attitudes (Nowicki & Sandieson, 2002), but are less accepted, have fewer peers, socialize less frequently, and report more loneliness than their typical peers (Bossaert, Colpin, Pijl & Petry, 2011). Various research studies note the importance of establishing learning standards which focus on the development of social skills and social competence skills, rather than focusing exclusively on the acquisition of academic competencies like literacy and mathematics (Scott, Little, Kagan & Freelow, 2006; National Research Council, 2001) in the classroom. Asher and Coie (1990) reveal that peer interactions are key ingredients towards developing social skills during childhood.

Already by preschool, children can form and enhance their repertoire of peer-related social skills (Odom et al., 2006). Unfortunately, even in high quality inclusion programs, children with disabilities appear less likely to get selected when children's play partner preferences are not predetermined by the instructors' planned activities or by the program structure (Guralnick, 1999). This aligns closely with research suggesting that typical children are more likely to select a typical doll as a play partner than a doll with a disability (Odom et al., 2006). Since preschool-aged children are already capable of identifying a child with a physical disability compared to a typically-developing peer (Diamond, 1994) and since children's experiences in preschool are likely to inform their reasoning about inclusion (Diamond & Stacey, 2000), it is critical that interventions enhance children's attitudes, intentions and knowledge of disabilities as early and as effectively as possible.

Stigma Towards Mental Illness (Anxiety and Depression)

Current statistics indicate that anxiety disorders occur in 32% of adolescents between the ages of 13 to 18 and depression occurs in approximately 13% of adolescents between the ages of 12 to 17 (NIMH, 2017; SAMHSA, 2017). Similar to disabilities, individuals who present with a mental illness often experience stigmatization, in the form of negative attitudes, which can have adverse effects on their health, social identity, and overall quality of life (Silton, Flannelly, Milestein, & Vaaler,

2011). Stigmatization directed at individuals with mental health disorders can be communicated in numerous ways and can result in the stigmatized individual being socially isolated and labeled with unwelcome attributes that separate them (Goffman, 1963). Social discrimination and stigma towards mental illness remains an issue among adolescents (Corrigan, 2004; Corrigan, Dremming, Goldman, Slopen, Medansani, & Phelan, 2004). In fact, a common barrier for adolescents seeking treatment is the stigma associated with mental illness (Clement, Schauman, Gram et al., 2015).

Mental health literacy is defined as having knowledge and an understanding of mental illnesses which assist in preventing or managing disorders (Jorm, Korten, Jacomb, Christensen, Rodgers, & Pollitt, 1997). Mental health literacy has five major components: 1) knowing how to prevent mental illness, 2) recognizing the development of a mental illness, 3) knowledge of treatment opportunities, 4) knowledge of self-coping mechanisms, and 5) first aid skills to support others with mental illness (Jorm, 2012). Jorm (2012) notes that an integral part of mental health literacy, is to connect knowledge to action in order to benefit oneself or others. This relates to adolescents since research has found that adolescents who recognize mental illness tend to be more successful at seeking help and finding treatment (Wright, Jorm, Harris, & McGorry, 2007). The present authors have used the theory of mental health literacy to expand the goals and content of *The Realabilities Comic Book Curriculum Series* by including new comics on mental health disorders for adolescents, rather than solely developing comics featuring disabilities for children. The researchers added *Got Talent* (which teaches about Anxiety and Depression) and *The Carnival* (which teaches about Generalized Anxiety Disorder, Obsessive Compulsive Disorder, and Specific Phobias) to *The Realabilities Comic Book Series* and to the adjoining companion manuals.

The Importance of Teaching Social Emotional Skills and Kindness to Children

Researchers have discovered that programming which aims to foster students' social-emotional skills can positively impact their academic, health and social outcomes. It is for this reason that school settings are now shifting towards teaching social and emotional and prosocial learning skills alongside traditional academics. Social Emotional Learning (SEL) involves identifying and managing emotions, caring about others, making good decisions, behaving ethically and responsibly, developing positive relationships and avoiding negative behaviors (Binfet & Schonert-Reichl, 2015). Similarly, prosocial behavior is important within school contexts, since schools are settings where frequent interpersonal interactions occur among individuals from diverse socioeconomic, social, and ethnic backgrounds and where interpersonal conflict can be prevalent (Binfet & Passmore, 2017).

More specifically, there appears to be an increased interest in examining the construct of kindness, since it is now deemed to be a "valuable socio-emotional skill" (Kaplan, DeBlois, Dominguez, & Walsh, 2016). For this reason, a variety of programs are now being developed to emphasize the importance of teaching kindness lessons in the school system. For instance, all of the following programs attempt to implement Kindness Education Programs: The Random Acts of Kindness in the Classroom Program (The Random Acts of Kindness Foundation, 2015), The Center for Investigating Healthy Minds' Mindfulness-based Kindness Curriculum (Flook, Goldberg, Pinger & Davidson, 2015) Think Kindness (Think Kindness, 2015), and The Ben's Bells Kindness Campus Program (Ben's Bells Project, 2015). More specifically, The Kind Campus Program, a widely-implemented school-based kindness education program that employs a bottom-up program framework, attempts to educate the full school community (students, families, faculty and staff) about the positive effects of kindness and to empower the community to cultivate kindness within and beyond the school walls. Using the Kind Campus Model, a study was conducted with a large number of school professionals and students from 50 schools in Tucson, Arizona to help develop school-based models to help teach kindness in schools. The research suggests that effective kindness education programs would afford students, faculty and staff a common language to discuss kindness and offer a framework that would encourage members of the school community to recognize acts of kindness occurring around the school and to practice kindness towards themselves and towards others (Kaplan et al., 2016).

An additional study specifically looked at the school kindness perceptions of 257 Kindergarten through twelfth grade teachers. Teachers were challenged to define kindness, to offer examples of kindness they had performed and received, to pinpoint key agents of kindness and to rate the quality of kind acts in their schools. Overall the findings revealed that teachers contend that they have a strong to moderate impact on shaping students' kindness and teachers' perceptions of school kindness tend to vary based on the grade they are teaching. Moreover, the research suggested that teachers' beliefs about prosocial behaviors, such as kindness, as well as practicing kindness as part of their professional role, may have far-reaching implications for teacher job satisfaction, and for teacher-student rapport, which could affect learning and the overall school climate (Binfet & Passamore, 2017)

Another study examined the psychometric properties of The School Kindness Scale (SKS) in a sample of 1,753 students from fourth through eighth grade, who were attending public schools in the large school district of Southern British Columbia, Canada. The researchers discovered that the School Kindness Scale (SKS) was significantly and positively associated with teacher reports on students' empathy, social skills and peer acceptance. With respect to gender and grade findings, girls perceived higher levels of kindness in school than boys and students' perceptions of kindness in school diminished from fourth to eighth grade, wherein fourth-grade students reported the highest perceptions of kindness in school compared to eighth graders, who reported the lowest levels of kindness. Moreover, the research revealed that the extent to which students perceive kindness as a commonly occurring aspect of school is a reflection of a broader learning context; wherein students' perceptions of kindness may indicate the level to which the school context fosters underlying conditions that support student development and learning (Binfet & Schonert-Reichl, 2015).

Moreover, a later study (Retnowati, Agoes Salim, & Saleh, 2017) examined whether or not picture books could help teach kindness to 31 five and six year old children from a Kindergarten in Bandung, Indonesia. The intervention was conducted by reading eight picture books to the 31 children over an eight day time frame. The storybooks helped describe kindness behaviors, including helping behaviors and cheering up friends. The storylines were simple, sequential, predictable, and offered clear examples of kind behaviors that could be performed every day. Kindness was measured by utilizing an instrument the researcher created, which involved showing nine colorful cards that described the kindness behaviors to children. Kindness was additionally assessed by reviewing the kindness tree and observation sheets the teachers filled out. Data analysis, employing the Wilcoxon Signed-Rank Test, revealed a significant positive change in the average score of kindness at the $p < .05$ level after the stories were read. Two weeks following the intervention, there were significant improvements on both the card test and on the kindness tree and observational sheets following the intervention (Retnowati et. al, 2017).

Similar to the success of the children's picture books in the aforementioned Retnowati et al. (2017) study, the present authors created the prosocial *Realabilities Comic Book Series Curriculum* to teach kindness and empathy to typical children and adolescents towards children with disabilities and towards individuals with mental health disorders, respectively. Pre and post-test assessments have been utilized at each stage of development to assess the efficacy of these literary interventions.

Key Ways to Enhance Kindness in Children

In addition to the benefits of literary resources, recent work by Harvard psychologist, Richard Weissbourd, who runs the *Making Caring Common Project*, suggests five key ways to raise kind children. A recent *Washington Post* article reviewed Weissbourd's work and shared his five essential ingredients for raising kind children, 1) Make caring for others a priority, 2) Provide opportunities for children to practice caring and gratitude, 3) Expand your child's circle of concern, 4) Be a strong moral role model and mentor, and 5) Guide children in managing destructive feelings.

With respect to the first ingredient, the research suggests that parents need to teach their children about the balance of their own desires and the desires of others. Parents should directly reinforce the importance of being kind and should ensure their children are acting respectfully, even when their children may be in angry or in upset moods. Parents can also visually express how to care for others by introducing children to additional adult figures in their lives.

In terms of the second ingredient of offering opportunities for children to practice caring and gratitude, the author suggests that children should practice being caring to others and showing others gratitude. A plethora of studies reveal that those who express gratitude are often more likely to be happier in life. Rather than rewarding children each time they do something positive, try to make "doing good" a daily activity and habit for children. Parents can also highlight expressions of kindness and caring on TV, in the movies and in books for their children.

With regard to the third ingredient of expanding your child's circle of concern, the author stresses how important it is for children to care about individuals beyond those in their immediate peer group. Encouraging children to look outside of their inner circle will afford them a better perspective of caring for others in the world around them. It is especially beneficial to encourage children to be helpful to those who are most vulnerable (Joyce, 2019). In fact, a renowned twentieth century philosopher, Emmanuel Levinas (1905-1995) suggests that individuals can reach their highest ethical authority when they help those who are most vulnerable, "the widow, the orphan, the stranger," or those with other vulnerabilities. Showing children TV news, periodicals or other stories can teach them about the diverse problems children may encounter around the world (Joyce, 2019). *The Realabilities Educational Comic Book Series Curriculum* seeks to employ an extended contact model through which to increase positive intergroup attitudes by teaching typical children and adolescents about disabilities and mental health disorders to enhance their knowledge, attitudes and behaviors towards those who may not initially be in their inner circle.

The fourth ingredient of encouraging parents to be strong moral role models and mentors for their children suggests the importance of observational learning and Social Learning Theory. Children learn a number of diverse behaviors and attitudes from observing adults, especially their parents. Parents have an opportunity to showcase honesty and fairness to their children and to model how to volunteer and give back to the community (Joyce, 2019).

Finally, the author suggests that parents should guide children in managing their destructive feelings. For instance, children may become overwhelmed by negative emotions like anger or envy and parents have an opportunity to teach their children helpful coping skills to best address these emotions (Joyce, 2019). One coping skill might be to teach children how to breathe and remain calm, for instance to tell children to "breathe in the roses and blow out the candles" to better help children relax and address head-on the struggles of the day.

Empathy

In addition to kindness, empathy, another critical social-emotional construct, relates to stepping into the shoes of another person and to perceiving and understanding the emotions that other individuals are experiencing (Dziobek, Rogers, Fleck, Bahnemann, Heekeren, Wolf, & Convit, 2008). Empathy involves both cognitive and affective components. *Cognitive Empathy* refers to how well one can *comprehend* another's emotions and *Affective Empathy* relates to how well one can *experience* another's emotions (Van Noorden, Haselager, Cillessen, and Bukowski, 2014). Empathy enables individuals to perceive the world through their peers' lenses. The ability to understand the attitudes and feelings of others is paramount toward establishing meaningful relationships and successful, prosocial behaviors with others (Dziobek et al., 2008). Individuals with higher levels of empathy are often more likely to help others or to pursue prosocial acts (Eisenberg, Eggum, & Di Giunta, 2010). It is therefore critical to cultivate empathy during childhood, since this critical period of development can lead to life-long behaviors.

However, empathy is a fundamental human characteristic that can impact both prosocial and antisocial behavior. Unfortunately, bullying has become one of the most common antisocial behaviors in children. It is thought that the principal motivation behind bullying is the power imbalance that exists between the bully and victim. Bullying can be manifested through verbal, physical or relational means or through cyberbullying. Many believe that those who bully, struggle with lower levels of empathy and therefore, many bullying prevention and intervention efforts have sought to include empathy training. For instance, individuals with disabilities are unfortunately two to three times more likely to be victimized by bullying behaviors than their typical peers. This increased vulnerability may be due to a lack of empathy and understanding of the differences associated with disabilities or of what causes these differences. When children glean a clearer awareness and understanding of differences, they are able to enhance their knowledge and sensitivity and to improve their attitudes and intentions towards individuals with disabilities, mental health disorders or other differences.

Aligned with this notion, Van Noorden, Haselager, Cillessen, and Bukowski (2014) conducted a study to determine the relationship between cognitive (mental) and affective (emotional) forms of empathy and bullying behaviors. After a search of 40 empathy studies (24 cognitive and 38 affective) associated with four forms of bullying (bullying, victimization, defending, and bystanding), there appeared to be a negative correlation between empathy and bullying (the higher the empathy, the lower the bullying behaviors). *Bullying* was found to be negatively correlated with both cognitive and affective forms of empathy. More specifically, *defending* was positively correlated with both cognitive and affective empathy, *victimization* was negatively correlated with cognitive empathy and *bystanding* had mixed results. While future studies in this field would be helpful, the current study offered a foundation for improving bullying prevention and intervention programs (Van Noorden et al., 2014).

As an intervention, *The Realabilities Comic Book Series* and the *Addy & Uno Off-Broadway Musical* were created to enhance children's knowledge and empathy towards the unique life circumstances of individuals with disabilities and now mental health disorders, as well. The *Realabilities Curriculum* attempts to increase a child's level of empathy through the engaging lessons incorporated into each storyline that accentuate prosocial values through each character's inner strengths and abilities. Children, as readers and as musical audience members, are able to empathize, since they can envision themselves within the characters and within the rich character experiences. These immersive, empathic opportunities are achieved through the creative media of musicals and graphic storytelling, which align closely with the strength and efficacy of the extended contact model.

Extended Contact Model

Since even high-quality inclusion may cause segregation among typical children and children with disabilities or children with mental health disorders in a classroom, it is useful to consider additional forms of instruction to enhance typical children's understanding, attitudes and intentions towards their peers with disabilities or mental health disorders.

The extended contact hypothesis posits that knowledge that an in-group member has established a close relationship with an out-group member may promote more positive intergroup attitudes (Wright, Aron, McLaughlin-Volpe, & Ropp, 1997). Typical children can benefit strongly from extended contact, since it offers them knowledge of individuals with disabilities or mental health disorders (the out-group) without the anxiety that initial, direct contact may introduce (Pettigrew & Tropp, 2000; Stephan & Stephan, 1985, as cited by Cameron & Rutland, 2006). Stated differently, extended contact can enhance typical children's ("the ingroup's") positive attitudes and knowledge of individuals with disabilities or mental health disorders ("the outgroup"), before children with differences enter the mainstream classroom. In fact, Favazza and Odom (1997) discovered that extended contact had a significant, positive effect on outgroup attitudes (improved attitudes of typical children towards children with disabilities) but not on in-group attitudes (typical children towards typical children). Therefore, learning about differences before students directly interact with their peers with special needs or mental health issues can be more beneficial than actual contact since it reduces the potential for a "backlash effect," if typical children experience anxiety when they first meet their new peers with differences (Paoloni et al., 2004).

Similarly, in England, Cameron and Rutland (2006) explored the efficacy of an extended contact prejudice-reduction intervention in enhancing typical children's attitudes towards children with disabilities. The researchers learned that when group boundaries are maintained and typicality or similarity is emphasized, the extended contact model was more effective and led to the most robust change in typical participants' attitudes towards children with disabilities (Cameron & Rutland, 2006). Therefore it appears that an Intergroup Extended Contact Model, wherein typical children are taught about the realities of disability through story-telling, role-playing or drama (Campbell et al., 2003) that emphasize the similarities and strengths of their peers with disabilities (Cameron & Rutland, 2006) may be a critical antidote to the increasingly negative relationship between age and attitudes towards children with disabilities (Campbell, Ferguson, Herzinger, Jackson, & Marino, 2004; Bell & Morgan, 2000; Morgan & Wisely, 1996). This aligns with research that reveals that story-time is a naturalistic strategy for providing information about individuals with disabilities since it is a typical feature of the kindergarten class routine (Favazaa & Odom, 1997). In addition, activities like roleplays, drama and storytelling help students empathize with the "outgroup" and makes them more likely to disapprove of bullying (Silton, Arucevic, Ruchlin, & Norkus, 2013; Pepler et al., 1993).

The Benefits of the *Realabilities* Comic Book Series Medium for Effective Storytelling

It is instructive to consider the appealing and creative medium of comic books for relaying critical messages related to disability awareness, mental health awareness, and a stop bullying platform in and out of the school environment. Comic books have differentiated themselves from traditional books due to their appealing and creative characteristics. Children may struggle with motivation or may experience difficulty focusing on reading, which can challenge their retention of information from the text (Versaci, 2001). This can often cause the child to feel defeated and frustrated about reading. Comic books offer an engaging alternative to traditional books, since they capitalize on visual aids to enhance the accompanying text. The combination of text and images within comic books provide the dual processing of images and words for the reader, which helps the reader to gain the valuable skill of formulating an inference to follow the storyline (Versaci, 2001).

Comic books are valuable tools in and outside of the classroom, since they help children establish a foundation on which to build their literacy and critical thinking skills (Versaci, 2001). In addition, comic books enable creators to channel their boundless creativity throughout the design and layout of the comic (Silton, 2016). The immersive and creative nature of comic books coupled with their storytelling capacity and literary appeal, prompted the creation of *The Realabilities Comic Book Series Educational Curriculum*. Sharing the adventures of the *Realabilities* characters through the visual form of comic books encourages children to empathize or to immerse themselves in the characters' experiences and enhances their disability and mental health knowledge. This nuanced understanding of disabilities and most recently mental health disorders ultimately leads to more positive cognitive attitudes and behavioral intentions towards the protagonists with disabilities and mental health disorders in the series. *The Comic Book Companion* and *Disability in Depth Manual,* the teaching manuals that supplement the *Realabilities Comic Book Series Curriculum*, further extend these important lessons about disabilities and mental health disorders in the classroom and offer richer learning experiences and positive outcomes for typical students and students with disabilities and mental health disorders, alike.

Previous Peer Education Programs

Beyond literary works, a variety of creative peer education programs have been developed over the years in order to enhance typical children's knowledge and positive attitudes towards children with disabilities through direct or indirect exposure using storytelling, role-playing or other techniques. Another form of storytelling, puppetry, has been identified as a potential promising approach toward improving attitudes and knowledge towards disabilities due to its capacity to inspire a large number of students and to be relatively cost-effective (Bernier, & O'Hare, 2005). Additionally, Trimingham (2010) suggests that puppetry also has a host of other benefits. She intimates that puppetry has been exceptionally useful in explaining the etiology of maladjustment in childhood and serves as a significant therapeutic technique through which children can learn to comprehend the complexities of deviating behaviors and to discover more successful solutions. The researchers also note that puppets can help children confront an externalization of themselves, wherein their focus can shift away from their closed, inner worlds and can accommodate another to share in their perception of the world (Trimingham, 2010; Woltmann, 1951). Additionally, Felisa Weiss (as cited in Trimingham, 2010) suggests that "The puppet acts as an intermediary, the projective object that absorbs both the interviewer and interviewee's vectors." (Trimingham, 2010; Weiss, 1998) Finally, Schummann suggests that the material nature of his puppets makes the puppets speak for themselves. Thus the object of the puppet speaks and there is no distortion by the intruding ego of the performer (Trimingham, 2010).

Limited Efficacy of Previous Puppet Show Interventions

Despite the unique strengths of puppetry, previous puppet show interventions have either shown no or minimal effects in transforming typical children's attitudes towards children with disabilities. Rosenbaum, Armstrong and King (1986) conducted a randomized-factorial-design study to evaluate the impact of two interventions, 1) *A Buddy Program-* offering direct exposure to children with disabilities, and 2) *The Kids-on-the-Block (KOB) Puppet Show Program-*wherein puppets are utilized to discuss disabilities to foster positive attitudes and intentions of typical children towards children with special needs. The researchers revealed that while the Buddy Program appeared efficacious, the KOB Program had no significant effect on any outcomes and actually appeared to reduce the impact of the Buddy Program when used in concert. The researchers noted that this might be a result of the dissonance between the puppets in the KOB intervention and the real-life children with disabilities in the Buddy program. In a later study, Baker (1991) discovered a short-term positive impact of the KOB intervention on elementary school children's attitudes in third through sixth grades, but there appeared to be only minimal long-term effects.

That same year, Thios and Foster (1991) assessed the efficacy of *The New Friends Program,* which utilized life-sized dolls with disabilities to relay important information about disabilities three times per week (25 minutes per session) over a three-week period. The intervention presented four units, including, an introductory unit on differences and similarities, and units on hearing impairment, physical impairment (cerebral palsy) and learning impairment. The researchers discovered that that the New Friends' Program enhanced attitudes and knowledge of disabilities but failed to show robust changes in social interaction patterns towards children with disabilities (Thios & Foster, 1991).

In 2014, Dunst conducted a metanalysis of 26 studies which explored the effects of the Kids on the Block (KOB) and/or *Count Me In Puppet Shows* on elementary school students' attitudes and knowledge of individuals with disabilities. The Kids on the Block (KOB) Puppet Troupe and Count Me In Puppet Troupes introduce puppets representing children with physical disabilities, intellectual disabilities, visual impairments, and hearing impairments. The forty-five-minute puppet shows included scripts to introduce each puppet in order to offer awareness of diverse disabilities and to correct common misconceptions of disability. The show also offered a fifteen-minute question-and-answer session after the show.

Dunst (2014) reviewed studies which included 5,302 participants in the intervention group and 2,642 student participants in the comparison group. The results suggested that the puppet shows had only a mild to medium impact on participants' knowledge and attitudes towards individuals with disabilities. More specifically, first and second grade students showed more robust changes in attitudes towards children with disabilities following the puppet show than their third through sixth grade peers and the effects of the puppet show were somewhat reduced over time. Moreover, students showed greater gains in their knowledge of disabilities than in their attitudes towards children with disabilities (Dunst, 2014). Finally, the researcher delineated the following study limitations, 1) There was a dearth of information pertaining to adherence or fidelity to the puppet show scripts, 2) There was minimal to no information regarding the schools or districts where the puppet show was performed, and 3) There was little description regarding the backgrounds of and manner in which the puppeteers performed the shows. Despite these limitations, similar to the notion of the extended contact model, Dunst (2014) intimated that puppet shows could be useful for transforming elementary students' knowledge of and attitudes towards individuals with disabilities, at least in terms of their initial exposure to individuals with disabilities before misconceptions and misunderstandings arise. Moreover, he recommended combining puppet shows with in-vivo or real-life, situated interactional opportunities with individuals with disabilities to offer an additive positive effect on typical students' knowledge and attitudes towards their peers with special needs.

The *Addy & Uno Musical* seeks to improve upon the Kids on the Block (KOB) and Count Me In Puppet Show Programs and research by offering real-life, situated interactional opportunities, information about adherence to the puppet show scripts, specific information pertaining to the location of the show performances, and a brief description of the puppeteers. *The Addy & Uno Musical* presents innovative, kid-friendly puppets with disabilities that are openly operated by the in-vivo, visible puppeteers, who are assuming the roles of individuals with disabilities. The *Addy & Uno Musical* also utilizes original music to foster children's understanding, recall and appreciation of their peers with disabilities. The puppeteers are also available after each show to answer a plethora of questions from audience members.

Moreover, researchers assessing the *Addy & Uno Musical* intervention and the *Realabilities Educational Comic Book Series Curriculum* are employing key valid, reliable and objective quantitative behavioral intention (The Shared Activities Questionnaire (SAQ); Morgan et al., 1996) and cognitive attitudinal (The Adjective Checklist (ACL); Siperstein & Bak, 1980) measures to evaluate the change in participants' perceptions from before and following the musical intervention and comic book series curriculum. They are also utilizing coding and other qualitative approaches to develop themes in order to attain a richer understanding of the program's impact on disability and mental health knowledge and sensitivity.

The four most recent *Realabilities* studies below include, 1) A qualitative study of 19 fourth grade students from an elementary school in Paramus, NJ, who viewed the *Addy & Uno Off Broadway Musical* and participated in the full *Realabilities Educational Comic Book Series Intervention*, 2) A qualitative study of 20 high school students with diverse disabilities, who participated in the full *Realabilities Comic*

Book Series Intervention, 3) A quantitative study of 76 students from a high school in Long Island City, NY, who read the first mental health-based *Realabilities* comic book and finally, 4) a quantitative study of 66 students from a high school in Long Island City, NY, who read the first and second mental health-based *Realabilities Comics.*

STUDY 1: ASSESSING THE EFFICACY OF *ADDY & UNO*, AN OFF-BROADWAY MUSICAL AND THE *REALABILITIES* EDUCATIONAL COMIC BOOK CURRICULUM IN ENHANCING CHILDREN'S SENSITIVITY AND INTEREST IN THEIR PEERS WITH DISABILITIES USING A QUALITATIVE METHODS APPROACH

Participants

Nineteen fourth grade students, 9 males and 10 females from a Jewish Day School in Paramus, New Jersey participated in the two-part disabilities intervention of *The Addy & Uno Musical* and *The Realabilities Educational Comic Book Curriculum.* All of the students self-reported that they were White and Jewish.

Procedure

The fourth grade students viewed the *Addy & Uno Musical* and participated in *The Realabilities Educational Comic Book Series.* Following the Musical, the students penned qualitative letters to the creators of the musical and reflected on the following: 1) What they enjoyed most about the Musical, 2) What they learned, 3) Whether they felt differently about disabilities and bullying following the Musical, 4) Whether they enjoyed the Musical and 5) Whether or not they would see the show again. Additionally, after reading the 11 *Realabilities Comics,* the students were asked to respond to the following questions: 1) Do you believe it's important for kids to stop bullying? 2) Who was your favorite character in the comic series and why? 3) Which comic book was your favorite and why? 4) What would you like the characters to do in the next *Realabilities Comic book* and finally, 5) Would you buy a Realabilities comic? The students responded to all of the aforementioned questions and the responses were collected, stored in a secure database, coded and analyzed (Please see APPENDIX A for images of the *Addy & Uno Musical* and APPENDIX B for images of *The Realabilities Comic Book Series*).

Results

With respect to appeal, the fourth grade students shared that they most enjoyed "the puppets and thought they were very interesting," "they liked when the bullies decided not to be mean," and "liked when (they) learned a sentence in sign language (during the show)." Moreover, the students "liked when Uno's friends helped him not be nervous" and "enjoyed the songs in the play." Following the Musical, the students noted that they learned "not to treat people differently just because they are different" and that "people aren't as different as we think they are." A large majority of students remarked that they would love to see the show again because it was "AMAZING!" Students also wondered if a second show would be made or if all of the comic books would be incorporated into the show. Finally, the students shared whether or not they enjoyed the Musical and whether or not they would like to view a TV show version of the show again. The lion's share of students said they enjoyed the Musical because it was "funny," "interesting," and "it was fun to watch the songs." Furthermore, students added that the Musical "taught me not to bully" and "helped me to be nice to be people who are different." When asked if they would watch an *Addy & Uno TV show*, the majority of students responded "yes" because they "love the play and (comic) books," they "like Addy and Uno," and "because you can learn a lot from it." One student mentioned that he/she would watch the TV show because "it teaches people to stop bullying" and another student said that the TV show "would make people who have disabilities happy."

Following the comic book series, the majority of students shared why they believe it is important to stop bullying. For instance, some students noted that "bullying can really hurt someone, even if it's not physical," "it affects how the kid being bullied feels about himself," and "because it can hurt people's feelings and (make) it like they're not important to the world." The students also discussed which characters from *The Realabilities Series* were their favorite characters and why. The majority of people liked Addy since she is "energetic and happy" and "she is really nice to people and her friends." Uno was the next highly-rated character since he is "smart" and "likes math." "Math Mania," the comic portraying Uno's preparation for a math competition and the comic that most closely relates to the Musical, was the most popular comic among the students. Students also enjoyed "Math Mania" because "it's about math," "Uno overcomes his fear," and "Uno's friends are helpful and supportive." The next most popular comic the students endorsed was "The Real Goal" because the characters are "kind" and "it involved sports." When asked what the students would like to see the characters do in a subsequent comic book, the students discussed a number of possibilities including "have a pool party and enjoy life," "go to Mars in a real rocket that RJ moves," and participate in more sports like baseball, snowboarding, and basketball." One student also wanted the characters to "tell us how they got their disabilities." Finally, when asked if the students would purchase a *Realabilities Comic Book*, the majority of student participants said they would, while a smaller minority said they would not. A reason for not wanting to purchase a comic was because they "don't like comics." Whereas reasons for wanting to purchase a comic book included "because they are funny," "it teaches kids to stop bullying," and "it could teach you to be nice to people who are different."

Principal Conclusions

Thus, the researchers found that the combination of *The Addy & Uno Off- Broadway Musical* and *The Realabilities Comic Book Series Curriculum* significantly enhanced typical students' nuanced knowledge, interest and understanding of disabilities as well as the importance of promoting a stop bullying platform in their schools. Overall, the study results confirm that an extended contact model, wherein appealing storylines, role-plays and other engaging media can be highly advantageous towards teaching about an outgroup (in this case disability), prior to or in addition to successfully interacting with children with disabilities in and outside of the classroom.

STUDY 2: THE IMPACT OF THE REALABILITIES COMIC BOOK SERIES CURRICULUM ON A SAMPLE OF STUDENTS WITH DIVERSE DISABILITIES

Participants

Twenty high school students <u>with</u> disabilities (fourteen males [70%] and six females [30%] from Manchester, New Jersey participated in *The Realabilities Educational Comic Book Intervention*. The majority of students identified as White (14; 70%), three (15%) as Other, two (10%) as Latino, and one (5%) as African American. Students presented with diverse disabilities, including autism, visual impairment, obsessive compulsive disorder (OCD), physical impairment, seizure disorders, intellectual disabilities, and/or with behavioral limitations.

Procedure

The students participated in the full *Realabilities Comic Book Series Curriculum* (11 comics featuring 11 disabilities, discussion questions and activities) and then responded to the following questions: 1) What did you learn from *The Realabilities Comic Book Series*? 2) Who was your favorite character in the comics and why? 3) Which comic was your favorite and why? 4) What would you like the characters to do in the next comic? and 5) Would you buy a *Realabilities Comic*? The students responded to all of the aforementioned questions and the responses were collected, stored in a secure database, coded and analyzed (Please see APPENDIX B for images of the comic series).

Results

Following the comic series, the students noted that they learned, "to never give up and to keep trying," "to not bully people," "to not judge people" and "that people have different strengths and weaknesses." In identifying their favorite characters, the majority of participants selected Beat, the African American character who stutters and dances, since she "resembles me," "is a good dancer," and is a "great singer." Uno, who presents with autism, was the next highly-rated character since he is "funny," "cool," and "smart." "Food Fight," the comic introducing Lexxy, a character with Down syndrome, and the comic that teaches about food allergies was rated the highest, because it "looks fun" and "teaches about allergies and shows there are ways to help." The next most popular comic the students endorsed was "Math Mania" because it was "funny," "cool," and "awesome." In a subsequent comic, the participants recommended that the characters "work on computers," "teach about the weather," "build a spaceship and go to the moon" "participate in basketball and football games" and do "more stuff that I can learn from." Finally, with respect to purchasing *Realabilities Comics*, the majority of students noted they would purchase them "because they were fun to read" and "are educational," while one participant remarked he wouldn't because he doesn't "read comics."

Principal Conclusions

Thus, the researchers found that *The Realabilities Comic Book Series* enhanced students' with disabilities nuanced knowledge of disabilities as well as the importance of promoting a stop bullying platform in their schools. Overall, the study results confirm that an extended contact model with appealing storylines and other engaging media can be highly advantageous towards teaching about diverse disabilities and that individuals with disabilities found the series both helpful and appealing.

STUDY 3: ASSESSING THE EFFICACY OF THE FIRST MENTAL HEALTH-BASED REALABILITIES COMIC AMONG A HIGH SCHOOL SAMPLE

Participants

Seventy-six students (44 males [61.1%] and 28 females [38.9%]) from an Information Technology High School in Long Island City, NY took pre and post-tests prior to and following the reading of the first comic book on mental health disorders in the *Realabilities Comic Book Series Curriculum.* In terms of grade, 71 (93.4%) of the students were enrolled in eleventh grade and five (6.6%) were enrolled in twelfth grade. The majority of students identified as Latino (50; 66.7%), nine (12.0%) identified as African American, five (6.7%) as Asian American, four (5.3%) as White and six (8.0%) as Other.

Procedure

The teachers administered brief Knowledge and Bullying Measures and Modified Pre and Post-Test Assessments of the Shared Activities Questionnaire (SAQ; Morgan et al., 1996), a behavioral intention measure, and The Adjective Checklist (ACL; Siperstein & Bak, 1980), a cognitive attitudinal measure, to students one day before and one day following the students reading through "Got Talent," the first mental health-focused comic of *The Realabilities Comic Book Series.* "Got Talent" introduces Celia with Anxiety and Kari with Depression. The students also noted whether they would view an episode of *Realabilities* or would purchase a comic. (Please see APPENDIX C for images of the new Mental Health-based comics).

Results

In terms of descriptive statistics, more than half of the participants (42; 56.8%) stated that they would purchase a *Realabilities Comic* and would watch an episode of the comic series (39; 50.6%) following the intervention.

Regarding principal study results, Paired Sample T-tests revealed that participants showed significantly more bullying knowledge, $t(76) = -2.296$, $p < .05$ and more stop bullying attitudes, $t(76) = -2.173$, $p < .05$ following the comic book intervention. The participants also showed more positive behavioral intentions (as measured via the Shared Activities Questionnaire [SAQ]) toward hypothetical peers with Anxiety on the SAQ Total, $t(76) = -2.514$, $p < .05$, on the SAQ Academic, $t(76) = -3.103$, $p < .01$ and on the SAQ Recreational, $t(76) = -2.164$, $p < .05$. Moreover, they showed more positive cognitive attitudes, as measured via The Adjective Checklist (ACL), towards hypothetical peers with Anxiety, $t(76) = -2.992$, $p < .01$ following the comic book intervention. Please see Tables 1 and 2 for Means, Standard Deviations and significance levels.

Principal Conclusions

Thus, the researchers discovered that students who read the "Got Talent" Comic, which discusses Anxiety and Depression and is the first comic to focus on Mental Health Disorders in the *Realabilities Series*, appeared to show more bullying knowledge and more positive stop bullying attitudes following the intervention. Additionally, the participants displayed more positive intentions and cognitive attitudes towards a hypothetical peer with Anxiety following the comic book intervention. This study was novel in not only showing the efficacy of a comic in enhancing attitudes toward Anxiety, but in successfully employing a high school population for this subject matter.

STUDY 4: EVALUATING THE EFFICACY OF THE FIRST AND SECOND MENTAL HEALTH-BASED REALABILITIES COMIC BOOKS AMONG A HIGH SCHOOL SAMPLE

Participants

Sixty-six students (45 males [68.2%], 20 females [30.3%], 1 Non-binary [1.5%]) from a High School in Long Island City, NY took pre and post-tests prior to and following the reading of the first two comic books on mental health disorders from the *Realabilities Comic Book Series*. The majority of students were in eleventh grade (59; 34.7%), one (1.6%) was in ninth grade, two (3.1%) in tenth grade, and two (3.1%) were in twelfth grade. Most students identified as Latino (43, 68.3%), seven as African American (11.1%) and as Asian American (11.1%), five (7.9%) as White, and one (1.6%) as Other.

Procedure

The high school teachers administered brief Knowledge Measures, Modified Pre and Post-Test Assessments of the Shared Activities Questionnaire (SAQ; Morgan et al., 1996), a behavioral intention measure, and The Adjective Checklist (ACL; Siperstein & Bak, 1980), a cognitive attitudinal measure both before and after students read the two Realabilities Mental Literacy-based comics.

Results

With regard to principal study results, Paired Sample T-tests revealed that participants showed significantly more knowledge about obsessive compulsive disorder (OCD), t (65) = -2.169, p <.05 and Phobias, t (64) = -2.408, p <.05 following the comic book intervention. After the comic book intervention, participants also displayed more positive behavioral intentions towards hypothetical peers with Anxiety on the SAQ Total, t (65) = -2.294, p <.05, SAQ Academic, t (65) = -2.288, p <.05, and on the SAQ Recreational, t (65) = -2.462, p < .05. Additionally, participants demonstrated improved intentions towards hypothetical peers with OCD on the SAQ Total, t (62) = -2.810, p <.01, SAQ Academic, t (65) = -2.558, p <.05, on the SAQ Social, t (63) = -2.149, p < .05, and on the SAQ Recreational, t (64) = -2.177, p <.05. Moreover, the participants showed more positive behavioral intentions towards hypothetical peers with Phobias on the SAQ Total, t (65) = -3.317, p <. 001, and on the SAQ Social, t (65) = - 3.753, p <.001. Finally, Participants showed significantly improved cognitive attitudes (via The ACL) towards hypothetical peers with Anxiety, t (64) = -6.527, p <.001, Depression, *t* (64) = -2.802, p < .01, and OCD, t (64) = - 3.648, p <.001 following the comic book intervention. Please see Table 3 for Means, Standard Deviations and significance levels.

Conclusions and Discussions

Thus, the researchers found that students who read the "Got Talent" and "Carnival" Comics, which discuss Anxiety, Depression, OCD, and Phobias, respectively, enhanced participants' knowledge of mental health literacy and improved participants' cognitive attitudes and behavioral intentions towards hypothetical peers with mental health disorders. Additionally, similar to the aforementioned study, the research revealed that the *Realabilities Mental Health Literacy Comics* could be effectively used with a high school population.

General Discussion

In summary, the first study found that a combination of the *Addy & Uno Off-Broadway Musical* and *The Realabilities Educational Comic Book Series Curriculum* significantly enhanced typical students' knowledge, interest and understanding of disabilities as well as the importance of promoting a stop bullying platform in school. The second study found that *The Realabilities Educational Comic Book Series* enhanced students with disabilities' nuanced knowledge of disabilities as well as the importance of promoting a stop bullying platform in their schools. The third study found that typical students who read the "Got Talent" Comic, which teaches about Anxiety and Depression, appeared to show more bullying knowledge and more positive stop bullying attitudes following the intervention. Furthermore, students displayed more positive behavioral intentions and cognitive attitudes towards a hypothetical peer with Anxiety after reading the "Got Talent" comic. Finally, the fourth study highlighted how participants increased their knowledge of mental health literacy and improved their cognitive attitudes and behavioral intentions towards hypothetical peers with mental health disorders after reading the "Got Talent" and "Carnival" Comics, which discuss Anxiety, Depression, OCD, and Phobias, respectively. Moreover, the research revealed that *The Realabilities Mental Health Literacy Comics* could be effectively utilized with a high school population. Overall, all four studies confirmed that an extended contact model with appealing storylines and other engaging media can be highly beneficial when teaching about diverse disabilities and mental health disorders.

With respect to study limitations, the aforementioned studies would benefit from even larger, diverse student samples in order to enhance the study's generalizability and external validity. Future studies would also benefit from observable behavioral data, to examine how student participants might actually act, behave or respond to students with disabilities following the research interventions, rather than solely relying on self-report measures of behavioral intentions and cognitive attitudes. While a limitation of earlier studies related to a failure to include participants with disabilities in the research intervention, our second study sought to rectify this earlier limitation, by recruiting students with diverse disabilities to participate in *The Full Realabilities Educational Comic Book Series Intervention*.

Finally with regard to future directions, the researchers hope to expand upon the Musical and Comic Book Series in multiple ways. Currently, a sequel to the *Addy & Uno Musical* is being created and the research team is in the process of developing two more comic books focusing on mental health disorders and an additional comic book featuring additional disabilities (facial deformities and differences). The research team is also currently designing a research-based, isometric, first-person adventure video game to offer typical junior high school viewers an opportunity to better empathize and comprehend the strengths and limitations associated with the everyday life experiences of individuals with disabilities (please see APPENDIX D for images of the video game).

Taken together, all of these interventions seek to enhance typical children and adolescents' knowledge, attitudes, behavioral intentions, empathy and kindness towards individuals with disabilities and mental health disorders. With more knowledge, understanding and recognition of the strengths and realities of these differences, rather than solely a focus on limitations, *The Addy & Uno Musical, The Realabilities Educational Comic Book Series Curriculum* and *The Realabilities First-Person Adventure Video Game* seek to enhance the positive intergroup attitudes towards individuals with disabilities and mental health disorders to reduce stigma and promote the socialization and success of individuals with disabilities, mental health disorders and typical individuals, alike.

REFERENCES

Asher, S. R., & Coie, J. D. (1990). *Peer Rejection in Childhood.* Cambridge University Press.

Baker, V.A. (1991). *Changing attitudes of children in grades three to six towards persons with disabilities via the 'Kids on the Block' program.* Academic Press.

Bell, S. K., & Morgan, S. B. (2000). Children's attitudes and behavioral intentions toward a peer pre- sented as obese: Does a medical explanation for the obesity make a difference? *Journal of Pediatric Psychology*, *25*(3), 137–145. doi:10.1093/jpepsy/25.3.137 PMID:10780140

Bernier, M., & O'Hare, J. (Eds.). (2005). *Puppetry in Education and Therapy: Unlocking the Doors to the Mind and Heart.* Bloomington, IN: AuthorHouse.

Binfet, J.-T., & Passmore, H.-A. (2017). Teachers' Perceptions of Kindness at School. *The International Journal of Emotional Education*, *9*(1), 37–53. https://files.eric.ed.gov/fulltext/EJ1137976.pdf

Binfet, J.T. & Schonert-Reichl, K. A. (2015). Measuring kindness at school: Psychometric properties of a school kindness scale for children and adolescents. *Psychology in the Schools, 0*, 1–16.

Bossaert, G., Colpin, H., Pijl, S. P., & Petry, K. (2011). Loneliness among students with special educational needs in mainstream seventh grade. *Research in Developmental Disabilities*, *33*(6), 1888–1897. doi:10.1016/j.ridd.2012.05.010 PMID:22705912

Cameron, L., & Rutland, A. (2006). Extended contact through story reading in school: Reducing children's prejudice toward the disabled. *The Journal of Social Issues*, *62*(3), 469–488. doi:10.1111/j.1540-4560.2006.00469.x

Campbell, J., Gilmore, L., & Cuskelly, M. (2003). Changing student teachers' attitudes towards disability and inclusion. *Journal of Intellectual & Developmental Disability, 28*(4), 369–379. doi:8250310001616407 doi:10.1080/1366

Campbell, J. M., Ferguson, J. E., Herzinger, C. V., Jackson, J. N., & Marino, C. A. (2004). Combined descriptive and explanatory information improves peers' perceptions of autism. *Research in Developmental Disabilities, 25*(4), 321–339. doi:10.1016/j.ridd.2004.01.005 PMID:15193668

Clement, S., Schauman, O., Graham, T., Maggioni, F., Evans-Lacko, S., Bezborodovs, N., & Thornicroft, G. (2015). What is the impact of mental health-related stigma on help-seeking? A systematic review of quantitative and qualitative studies. *Psychological Medicine, 45*(1), 11–27. doi:10.1017/S0033291714000129 PMID:24569086

Corrigan, P. (2004). How stigma interferes with mental health care. *The American Psychologist, 59*(7), 614–625. doi:10.1037/0003-066X.59.7.614 PMID:15491256

Corrigan, P. W., Lurie, B. D., Goldman, H. H., Slopen, N., Medasani, K., & Phelan, S. (2005). How adolescents perceive the stigma of mental illness and alcohol abuse. *Psychiatric Services, 56*(5), 544–550. doi:10.1176/appi.ps.56.5.544 PMID:15872162

Diamond, K. E. (1994). Evaluating preschool children's sensitivity to developmental differences. *Topics in Early Childhood Special Education, 14*(1), 49–63. doi:10.1177/027112149401400107

Diamond, K. E., & Stacey, S. (2000). The other children at preschool: Experiences of typically developing children in inclusive programs. In S. Sandall & M. Ostrosky (Eds.), *Natural Environments and Inclusion* (pp. 59–68). Frederick, CO: Sopris West.

Dunst, C. J. (2014). Meta-analysis of the effects of puppet shows on attitudes toward and knowledge of individuals with disabilities. *Exceptional Children, 80*(2), 136–148. doi:10.1177/001440291408000201

Dziobek, I., Rogers, K., Fleck, S., Bahnemann, M., Heekeren, H. R., Wolf, O. T., & Convit, A. (2008). Dissociation of cognitive and emotional empathy in adults with Asperger syndrome using the Multifaceted Empathy Test (MET). *Journal of Autism and Developmental Disorders, 38*(3), 464–473. doi:10.100710803-007-0486

Eisenberg, N., Eggum, N. D., & Di Giunta, L. (2010). Empathy-related responding: Associations with prosocial behavior, aggression, and intergroup relations. *Social Issues and Policy Review, 4*(1), 143–180. doi:10.1111/j.1751-2409.2010.01020.x PMID:21221410

Favazaa, P. C., & Odom, S. L. (1997). Promoting Positive Attitudes of Kindergarten-Age Children toward People with Disabilities. *Exceptional Children, 63*(3), 405–418. doi:10.1177/001440299706300308

Goffman, E. (1963). *Stigma: Notes on the management of spoiled identity*. New York: Simon and Schuster.

Guralnick, M. J. (1999). Family and child influences on the peer-related social competence of young children with developmental delays. *Mental Retardation and Developmental Disabilities Research Reviews, 5*(1), 21–29. doi:<2 doi:10.1002/(SICI)1098-2779(1999)5:1

Jorm, A. F. (2012). Mental health literacy: Empowering the community to take action for better mental health. *The American Psychologist, 67*(3), 231–243. doi:10.1037/a0025957 PMID:22040221

Jorm, A. F., Korten, A. E., Jacomb, P. A., Christensen, H., Rodgers, B., & Pollitt, P. (1997). "Mental health literacy": A survey of the public's ability to recognize mental disorders and their beliefs about the effectiveness of treatment. *The Medical Journal of Australia, 166*(4), 182–186. doi:10.5694/j.1326-5377.1997.tb140071.x PMID:9066546

Joyce, A. (2019, April 21). *Are you raising nice kids? A Harvard psychologist gives 5 ways to raise them to be kind.* Retrieved from: https://www.washingtonpost.com/news/parenting/wp/2014/07/18/are-you-raising-nice-kids-a-harvard-psychologist-gives-5-ways-to-raise-them-to-be-kind/

Kaplan, D. M., DeBlois, M., Dominguez, V., & Walsh, M. E. (2016). Studying the teaching of kindness: A conceptual model for evaluating kindness education programs in schools. *Evaluation and Program Planning, 58*, 160–170.

Morgan, S. B., & Wisely, D. W. (1996). Children's attitudes and behavioral intentions toward a peer presented as physically handicapped: A more positive view. *Journal of Developmental and Physical Disabilities, 8*(1), 29–42. doi:10.1007/BF02578438

National Center for Education Statistics. (2016). *Children and youth with disabilities*. Author.

National Research Council. (2001). *Eager to Learn: Educating Our Preschoolers*. Washington, DC: National Academy Press.

Nowicki, E. A., & Sandieson, R. (2002). A meta-analysis of school-age children's attitudes towards persons with physical or intellectual disabilities. *International Journal of Disability Development and Education*, *49*(3), 243–265. doi:10.1080/1034912022000007270

Odom, S., Zercher, C., Li, S., Marquart, J., Sandall, S., & Brown, W. (2006). Social acceptance and rejection of preschool children with disabilities: A mixed-method analysis. *Journal of Educational Psychology*, *98*(4), 807–823. doi:10.1037/0022-0663.98.4.807

Okoro, C. A., Hollis, N. D., Cyrus, A. C., & Griffin-Blake, S. (2018). Prevalence of disabilities and health care access by disability status and type among adults—United States, 2016. *Morbidity and Mortality Weekly Report*, *67*(32), 882–887. doi:10.15585/mmwr.mm6732a3 PMID:30114005

Paolini, S., Hewstone, M., Cairns, E., & Voci, A. (2004). Effects of direct and indirect cross-group friendships on judgments of Catholics and Protestants in Northern Ireland: The mediating role of an anxiety-reduction mechanism. *Personality and Social Psychology Bulletin*, *30*(6), 770–786. doi:10.1177/0146167203262848 PMID:15155040

Pettigrew, T. F., & Tropp, L. R. (2000). Does inter-group contact reduce prejudice: Recent meta-analytic findings. In S. Oskamp (Ed.), *Reducing prejudice and discrimination. The Claremont Symposium on Applied Social Psychology* (pp. 93–114). Mahwah, NJ: Lawrence Erlbaum Associates, Publishers.

RespectAbility, Fighting Stigmas, Advancing Opportunities. (2018). Retrieved from www.respectability.org

Retnowati, G. M., Agoes Salim, R. Y., & Saleh, A. (2017). Effectiveness of Picture Story Books Reading To Increase Kindness In Children Aged 5-6 Years. *Lingua Cultura, 12*(1), 89–95.

Rosenbaum, P. L., Armstrong, R. W., & King, S. M. (1986). Improving attitudes toward the disabled: A randomized controlled trial of direct contact versus Kids-on-the-Block. *Journal of Developmental and Behavioral Pediatrics*, *7*(5), 302–307. doi:10.1097/00004703-198610000-00005 PMID:2945833

Scott-Little, C., Kagan, S. L., & Frelow, V. S. (2006). Conceptualization of readiness and the content of early learning standards: The intersection of policy and research? *Early Childhood Research Quarterly*, *21*(2), 153–173. doi:10.1016/j.ecresq.2006.04.003

Silton, N. R., Flannelly, K. J., Milstein, G., & Vaaler, M. L. (2011). Stigma in America: has anything changed?: Impact of perceptions of mental illness and dangerousness on the desire for social distance: 1996 and 2006. *The Journal of Nervous and Mental Disease, 199*(6), 361–366. doi:10.1097/NMD.0b013e31821cd112 PMID:21629012

Siperstein, G. N. (1980). *Development of the Adjective Checklist: An instrument for measuring children's attitudes toward the handicapped* (Unpublished manuscript). University of Massachusetts, Boston, MA.

Siperstein, G. N., & Bak, J. (1977). *Instruments to measure children's attitudes toward the handicapped: Adjective Checklist and Activity Preference List* (Unpublished manuscript). University of Massachusetts, Boston, MA.

Thios, S. J., & Foster, S. B. (1991). *Changing Preschoolers' Attitudes toward Children with Disabilities.* Paper presented at the Annual Meeting of the American Psychological Association, San Francisco, CA.

Trimingham, M. (2010). Objects in transition: The puppet and the autistic child. *Journal of Applied Arts & Health, 1*(3), 251–265. doi:10.1386/jaah.1.3.251_1

U.S. Department of Health and Human Services, National Institute of Mental Health. (2017). *Any anxiety disorder.* Retrieved from https://www.nimh.nih.gov/health/statistics/any-anxiety-disorder.shtml

U.S. Department of Health and Human Services, Substance Abuse and Mental Health Administration. (2017). *Key substance use and mental health indicators in the United States: Results from the 2016 National Survey on Drug Use and Health.* Retrieved from https://www.samhsa.gov/data/sites/default/files/NSDUH-FFR1-2016/NSDUH-FFR1-2016.pdf - PDF

Van Noorden, T. H. J., Haselager, G. J. T., Cillessen, A. H. N., & Bukowski, W. M. (2014). Empathy and Involvement in Bullying in Children and Adolescents: A Systematic Review. *Journal of Youth and Adolescence*, 1–22.

Versaci, R. (2001). How Comic Books Can Change the Way Our Students See Literature: One Teacher's Perspective. *English Journal, 91*(61), 61–67. doi:10.2307/822347

Vignes, C., Godeau, E., Sentenac, M., Coley, N., Niavarro, F., & Grandjean, H. (2009). Determinants of students' attitudes towards peers with disabilities. *Developmental Medicine and Child Neurology, 51*(6), 473–479. doi:10.1111/j.1469-8749.2009.03283.x PMID:19416319

Weiss, F. (1998). The Field of Wings, Puppetry as Therapy from an Object Relations Point of View and Incorporating Field Psychology. In A. Robbins (Ed.), *Therapeutic Presence* (pp. 219–243). London: Jessica Kingsley.

Woltmann, A. (1951). The Use of Puppetry as a Projective Method in Therapy. In H. Anderson & G. Anderson (Eds.), *Introduction to Projective Techniques* (pp. 606–637). New York: Prentice Hall.

Wright, A., Jorm, A. F., Harris, M. G., & McGorry, P. D. (2007). What's in a name? Is accurate recognition and labelling of mental disorders by young people associated with better help-seeking and treatment preferences? *Social Psychiatry and Psychiatric Epidemiology*, *42*(3), 244–250. doi:10.100700127-006-0156-x PMID:17450404

Wright, S. C., Aron, A., McLaughlin-Volpe, T., & Ropp, S. A. (1997). The extended contact effect: Knowledge of cross-group friendships and prejudice. *Journal of Personality and Social Psychology*, *73*(1), 73–90. doi:10.1037/0022-3514.73.1.73

KEY TERMS AND DEFINITIONS

Behavioral Intentions: A person's perceived likelihood or subjective probability that he/she will engage in a given behavior.

Bullying: Seeking to harm, intimidate, or coerce (someone perceived as vulnerable).

Cognitive Attitudes: The beliefs, thoughts, and attributes that we would associate with a person or object.

Empathy: Stepping into the shoes of another person and perceiving and understanding the emotions that other individuals are experiencing.

Extended Contact Hypothesis: Coined by Wright and colleagues in 1997, postulates that knowledge that an in-group member has established a close relationship with an out-group member may promote more positive intergroup attitudes.

Kindness: The quality of being friendly, generous, and considerate.

Mental Health Literacy: The ability to identify specific disorders; knowing how to seek mental health information; knowledge of risk factors and causes, of self-treatments, and of access to professional assistance; and attitudes that promote recognition and appropriate help-seeking.

Social and Emotional Learning (SEL): Identifying and managing emotions, caring about others, making good decisions, behaving ethically and responsibly, developing positive relationships and avoiding negative behaviors.

APPENDIX A: IMAGES FROM *ADDY & UNO* OFF-BROADWAY MUSICAL

Figure 1.

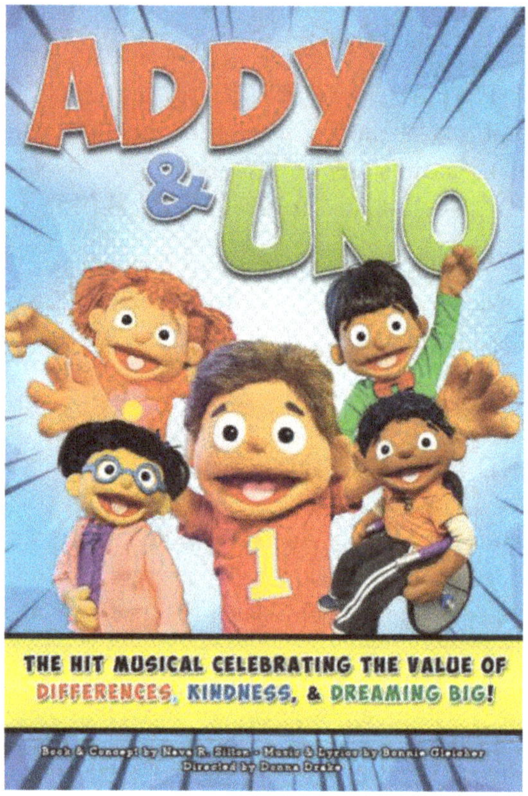

Figure 2.

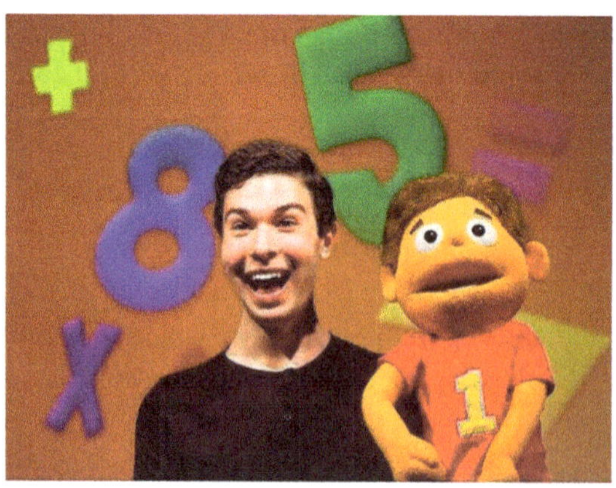

Figure 3.

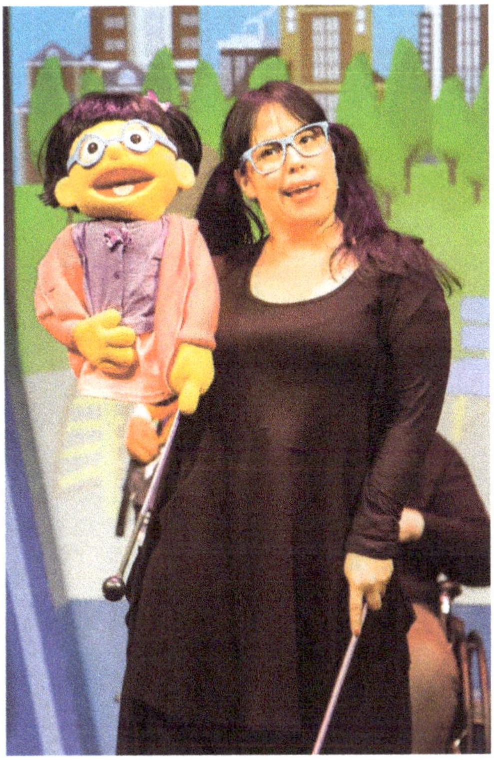

Figure 4.

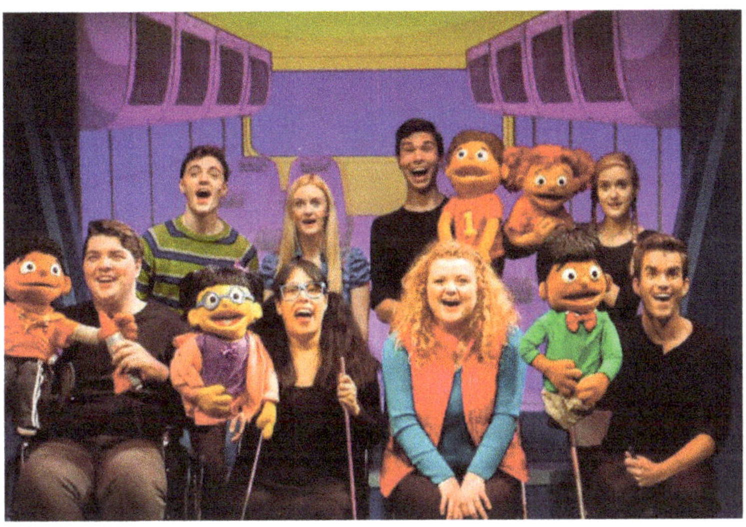

APPENDIX B: IMAGES OF *REALABILITIES* COMIC BOOK SERIES CURRICULUM

Figure 5.

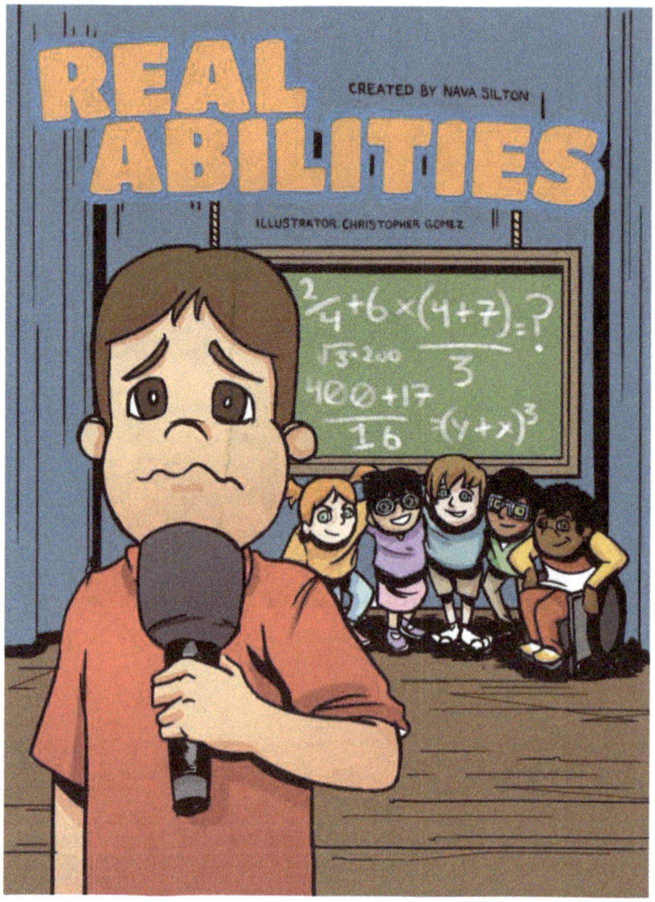

Figure 6.

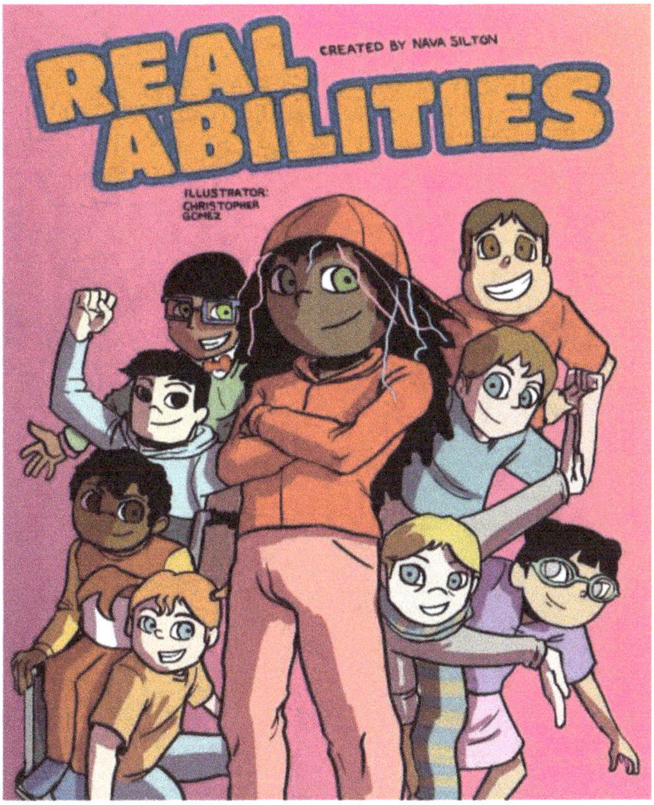
CREATED BY NAVA SILTON
REAL ABILITIES
ILLUSTRATOR: CHRISTOPHER GOMEZ

Figure 7.

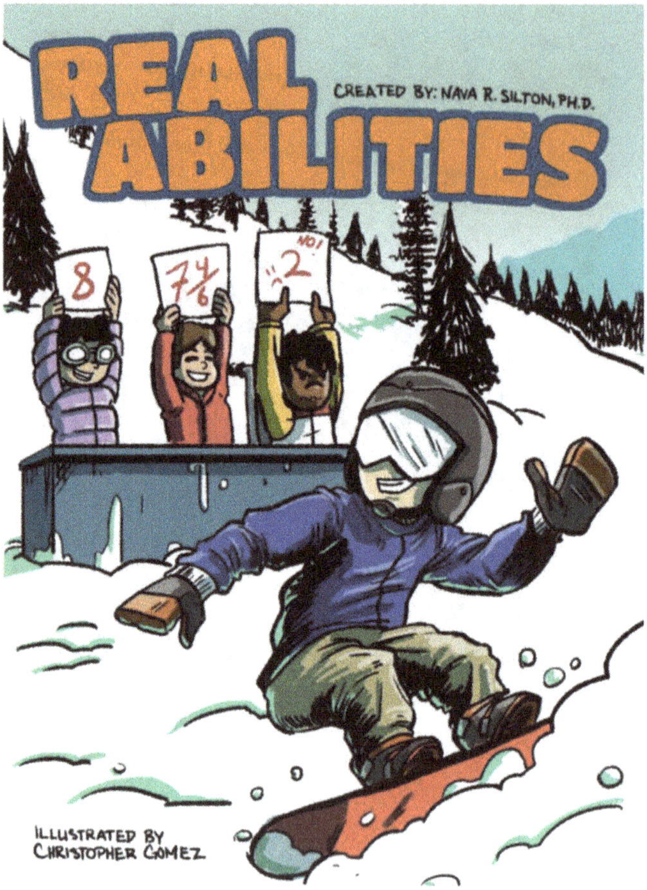
REAL ABILITIES
CREATED BY: NAVA R. SILTON, PH.D.
8
7 4/6
2
NO!
ILLUSTRATED BY
CHRISTOPHER GOMEZ

Figure 8.

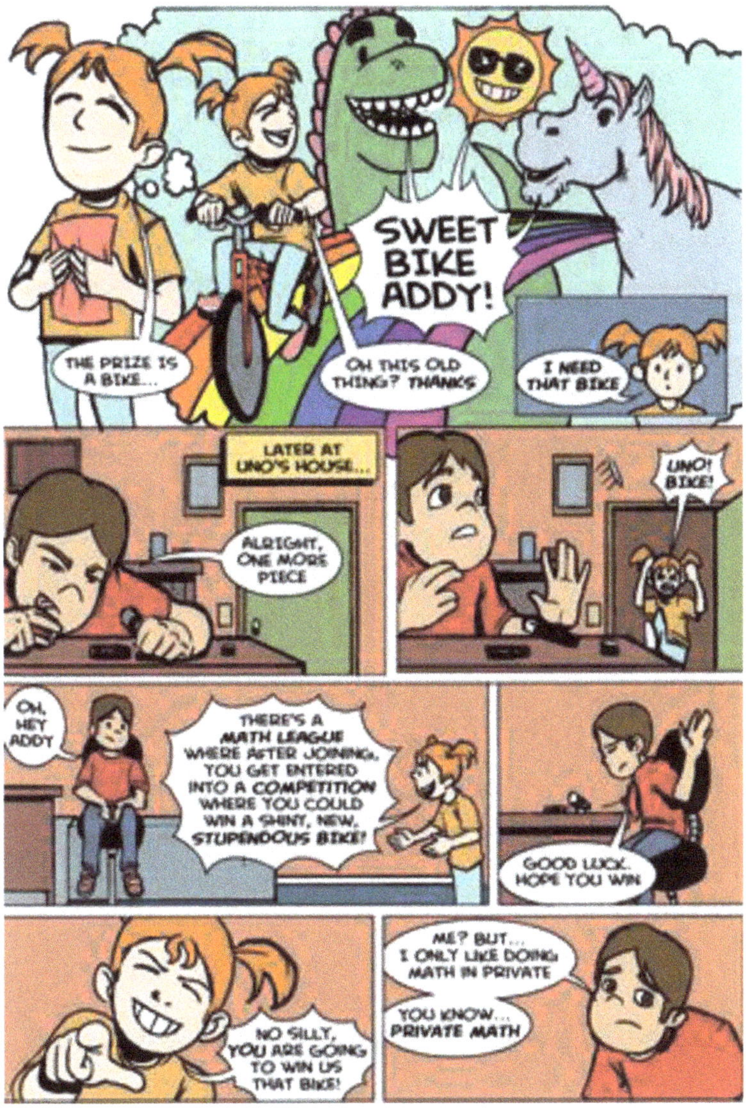

THE PRIZE IS A BIKE...
SWEET BIKE ADDY!
OH THIS OLD THING? THANKS
I NEED THAT BIKE
LATER AT UNO'S HOUSE...
ALRIGHT, ONE MORE PIECE
UNO! BIKE!
OH, HEY ADDY
THERE'S A MATH LEAGUE WHERE AFTER JOINING, YOU GET ENTERED INTO A COMPETITION WHERE YOU COULD WIN A SHINY, NEW, STUPENDOUS BIKE!
GOOD LUCK. HOPE YOU WIN
NO SILLY, YOU ARE GOING TO WIN US THAT BIKE!
ME? BUT... I ONLY LIKE DOING MATH IN PRIVATE
YOU KNOW... PRIVATE MATH

Figure 9.

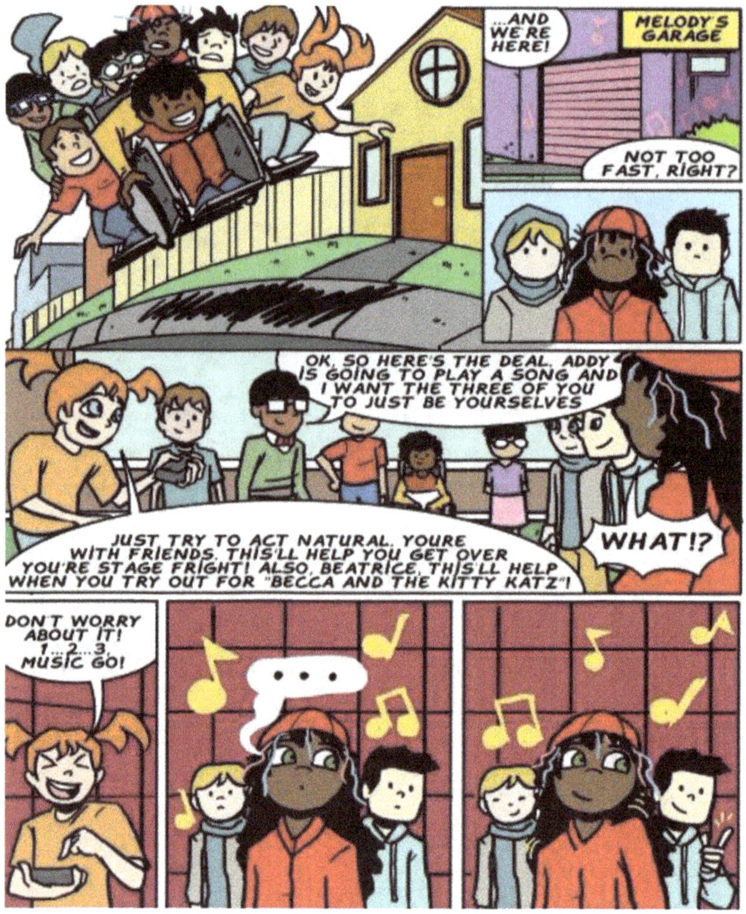
...AND WE'RE HERE!
MELODY'S GARAGE
NOT TOO FAST, RIGHT?
OK, SO HERE'S THE DEAL. ADDY IS GOING TO PLAY A SONG AND I WANT THE THREE OF YOU TO JUST BE YOURSELVES
WHAT!?
JUST TRY TO ACT NATURAL. YOURE WITH FRIENDS. THIS'LL HELP YOU GET OVER YOU'RE STAGE FRIGHT! ALSO, BEATRICE, THIS'LL HELP WHEN YOU TRY OUT FOR "BECCA AND THE KITTY KATZ"!
DON'T WORRY ABOUT IT! 1...2...3, MUSIC GO!

Figure 10.

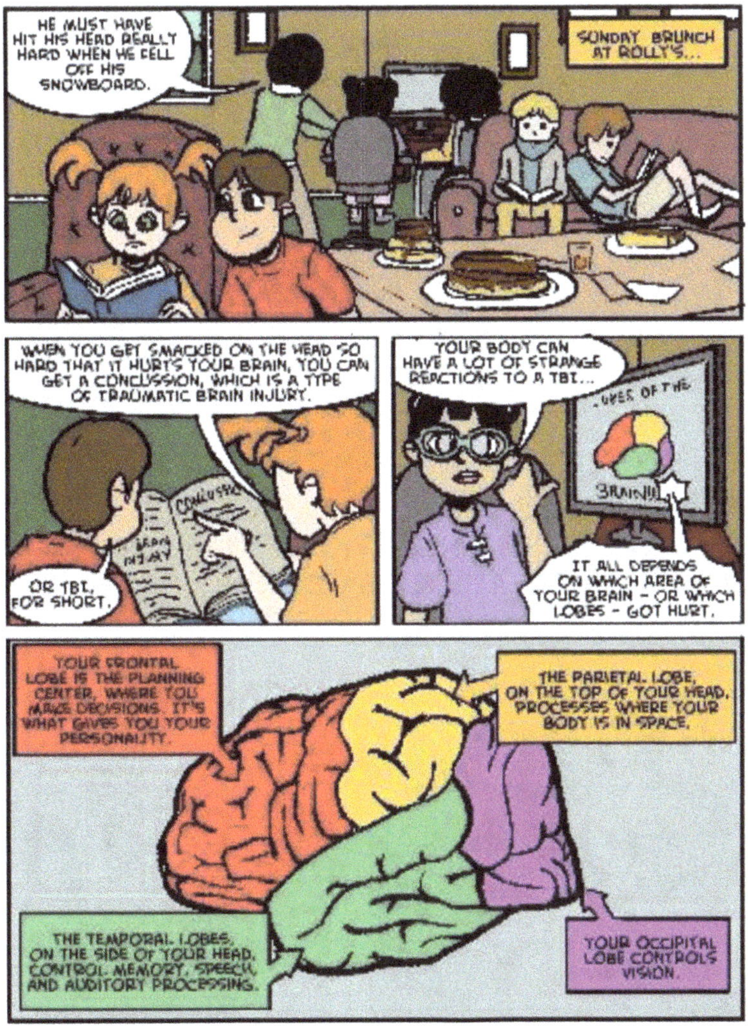
SUNDAY BRUNCH AT ROLLY'S...
HE MUST HAVE HIT HIS HEAD REALLY HARD WHEN HE FELL OFF HIS SNOWBOARD.
WHEN YOU GET SMACKED ON THE HEAD SO HARD THAT IT HURT'S YOUR BRAIN, YOU CAN GET A CONCUSSION, WHICH IS A TYPE OF TRAUMATIC BRAIN INJURY.
OR TBI, FOR SHORT.
YOUR BODY CAN HAVE A LOT OF STRANGE REACTIONS TO A TBI...
BRAIN!!!
IT ALL DEPENDS ON WHICH AREA OF YOUR BRAIN – OR WHICH LOBES – GOT HURT.
YOUR FRONTAL LOBE IS THE PLANNING CENTER, WHERE YOU MAKE DECISIONS. IT'S WHAT GIVES YOU YOUR PERSONALITY.
THE PARIETAL LOBE, ON THE TOP OF YOUR HEAD, PROCESSES WHERE YOUR BODY IS IN SPACE.
THE TEMPORAL LOBES, ON THE SIDE OF YOUR HEAD, CONTROL MEMORY, SPEECH, AND AUDITORY PROCESSING.
YOUR OCCIPITAL LOBE CONTROLS VISION.

Figure 11.

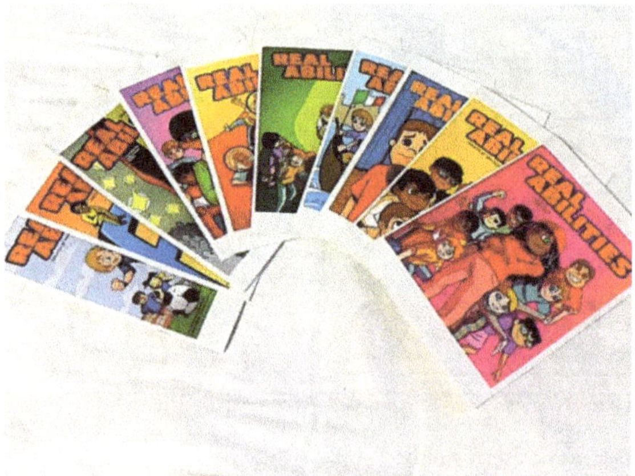

APPENDIX C: IMAGES OF THE "GOT TALENT" AND "CARNIVAL" (THE FIRST TWO MENTAL HEALTH-BASED REALABILITIES COMICS)

Figure 12.

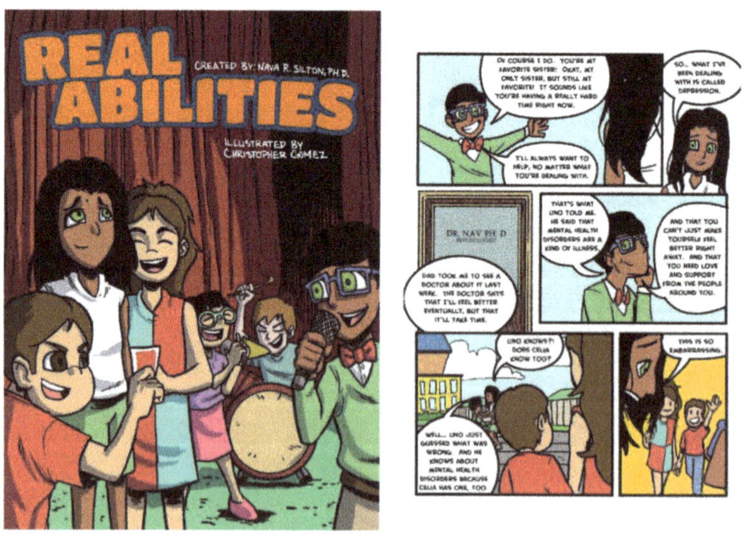
REAL ABILITIES
CREATED BY: NAVA R. SILTON, PH.D.
ILLUSTRATED BY CHRISTOPHER GOMEZ
OF COURSE I DO. YOU'RE MY FAVORITE SISTER! OKAY, MY ONLY SISTER, BUT STILL MY FAVORITE! IT SOUNDS LIKE YOU'RE HAVING A REALLY HARD TIME RIGHT NOW.
I'LL ALWAYS WANT TO HELP, NO MATTER WHAT YOU'RE DEALING WITH.
SO... WHAT I'VE BEEN DEALING WITH IS CALLED DEPRESSION.
DR. NAV PH.D
DAD TOOK ME TO SEE A DOCTOR ABOUT IT LAST WEEK. THE DOCTOR SAYS THAT I'LL FEEL BETTER EVENTUALLY, BUT THAT IT'LL TAKE TIME.
THAT'S WHAT UNO TOLD ME. HE SAID THAT MENTAL HEALTH DISORDERS ARE A KIND OF ILLNESS.
AND THAT YOU CAN'T JUST MAKE YOURSELF FEEL BETTER RIGHT AWAY. AND THAT YOU NEED LOVE AND SUPPORT FROM THE PEOPLE AROUND YOU.
UNO KNOWS?! DOES CELIA KNOW TOO?
WELL... UNO JUST GUESSED WHAT WAS WRONG. AND HE KNOWS ABOUT MENTAL HEALTH DISORDERS BECAUSE CELIA HAS ONE, TOO.
THIS IS SO EMBARRASSING.

Figure 13.

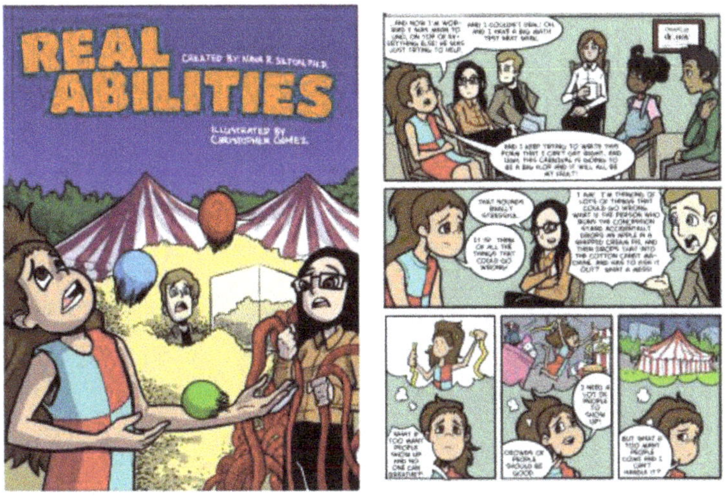

APPENDIX D: IMAGES OF THE RESEARCH-BASED, ISOMETRIC, FIRST-PERSON REALABILITIES ADVENTURE VIDEO GAME

Figure 14.

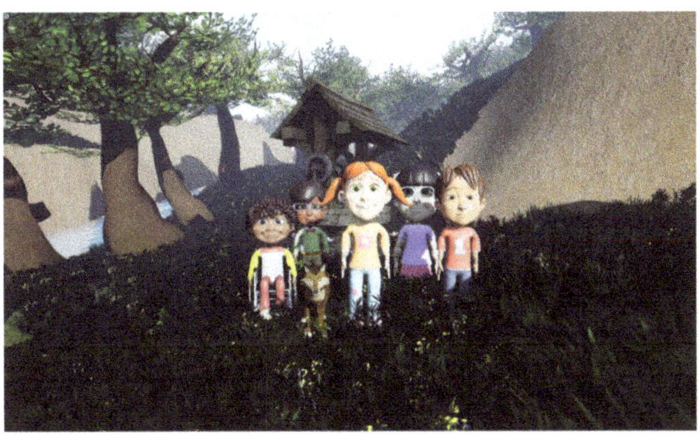

Figure 15.

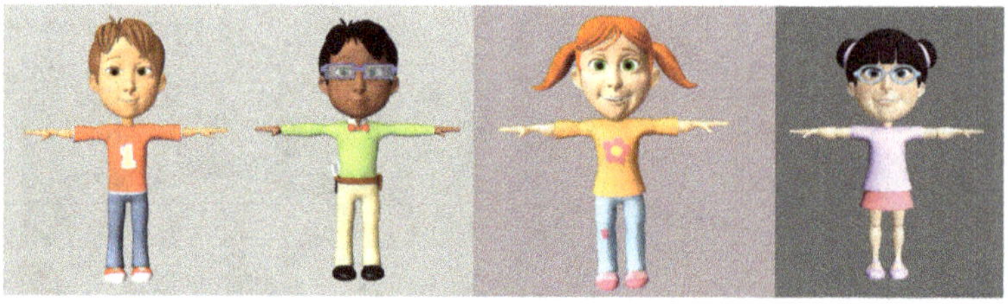

Figure 16.

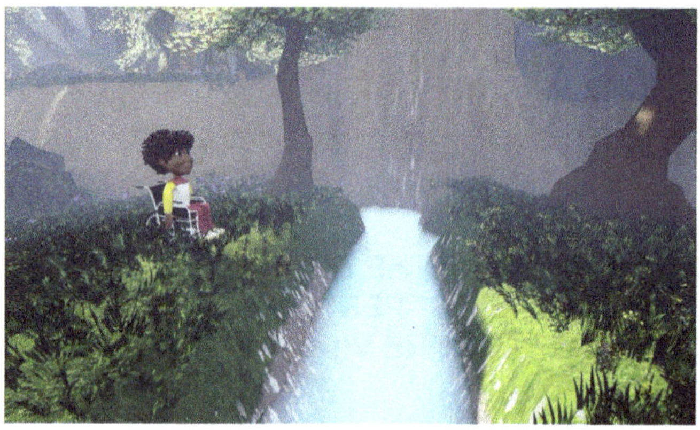

Figure 17.

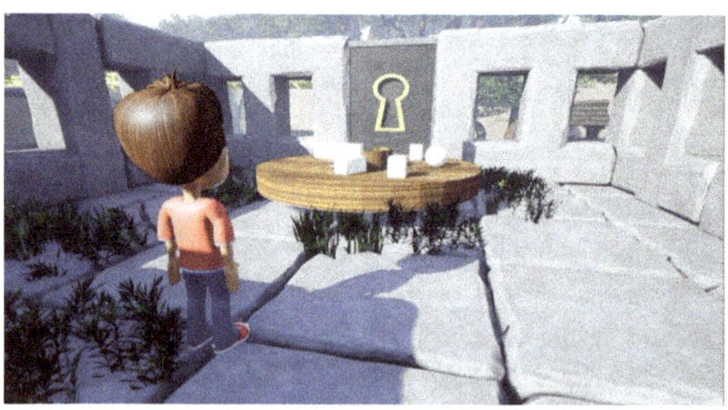

APPENDIX E: TABLES

Table 1. SAQ and ACL Paired Sample T-test Results of The Got Talent Comic Book Intervention.

	SAQ Total		SAQ Academic Subtest		SAQ Social Subtest		SAQ Recreational Subtest		ACL	
	Pre	Post	Pre	Post	Pre	Post	Pre	Post	Pre	Post
Anxiety (mean ± SD)	18.79± 3.98	19.87 ± 4.75*	7.03 ± 1.62	7.57± 1.84**	7.34± 1.75	7.64± 1.78	4.25± 1.29	4.59± 1.51*	6.04± 2.66	6.96± 2.89**
Depression (mean ± SD)	18.86± 4.77	19.55± 5.19	7.26± 1.76	7.49± 1.94	7.23± 1.95	7.52± 1.96	4.27± 1.49	4.53± 1.53	4.69± 2.31	4.79± 2.36

Asterisks indicate significance of pre- versus post-test results: $*p<.05$, $** p < 0.01$; $*** p < 0.001$

Table 2. Bullying Knowledge and Bullying Attitudes Samples T-test Results of The Got Talent Comic Book Intervention.

	Pre	Post
Bullying: Knowledge (mean ± SD)	3.66± .66	3.78 ± .41*
Bullying: Attitudes (mean ± SD)	8.08± 1.73	8.80± 3.13*

Asterisks indicate significance of pre- versus post-test results: $*p<.05$, $** p < 0.01$; $*** p < 0.001$

Table 3. SAQ and ACL Paired Sample T-test Results of The Got Talent and Carnival Comic Book Intervention.

	SAQ Total		SAQ Academic Subtest		SAQ Social Subtest		SAQ Recreational Subtest		ACL	
	Pre	Post	Pre	Post	Pre	Post	Pre	Post	Pre	Post
Anxiety (mean ± SD)	17.62± 4.49	18.74 ± 4.90*	6.86 ± 1.84	7.30 ± 1.92*	6.92± 1.88	7.23± 1.99	3.83± 1.30	4.21± 1.48*	5.51± 2.34	7.31± 2.46***
Depression (mean ± SD)	18.82± 4.51	19.25± 4.65*	7.30± 1.68	7.52± 1.75*	7.22± 1.87	7.29± 1.83	4.33± 1.46	4.47± 1.41	4.28± 1.94	4.98± 2.15**
OCD (mean ± SD)	17.60 ± 4.71	18.83 ± 5.08**	6.85 ± 1.84	7.38± 1.94*	6.83 ± 1.92	7.19 ± 1.97*	3.91± 1.52	4.25 ± 1.57*	6.72± 2.57	7.71± 2.08***
Phobia (mean ± SD)	17.62± 5.06	18.97 ± 4.69***	7.00± 2.09	7.38 ± 1.94	6.68± 2.02	7.30 ± 1.78***	3.94 ± 1.46	4.21 ± 1.49	6.08± 2.20	6.72± 2.57

Asterisks indicate significance of pre- versus post-test results: $*p<.05$, $** p < 0.01$; $*** p < 0.001$

Chapter 7
The Art of Consumption:
Cultivating a Healthy Food and Media Diet in Children

Lauren G. Ashbrook
Marymount Manhattan College, USA

ABSTRACT

This chapter addresses the many different ways children consume both food and media, and the diverse effects these consumption habits have. This chapter also addresses how the consumption of these two variables are related and have reciprocal effects, which can be damaging, to one another. The negative effects of certain consumption habits can be detrimental for the child and family as a whole. Furthermore, the author discusses the most beneficial practices for children to cultivate in order to develop an overall healthy food and media diet.

INTRODUCTION

The way a child consumes both food and media is crucial for the child's further development and overall health. These two variables can affect the child in different ways; however, food and media often have intertwining effects. For example, being exposed to media that consistently promotes a thin body ideal may lead a child to want to eat less to achieve that ideal. Conversely, having a high-fat and high calorie diet may contribute to a child living a fairly sedentary lifestyle, typically leading to a higher consumption of media.

No matter what, children will be exposed to both food and media, so it is important to instill healthy habits regarding the two as early as possible in today's youth. This

DOI: 10.4018/978-1-7998-2940-9.ch007

chapter will discuss the positive and negative effects of the different ways in which food and media are commonly consumed by children. This chapter will also address how parents can establish the healthiest food and media diet for their children.

A Child's Food Diet

What defines a healthy food diet? There is no perfect answer, since it is different for each individual. However, there are some simple behavioral changes that can be made to help improve a child's diet. A healthy diet, along with sufficient physical activity and limited sedentary behavior, have been shown to help prevent being overweight and obese, cardiovascular diseases, depression, fear, stress, poor self-image, and contribute to improving the overall quality of life (De Lepeleere, DeSmet, Verloigne, Cardon, & De Bourdeaudhuij, 2013). A healthy diet during childhood and adolescence promotes optimal health, growth, and cognitive development of the child and adolescent, and may contribute to the prevention of chronic disease in later life (Van Cauwenberghe, Maes, Spittaels, Van Lenthe, Brug, Oppert, & De Bourdeaudhuij, 2010).

Evidence suggests that eating habits adopted early in life will most likely extend into adulthood; however, the transition from childhood into adolescence can often usher in unhealthy dietary choices (Van Cauwenberghe et al., 2010). Therefore, it is important to establish healthy eating behaviors early in life, and focus particularly on the transition from childhood to adolescence to ensure the most stable diet over time. Parents play an important role in a child's eating patterns, and it is encouraged that interventions aimed at improving a child's nutrition involve parents and/or the entire family in some way.

A Dietary Epidemic

One of the largest nutritional issues facing children and adolescents today is obesity. In fact, almost 80% of 11–15 years olds have multiple dietary and physical activity risk factors of being overweight or obese (Leech, McNaughton, & Timperio, 2014). There are eight early life risk factors correlated with the development of obesity: birth weight, parental obesity, sleep duration, television viewing, size in early life, weight gain in infancy, catch-up growth, and body mass index rebound (Pocock, Trivedi, Wills, Bunn, & Magnusson, 2010). Research also states that patterns of obesity and physical activity levels were found to differ according to age, gender, and socio-economic status. A consistent finding stated that mostly girls, older children/adolescents, and children/adolescents of a lower socio-economic status had high levels of obesity and low levels of physical activity (Leech, McNaughton, & Timperio, 2014).

Fortunately, parents are becoming more aware of what causes obesity and how they can help their children, but it is not always so clear-cut. While it has been shown that parental support of health promoting behaviors can positively impact children, research shows that parents may not recognize the negative health consequences of their children being overweight, and even when they do, may feel confused by the vast array of messages about strategies for addressing the problem (Leech, McNaughton, & Timperio, 2014). Parents typically find that there are various factors that impact their child's behaviors associated with being overweight or obese, particularly preference for certain foods. Children disliking new foods and being 'picky eaters' are considered common barriers to healthy eating (Leech, McNaughton, & Timperio, 2014). Some parents also tend to rely on "fast foods," because they are concerned that their children will eat nothing else. Parents commonly perceive that the cost of food is also a barrier to a healthy diet (Leech, McNaughton, & Timperio, 2014).

Effects of Parenting Styles on Diet

Parents' involvement in a child's nutritional curriculum or intervention is not the only way they can help improve their child's diet. Parenting styles can also have an effect on diet and lifestyle. Evidence suggests that parents who enhance their children's self-efficacy in an overall healthy manner can be very beneficial in the long run toward a healthy diet and lifestyle (De Lepeleere et al., 2013).

Regarding diet, both general and specific parenting styles are important and have an effect on the child. Based on the research of Maccoby and Martin (1983), the general parenting styles are categorized under two umbrellas: responsiveness of parents to a child's needs through affectionate and sensitive interactions (i.e. involvement), and attempting to control a child's behavior through discipline and expectations (i.e. strictness) (De Lepeleere et al., 2013). Specific parenting styles include when a parent influences a child's specific behavior, such as diet, through modeling, social support, parental control, rules, and agreements. Maccoby and Martin (1983) suggest that the combination of a general parenting style with specific parenting interactions is the best method for helping children become accustomed to the best diet for themselves (De Lepeleere et al., 2013). This can also be defined as an authoritative parenting style. This style reflects parents who are motivating, empathic when they increase the intrinsic value of activities, apply clear rules and agreements, are consistent, model and monitor behavior, and offer alternative activities with as much choice for the child as possible (Lepeleere et al., 2013). On top of this, offering an immediate reward after a child engages in a healthy behavior provides even more of an incentive for the child to repeat the behavior, thus hopefully creating a habit.

A Child's Media Diet

It is no secret that children, particularly adolescents, spend a good portion of their days engaging with media in some way. In fact, the American Academy of Pediatrics (AAP) states that American children and adolescents from age 2 to 18 years spend on average, more than four hours using electronic media daily; this is more time than they spend on any other activity other than sleep (Barkin, Richardson, Klinepeter, Finch, & Krcmar, 2006). Recent data also indicates that 95% of teenagers in the United States aged 12–17 use the internet and spend up to 7 hours a day on screen-based activities (Boniel-Nissim, Tabak, Mazur, Borraccino, Brooks, Gommans, & Finne, 2015). This extensive media exposure can have significant cognitive and behavioral impacts on children.

EFFECTS OF MEDIA EXPOSURE

Negative Effects

Media exposure has been associated with aggressive behavior, poor moral reasoning, desensitization, obesity, and decreased attention span (Barkin et al., 2006). There is also strong evidence that electronic media use may be related to a variety of problem behaviors in adolescence such as internet addiction, shortened sleep duration, poor diet quality, lower physical activity levels, poor school performance, loneliness, depression, social anxiety, and an increased likelihood of physical complaints (Boniel-Nissim et al., 2015).

Another study examined the impact of technology on four areas: psychological issues, behavior problems, attention problems, and physical health among children (aged 4–8), preteens (9–12), and teenagers (13–18) (Rosen, Lim, Felt, Carrier, Cheever, Lara-Ruiz, & Rokkum, 2014). The research found that: (i) more television viewing at 2-3 years of age predicted more attention problems at 10 years of age, (ii) more TV viewing at 2.5 years predicted more behavior problems at 5 years of age, (iii) more television viewing at age 5 predicted more psychosocial adjustment problems at age 7, (iv) more television at ages 1-3 predicted more attention problems at age 7, and (v) more television in middle school predicted more attention problems in late adolescence (Rosen et al., 2014).

Heavy video game usage, regardless of the content, has been shown to predict depression among adolescents and young adults (Rosen et al., 2014). Additional research has shown that the impact of video gaming depends on with whom one is playing (i.e. if with new people, the result is increased loneliness; however, if with family or friends, the impact can enhance a sense of positive well-being) (Rosen et al., 2014).

Positive Effects

Media has also been associated with positive social interactions, improved intelligence scores, improved problem-solving skills, accelerated language acquisition, and enhanced school performance. Electronic media in particular can positively influence factors such as ease of communication with peers and number of friends, as well as have a positive impact on spatial skills, cognitive development, reading skills, and can even contribute to the development of resilience (Boniel-Nissim et al., 2015). Frequent play of digital games, aside from those violent in nature, have also been associated with enhanced inductive reasoning, mental rotation and spatial visualization skills, metacognition, memory, and spatial distribution of attention and visual selective attention (Blumberg, Blades, & Oates, 2015). This difference exists in the content of the programming and the time spent engaged in media use.

Parental Involvement

Parents need to be aware of the potentially harmful effects of technology and need to implement strategies to help their children moderate their own usage to reduce their overall screen time (Rosen et al., 2014). The American Academy of Pediatrics (AAP) recommends that parents use the media's influence in a positive manner by helping their children to be intelligent media viewers, restricting their media exposure, co-viewing with their children, explaining what the child sees, and creating an electronic media–free environment in children's rooms (Barkin et al., 2006). Parents play a key role in shaping how their children use the media. Recent research has identified that the quality of communication between adolescents and parents remains significant and operates as an important protective health asset (Boniel-Nissim et al., 2015).

In a previous study, the majority (59%) of parents reported using a variety of media mediation strategies with their child (ren) (Barkin et al., 2006). Only 7% allowed unlimited media use and engaged in no mediation. A third of the sample reported using a single active media strategy, including 11% who used instructive mediation and 23% who used restrictive mediation. Each media strategy demonstrated varying degrees of reported media exposure; not surprisingly, the restrictive approach was associated with the least amount of exposure (Mean: 2.4 hours) and the unlimited approach was associated with the highest amount of exposure (Mean: 4.1 hours). That being said, the more involved parents are with their child's media exposure, the more control they can have over the amount of media they are viewing.

How Media Affects Food

Food and media are two variables that are related to consumption; in this day and age, it is almost impossible to avoid consuming both. While food and media's impact and effects need to be looked at separately, it is critical that they are also analyzed together. These two variables are often intertwined and influence one another in many different ways.

Food Advertising

Many social and environmental contexts have an impact on food choices. Mass media and advertising in particular have an influence on eating behavior and body image, especially due to the mass exposure of media to children and adolescents (Story, Neumark-Sztainer, & French, 2002). Food advertising and promotion are essential to the marketing of the United States food supply. The U.S. food system is the second-largest industry that is advertised, and is often showcased on all media platforms and via various distributors (Story, Neumark-Sztainer, & French, 2002).

Excessive Consumption and Obesity

The food industry spends approximately $11 billion annually on advertising; food manufacturers spend $7 billion, and food establishments, particularly fast-food establishments, spend around $3 billion (Story, Neumark-Sztainer, & French, 2002). Most of the advertising focuses mainly on packaged and processed foods. This vast exposure to unhealthy foods can be dangerous, particularly for vulnerable, impressionable populations such as children and adolescents. Exposure to food advertising, especially commercials for fast food, may influence viewers to select more higher-fat and higher calorie content foods. Previous research has consistently shown a positive association between television viewing and child and adolescent obesity (Story, Neumark-Sztainer, & French, 2002). The impact of television on obesity is believed to be a result of two variables: reduced calorie loss due to the lack of physical activity, and increased dietary energy intake, either during viewing or as a result of food advertising. Studies with young children have shown that the greater number of hours of television watched, the more children request, purchase, and consume those advertised foods (Story, Neumark-Sztainer, & French, 2002).

Negative Body Image and Dieting

However, the media can also have an effect on eating and weight concerns on the other end of the spectrum. There is increasing evidence that advertising has an effect on adolescents' health behaviors in regard to losing weight (Story, Neumark-Sztainer, & French, 2002). Mass media is considered to be an important influence on how adolescents, girls in particular, view their bodies. Studies have shown that as many as 50% to 75% of adolescent girls are dissatisfied with their weight and body image (Story, Neumark-Sztainer, & French, 2002). The widening gap between women's actual body sizes and the media's use of unrealistic thin ideals make women feel bad about their bodies and pressure them to lose weight (Anschutz, Van Strien, & Engels, 2011).

Previous research has found that adolescent girls' discontentment with body weight and shape was related to the frequency of viewing images of the "ideal body type," whether these images were communicated through social media, television, movies, or fashion magazines (Story, Neumark-Sztainer, & French, 2002). Frequency of exposure to these mediums was also positively associated with the prevalence of having dieted to lose weight and/or having gone on a diet to lose weight specifically because of the images they have viewed. In addition to print media, television and internet exposure have also been found to be associated with a drive for thinness among adolescent girls (Story, Neumark-Sztainer, & French, 2002).

Using Media Characters for Good

While media has been known to affect food consumption negatively, there is the possibility of using media in a way that has a positive outcome. Research has suggested that popular characters can make a difference in encouraging children to select one food over another (Kotler, Schiffman, & Hanson, 2012). Children were more likely to prefer one food over another when it was associated with characters that they liked and were familiar with. In a previous study, when foods within the same category (i.e., two vegetables, two fruits, or two grains) were asked to compete against each other, character branding strongly influenced the child's food choice (Kotler, Schiffman, & Hanson, 2012). However, "healthy" options as a whole were not seen as more appealing than sugary or salty snacks just because a character the child knows or favors is endorsing it. While it can be seen as almost impossible to make a child prefer a vegetable over candy when presented with the two choices, overall perceptions of food can still be altered in the right direction.

The Kaiser Family Foundation suggests that one way to decrease the obesity epidemic is for media producers to use popular media characters to promote healthy food alternatives. In a recent study, researchers found that 4 to 6 year-old children claimed that snack foods tasted better when they were branded with a licensed character on the packaging than when the same snacks were presented without the licensed character on the packaging (Kotler, Schiffman, & Hanson, 2012). That being said, popular characters endorsing healthy food options without the presence of an unhealthy food option may make these options more appealing to children, making them more willing to try and enjoy them.

A Potential Dangerous Outcome Regarding Food and Media

While food and media have varying effects on different children, some effects may be more serious for some children, rather than others. Media has been known to lead to severe difficulties regarding food consumption, particularly resulting in disordered eating, or possibly even eating disorders (Harrison & Cantor, 1997). While these are more extreme cases, they are still very prevalent and are increasing in numbers, mainly for adolescents and children.

Types of Eating Disorders

Eating disorders are serious psychological illnesses that affect the way one eats and relates to food on a daily basis (NEDA, 2018). Approximately 20 million women and 10 million men in the United States will suffer from an eating disorder at some point in their lives. The three main eating disorders are anorexia nervosa, bulimia nervosa, and binge eating disorder (NEDA, 2018). Eating disorders are often strongly correlated with low self-esteem, depression, suicidal ideation, and substance use (Pratt & Woolfenden, 2002).

Anorexia Nervosa (AN)

Anorexia nervosa (AN) is an eating disorder characterized by weight loss, difficulty maintaining an appropriate body weight for height and age, and commonly but not in all cases, a poor body image (NEDA, 2018). People with anorexia typically restrict the number of calories they consume, as well as the types of food they eat, usually avoiding high fat and sugar contents. Those with anorexia usually begin to first show symptoms during adolescence; however, an increasing number of children are being diagnosed with anorexia, as well (NEDA, 2018). Despite common beliefs, a person does not need to be underweight in order to be struggling with anorexia. One cannot judge if a person has an eating disorder just by looking at him/her. Studies have found that larger-bodied individuals can have anorexia; however, they are less likely to be diagnosed due to the normalized discrimination against obesity and overweight individuals (NEDA, 2018).

Bulimia Nervosa (BN)

Bulimia nervosa (BN) is another very serious, potentially dangerous eating disorder. Those who suffer with bulimia secretly binge (eat large amounts of food with a loss of control over the eating), and then purge what they ate in order to get rid of the calories they consumed (Mayo Clinic, 2018). There are several different ways individuals with bulimia purge the calories they consumed; some may use one or many different methods of purging. Common examples include self-induced vomiting, misuse of laxatives, weight-loss supplements, or diuretics after bingeing (Mayo Clinic, 2018). Those with bulimia are typically just as body and weight-conscious as individuals with anorexia.

Binge Eating Disorder (BED)

Binge eating disorder (BED) is one of the new diagnoses of eating disorders as a whole; however, it is actually more common than both anorexia and bulimia. With BED, an individual consumes an abnormally large amount of food in a short period of time, typically feeling a loss of control and an inability to stop eating (Real Stories, Real People, 2019). People with BED usually feel significant disgust, guilt, and depression after a binge (Real Stories, Real People, 2019).

Causes and Vulnerabilities of Eating Disorders

The prevalence of eating disorders has increased significantly in both children and adolescents over the past few decades (Rosen, 2010). Therefore, it is crucial for healthcare providers and parents alike to be aware of the symptoms and warning signs in order to help their children as soon as possible. It is particularly important to know the possible genetic and environmental vulnerabilities that may later influence the development of an eating disorder in children and adolescents.

Prevalence Rates

A recent analysis by the Agency for Healthcare Research and Quality revealed that from 1999 to 2006, hospitalizations for eating disorders increased approximately 119% for children younger than 12 years of age (Rosen, 2010). Research states that approximately 0.5% of adolescent girls in the United States have AN, approximately 1% to 2% suffer from BN, and up to 5% to 10% of all cases of eating disorders in children or adolescents occur in males (Rosen, 2010). The lifetime prevalence of AN is between 0.5% to 2%, with the peak age of onset being around 13 to 18 years (Campbell & Peebles, 2014). Due to the nature of the illness, AN has a mortality rate of at least 5% to 6%, the highest of any psychiatric illness. The lifetime prevalence of BN is a bit higher, falling anywhere from 0.9% and 3%; BN also has an older age of onset-around 16 to 17 years (Campbell & Peebles, 2014).

As females reach adolescence, unhealthy eating behaviors and eating disorders come to represent major health concerns (Pratt & Woolfenden, 2002). Previous research has shown that there is a high prevalence of disordered eating behaviors (33%), unhealthy dieting practices (57%), and a distorted body image (12%) among adolescents. In addition, a study claimed that the majority of adolescents want to lose weight (77%) and half have attempted to lose weight in the past month (51%) (Pratt & Woolfenden, 2002).

Biological and Genetic Vulnerabilities

Evidence continues to abound stating that eating disorders are heritable; in fact, if an individual has a relative suffering from an eating disorder, they are 7 to 12 times more likely to develop one, as well (Campbell & Peebles, 2014). A genetic predisposition to various trait disturbances, including, behavioral rigidity, perfectionism, or harm avoidance, are typically associated with developing an eating disorder, as well (Rosen, 2010). These genetic effects seem to be most prominent and begin to show during puberty. Younger patients (prepubescent) with eating disorders are more likely to suffer from depression, obsessive-compulsive disorder, or other anxiety disorders, and are less likely to have binge/purge behaviors associated with their illness (Rosen, 2010). Adolescents with chronic illnesses, especially insulin-dependent diabetes, are also at a higher risk of developing eating disorder behaviors (Campbell & Peebles, 2014).

Environmental Vulnerabilities

Athletes and performers, particularly those who participate in sports and activities that reward a lean body (i.e. gymnastics, running, wrestling, dance, modeling) are often more susceptible to developing eating disorders and/or disordered eating behaviors (Rosen, 2010). Similarly, research has shown that female adolescents who diet at a severe level are 18 times more likely to develop an eating disorder within 6 months than those who did not diet; additionally, those who diet at a moderate level are five times more likely to develop an eating disorder than those who do not diet (Pratt & Woolfenden, 2002). For BN in particular, common environmental contributors include parental obesity, childhood obesity, critical comments by family about shape/weight/eating, early onset of menstrual cycle, parental psychiatric disorder(s), and certain parental problems, such as low contact, high expectations, and alcohol use (Pratt & Woolfenden, 2002).

Online Communities

Food and media have come together in an even more dangerous way since the birth of online pro-eating disorder websites, blogs, and communities. These sites are designed as a way to motivate and prolong the symptoms of those suffering with eating disorders. These sites also tend to support self-harm behaviors and suicidality (Borzekowski, Schenk, Wilson, & Peebles, 2010). Given the secretive nature of eating disorders, individuals who suffer, particularly adolescents, may seek social support or resources online. Pro-eating disorder online communities emerged in the early 2000s to support the illness as a lifestyle (Arseniev-Koehler, Lee, McCormick, & Moreno, 2016). Previous studies have illustrated that Pro-ED cyberspaces often exacerbate eating disorder risk factors such as poor body image and learning new unhealthy weight loss methods; these sites are also used as a tool to reinforce an individual's "eating disorder identity" (Arseniev-Koehler et al., 2016).

In a recent content analysis of 180 pro-eating disorder websites, the researchers found that just about all (91%) of the websites were open to the public; the majority (84%) of them offered pro-anorexia content, and 64% showcased pro-bulimia content (Borzekowski et al., 2010). Thinspiration (photos of extremely thin individuals used for weight loss motivation) appeared on 85% of the sites, and 83% provided suggestions on how to engage in eating-disordered behaviors (Borzekowski et al., 2010). The main themes found on the sites were perfection, control, and success. These communities can be extremely inviting and dangerous for young, impressionable individuals who may have already developed or have the potential to develop an eating disorder. Therefore, it's important to be mindful and aware of these media sites.

Helpful Screening and Treatment Methods

Pediatricians should screen for eating disorders as part of annual health supervision or during pre-participation sports examinations by monitoring weight and height longitudinally and paying careful attention to potential signs and symptoms of disordered eating (Rosen, 2010). Any evidence of excessive weight concern, inappropriate dieting, or a pattern of weight loss requires further attention. It is also important to look out for amenorrhea (the loss of one's menstrual period) or a failure to achieve appropriate increases in weight or height that are suitable for a child's age (Rosen, 2010). In addition, it may be a warning sign if an adolescent girl consistently seeks physician care for weight, shape, or eating concerns, since this is a warning sign for the development of AN.

An eating disorder may be suspected in a patient with weight loss, unexplained delay in puberty, restrictive or abnormal eating behaviors, recurrent vomiting, excessive exercise, trouble gaining weight, or body image concerns (Campbell &

Peebles, 2014). Particular habits regarding food are also important to notice. This includes restriction of entire food groups (ie, new-onset vegetarianism or veganism) or calories, as well as the development of food rituals. Individuals with AN often refuse to eat foods they once enjoyed, avoid meals with family and friends, and over-exercise in a rigid manner (Campbell & Peebles, 2014).

Evidence for effective treatments for eating disorders in children and adolescents is growing, but still remains limited. When an eating disorder is officially present, it is recommended that children and adolescents seek outpatient treatment, partial hospitalization, residential programs, or inpatient hospitalization, depending on the severity of the illness, how long the child has had the illness, and what is best for the individual and his/her family overall (Campbell & Peebles, 2014). Treating patients in a home setting is preferred, but other models of care may be necessary and more appropriate for long-term recovery, especially if the home is a more triggering environment. Common treatment models for pediatric AN, BN, and BED include individual therapy, CBT (Cognitive Behavioral Therapy), and FBT (Family-Based Therapy) (Campbell & Peebles, 2014). FBT has the largest evidence base of any treatment of being effective for adolescents and young adults with eating disorders. There is also growing evidence that it is useful for children under age 12 with restrictive eating disorders (Campbell & Peebles, 2014).

BEST PRACTICES FOR FOOD AND MEDIA CONSUMPTION

Best Food Practices

As previously mentioned, both obesity and eating disorders are common issues that are facing today's children. Obesity, in particular, is very much on the rise; while some aspects of body shape are uncontrollable, there are still a number of steps that can be put in place for the benefit of not only children, but the whole family. When children go through the transition period to adolescence, most of their days are spent in school; that being said, the school environment can be used as a tool to help improve overall diets. There is strong evidence that interventions that combine increased availability of fruit and vegetables with a nutritionally-based curriculum in schools, with some parental involvement, can help increase the intake of fruits and vegetables (Van Cauwenberghe et al., 2010).

Genetic predispositions to obesity, that are partially mediated by specific eating traits and food preferences, can be modified by parental behaviors (i.e. modeling healthy eating habits) and the home environment (i.e. having access to healthy foods) (Kral, & Rauh, 2010). Interventions targeting healthy eating in children have the potential to achieve more of an impact if the healthy foods are often available and easily accessible in the home. It is also beneficial if the healthy foods are also consumed by their mothers and/or other family members in the household (Kral, & Rauh, 2010).

Within the eating disorder prevention field, the need for more socio-environmental approaches has been stressed, given that children's body image, self-esteem, weight bias, and eating behaviors are influenced by parents, peers, teachers, the school environment, as well as their community and culture (Sánchez-Carracedo, Neumark-Sztainer, & López-Guimera, 2012).

According to the research, greater efforts should be dedicated to modifying the factors that shape our physical and social environment by means of: (i) encouraging parents to refrain from making comments that contribute to body dissatisfaction and disordered eating behaviors, as well as by promoting healthy norms with regard to eating, weight, body shape. and how to deal adequately with stress; (ii) working with groups of peers to promote healthy norms with regard to weight-related teasing; (iii) educating teachers in relation to prejudices about weight and eating disorders to help facilitate changes in the school environment, as well as to promote healthy norms on eating and physical activity, while encouraging the acceptance and tolerance of different body shapes, and (iv) training health professionals to take into account shared risk factors for not just obesity, but for other eating disturbances and eating disorders as well. This will help them correctly manage different types of problems while avoiding a possible negative impact on the individual (Sánchez-Carracedo, Neumark-Sztainer, & López-Guimera, 2012).

Best Media Practices

Regarding television, it is critical for parents to decide which technology and content is best for their children and how they plan to monitor and set rules for use. Violence on mobile media should be avoided, and when children encounter it, they should be guided on how to understand it. It is recommended to show age-appropriate, educational content and to use resources such as PBS Kids, Sesame Workshop, or Common Sense Media to help guide media choices (Radesky, Schumacher, & Zuckerman, 2015). Parents should be encouraged to try a game or app first, play it with the child, and ask the child about it afterward to see what he or she is learning. There are significant benefits of parents and children using interactive media together to help enhance its educational value (Radesky, Schumacher, & Zuckerman, 2015). It is also important for parents to help children find developmentally appropriate activities to pursue, and provide alternative strategies besides just media to help a child self-regulate when distressed or bored. In general, pediatric providers advise parents to preserve quality, connected family interactions, whether it's through "unplugged time" or a designated family hour, and how to establish healthy childhood media habits from early childhood (Radesky, Schumacher, & Zuckerman, 2015).

Encouraging Prosocial Behavior

Significant effects of prosocial media on helping others have been demonstrated for a variety of media, including television shows, video games, and music lyrics (Prot, Gentile, Anderson, Suzuki, Swing, Lim, & Liau, 2014). For example, previous research found that adolescents' greater use of prosocial video games was related to more frequent helping, cooperation, and sharing. Media content determines much of what is learned. Prosocial media is expected to decrease the likelihood of aggression and increase the likelihood of positive, beneficial, behavior (Prot et al., 2014). Children who watched educational programs were also more likely to imitate positive behavior than those who watched more entertainment-based television (Hogan & Strasburger, 2008).

Socially desirable outcomes after prosocial television can be amplified by combining prosocial programs with other experiences," specifically role-playing (puppets and dialogue) or verbal labeling (discussion) (Hogan & Strasburger, 2008). Researchers have also found that the prosocial effect is twice as strong as the antisocial effect. Antisocial outcomes included aggression, criminality, and stereotyping while prosocial outcomes included friendly interaction, aggression reduction, altruism, and stereotype reduction (Hogan & Strasburger, 2008). Not only are prosocial effects stronger, but they have also been shown to be more enduring, both in laboratory and natural settings (Hogan & Strasburger, 2008).

CONCLUSION

The quality of food and media consumption is crucial to a child's physical and mental health. The consumption of these two variables can lead to both positive and negative outcomes. Fortunately, parents have the capability to alter their child's consumption habits to lead him or her towards a healthy lifestyle.

Trying to take control of your child's food and media diet can seem daunting, since there are many uncontrollable, external factors that may come into play- there is still the possibility for enhancement in this area. With food, it is best to establish a non-rigid, balanced diet, particularly one that encourages a child to listen to his or her body and follow hunger cues. With media, it is encouraged to have children view programs that showcase positive behavior, and reduce the consumption of media that showcases negative behavior. These habits can lead to long-term benefits for one's child and family as a whole.

LIMITATIONS AND FUTURE RESEARCH

There are several limitations in the research of different food and media diets in children. Particularly, there is very little research regarding the long-term effects of certain practices that are said to be beneficial for children. For example, while more exposure to fruits and vegetables in schools may be helpful for a period of time, it is unclear whether that will continue to establish healthy habits as adults. Likewise, the research does not examine whether or not too much emphasis on healthy foods has the potential to lead to negative views about oneself and about one's body as an adult.

An opportunity for future research is to conduct longitudinal studies of various food and media practices, examining whether these practices are beneficial as they develop into adults, as well. These studies can then examine the different effects from food and media that individuals experience as they develop into adolescence and adulthood. The extraneous variables of adolescence and adulthood also change the way an individual is able to look at and take control over his or her food and media diets.

REFERENCES

Anschutz, D. J., Van Strien, T., & Engels, R. C. (2011). *Exposure to slim images in mass media: Television commercials as reminders of restriction in restrained eaters*. Academic Press.

Arseniev-Koehler, A., Lee, H., McCormick, T., & Moreno, M. A. (2016). # Proana: Pro-eating disorder socialization on Twitter. *The Journal of Adolescent Health, 58*(6), 659–664. doi:10.1016/j.jadohealth.2016.02.012 PMID:27080731

Barkin, S., Ip, E., Richardson, I., Klinepeter, S., Finch, S., & Krcmar, M. (2006). Parental media mediation styles for children aged 2 to 11 years. *Archives of Pediatrics & Adolescent Medicine, 160*(4), 395–401. doi:10.1001/archpedi.160.4.395 PMID:16585485

Blumberg, F. C., Blades, M., & Oates, C. (2015). Youth and new media. *Zeitschrift fur Psychologie mit Zeitschrift fur Angewandte Psychologie*.

Boniel-Nissim, M., Tabak, I., Mazur, J., Borraccino, A., Brooks, F., Gommans, R., ... Finne, E. (2015). Supportive communication with parents moderates the negative effects of electronic media use on life satisfaction during adolescence. *International Journal of Public Health, 60*(2), 189–198. doi:10.100700038-014-0636-9 PMID:25549611

Borzekowski, D. L., Schenk, S., Wilson, J. L., & Peebles, R. (2010). e-Ana and e-Mia: A content analysis of pro–eating disorder websites. *American Journal of Public Health, 100*(8), 1526–1534. doi:10.2105/AJPH.2009.172700 PMID:20558807

Bulimia nervosa. (2018, May 10). Retrieved from https://www.mayoclinic.org/diseases-conditions/bulimia/symptoms-causes/syc-20353615

Campbell, K., & Peebles, R. (2014). Eating disorders in children and adolescents: State of the art review. *Pediatrics, 134*(3), 582–592. doi:10.1542/peds.2014-0194 PMID:25157017

De Lepeleere, S., DeSmet, A., Verloigne, M., Cardon, G., & De Bourdeaudhuij, I. (2013). What practices do parents perceive as effective or ineffective in promoting a healthy diet, physical activity, and less sitting in children: Parent focus groups. *BMC Public Health, 13*(1), 1067. doi:10.1186/1471-2458-13-1067 PMID:24219513

Harrison, K., & Cantor, J. (1997). The relationship between media consumption and eating disorders. *Journal of Communication, 47*(1), 40–67. doi:10.1111/j.1460-2466.1997.tb02692.x

Hogan, M. J., & Strasburger, V. C. (2008). *Media and prosocial behavior in children and adolescents. In Handbook of Moral and Character Education* (pp. 537–553). Mahwah, NJ: Lawrence Erlbaum.

Kotler, J. A., Schiffman, J. M., & Hanson, K. G. (2012). The influence of media characters on children's food choices. *Journal of Health Communication, 17*(8), 886–898. doi:10.1080/10810730.2011.650822 PMID:22475307

Kral, T. V., & Rauh, E. M. (2010). Eating behaviors of children in the context of their family environment. *Physiology & Behavior, 100*(5), 567–573. doi:10.1016/j.physbeh.2010.04.031 PMID:20457172

Leech, R. M., McNaughton, S. A., & Timperio, A. (2014). The clustering of diet, physical activity and sedentary behavior in children and adolescents: A review. *The International Journal of Behavioral Nutrition and Physical Activity, 11*(1), 4. doi:10.1186/1479-5868-11-4 PMID:24450617

Pocock, M., Trivedi, D., Wills, W., Bunn, F., & Magnusson, J. (2010). Parental perceptions regarding healthy behaviours for preventing overweight and obesity in young children: A systematic review of qualitative studies. *Obesity Reviews, 11*(5), 338–353. doi:10.1111/j.1467-789X.2009.00648.x PMID:19780989

Pratt, B. M., & Woolfenden, S. (2002). Interventions for preventing eating disorders in children and adolescents. *Cochrane Database of Systematic Reviews*, 2. PMID:12076457

Prot, S., Gentile, D. A., Anderson, C. A., Suzuki, K., Swing, E., Lim, K. M., ... Liau, A. K. (2014). Long-term relations among prosocial-media use, empathy, and prosocial behavior. *Psychological Science*, *25*(2), 358–368. doi:10.1177/0956797613503854 PMID:24335350

Radesky, J. S., Schumacher, J., & Zuckerman, B. (2015). Mobile and interactive media use by young children: The good, the bad, and the unknown. *Pediatrics*, *135*(1), 1–3. doi:10.1542/peds.2014-2251 PMID:25548323

Rosen, D. S. (2010). Clinical report—identification and management of eating disorders in children and adolescents. *Pediatrics*.

Rosen, L. D., Lim, A. F., Felt, J., Carrier, L. M., Cheever, N. A., Lara-Ruiz, J. M., ... Rokkum, J. (2014). Media and technology use predicts ill-being among children, preteens and teenagers independent of the negative health impacts of exercise and eating habits. *Computers in Human Behavior*, *35*, 364–375. doi:10.1016/j.chb.2014.01.036 PMID:25717216

Sánchez-Carracedo, D., Neumark-Sztainer, D., & López-Guimera, G. (2012). Integrated prevention of obesity and eating disorders: Barriers, developments and opportunities. *Public Health Nutrition*, *15*(12), 2295–2309. doi:10.1017/S1368980012000705 PMID:22455792

Story, M., Neumark-Sztainer, D., & French, S. (2002). Individual and environmental influences on adolescent eating behaviors. *Journal of the American Dietetic Association*, *102*(3), S40–S51. doi:10.1016/S0002-8223(02)90421-9 PMID:11902388

Types of Eating Disorders. (2019). Retrieved from http://www.reelstoriesrealpeople.org/educational-films/types-of-eating-disorders/? gclid=EAIaIQobChMI4NziuN-W4gIVBqSzCh3w9g3qEAAYAyAAEgIx9vD_BwE

Van Cauwenberghe, E., Maes, L., Spittaels, H., van Lenthe, F. J., Brug, J., Oppert, J. M., & De Bourdeaudhuij, I. (2010). Effectiveness of school-based interventions in Europe to promote healthy nutrition in children and adolescents: systematic review of published and 'grey' literature. *British Journal of Nutrition, 103*(6), 781-797.

What are Eating Disorders? (2018, August 7). Retrieved from https://www.nationaleatingdisorders.org/what-are-eating-disorders

KEY TERMS AND DEFINITIONS

Anorexia Nervosa: An eating disorder characterized by weight loss (or lack of appropriate weight gain in growing children); difficulties maintaining an appropriate body weight for height, age, and stature; and, in many individuals, distorted body image.

Binge Eating Disorder: An eating disorder characterized by recurrent episodes of eating large quantities of food (often very quickly and to the point of discomfort); a feeling of a loss of control during the binge; experiencing shame, distress or guilt afterwards; and regularly using unhealthy compensatory measures (e.g., purging) to counter the binge eating.

Bulimia Nervosa: An eating disorder characterized by a cycle of bingeing and compensatory behaviors such as self-induced vomiting designed to undo or compensate for the effects of binge eating.

Cardiovascular: Relating to the heart and blood vessels.

Depression: A common and serious medical illness that negatively affects how you feel, the way you think, and how you act. Depression causes feelings of sadness and/or a loss of interest in activities once enjoyed. It can lead to a variety of emotional and physical problems and can decrease a person's ability to function at work and at home.

Desensitization: A process that diminishes emotional responsiveness to a negative, aversive or positive stimulus after repeated exposure to it.

Genetic Predisposition: An increased likelihood of developing a particular disease based on a person's genetic makeup; results from specific genetic variations that are often inherited from a parent.

Metacognition: Awareness and understanding of one's own thought processes.

Psychosocial: Relating to the interrelation of social factors and individual thought and behavior.

Selective Attention: The capacity for or process of reacting to certain stimuli selectively when several occur simultaneously.

Self-Efficacy: One's belief in one's ability to succeed in specific situations or to accomplish a task.

Chapter 8
Conduct Disorder and Oppositional Defiant Disorder:
Their Effect on Development

Ingrid Carla Brussier
Marymount Manhattan College, USA

ABSTRACT

This chapter investigates the psychological, physiological, and social aspects of conduct disorder (CD) and oppositional defiant disorder (ODD). These disorders are classified in the disruptive, impulse-control, and conduct disorders class in the fifth edition of the Diagnostic and Statistical Manual of Mental Disorders (2013). This chapter will consider the symptoms of ODD and CD and their effect on a child's social and biological development. The most common consequences of the disorders will be discussed: for example, the risk for other psychopathologies, social adversities, delinquency, and aggression. These severe outcomes signal the need for therapy options for children and adolescents and the assessment of their efficacy.

INTRODUCTION

This chapter investigates Oppositional Defiant disorder (ODD) and Conduct disorder (CD) based on their similarities, differences, and controversies. Both of these disorders can develop during childhood and adolescence. Oppositional defiant disorder's symptomatology includes hostile, uncontrollable anger, vindictiveness, and defying others. This chapter will investigate the environmental and biological factors that can influence its development as well as its psychosocial components. Conduct disorder will be largely discussed throughout this chapter due to its complex

DOI: 10.4018/978-1-7998-2940-9.ch008

symptomatology and subtypes. The DSM-V (APA 2013) states that aggressivity, destruction of property, cruelty, and violation of rules are criteria of CD. Many researchers note that there is a covert and overt subtype as well as an aggressive and non-aggressive type (Loeber, Burke, Lahey, Winters & Zera 2000) which can lead to misdiagnosis and will also be investigated throughout this review. CD and ODD can also strongly impact a child's academic performance and relationships with others due to their associated externalized, disruptive behaviors. The chapter will discuss the social adversities with peers and the negative parent-child relationships that are often related to the disorders.

Many psychologists have investigated the roots of disruptive behaviour disorders, questioning whether they are hereditary, due to environmental factors or both. This chapter also looks into the predictors of these disorders as well as their outcomes. Oppositional defiant disorder and conduct disorder can lead to the development of antisocial personality disorder (ASPD) and psychopathy in the adult years. These psychopathologies can be extremely detrimental to one's life, which is the reason why signs of ODD and CD need to be detected and treated early. Similarities in the disorders' symptoms cause many psychologists to believe that ODD should be described as a milder version of CD. While the Diagnostic and Statistical Manual of Mental Disorders (DSM) (APA 2013) separates the disorders; CD includes a vast majority of ODD's symptomatology. The DSM-V have them registered in the disruptive, impulse-control, and conduct disorders class (APA 2013). This chapter will be investigating, through a comprehensive literature review, different perspectives and findings on this controversy.

Finally, four different types of therapy will be discussed, since conduct disorder and oppositional defiant disorder can affect children and adolescents with varying levels of severity. Each form of intervention has its target and techniques. Parent-child interaction, Cognitive Behavioral, Multisystemic and Mindfulness Therapy will be discussed to conclude this chapter. Conduct and oppositional defiant disorder are to be taken seriously and seeking treatments critical towards helping individuals avoid any life-long consequences.

Background

Oppositional Defiant Disorder

Oppositional Defiant Disorder (ODD) affects children and adolescents during their developmental years. The disorder manifests through externalized maladaptive behaviors towards others and more specifically, toward authoritative figures. Maladaptive behaviour in children is shown through tantrums, misconduct and actions that do not fit societal norms. The DSM-V (American Psychiatric Association

2013) describes the symptoms as irritable moods, defiant behaviors, hostility, and vindictiveness. Arguing with others, defying rules, and being spiteful are some examples of specific behaviors recognized as signs of ODD. The frequency of the behavioral pattern is taken into account during the diagnosis. A child younger than five years old will need to externalize disruptive behavior more often than an older child to fit the criteria to be diagnosed with ODD. Oppositional defiant disorder is detrimental to a child's ability to have a healthy social life and to succeed in an educational environment, both of which can negatively impact his/her future as an adolescent or even as an adult. These factors are the reason why it is essential to proceed with treatment methods as soon as possible to avoid irreversible impacts on the individual's life.

Many researchers have investigated the predictors of a child developing oppositional defiant disorder. The individual's environment can have a substantial impact on a child's likelihood of developing ODD such as low social-economic status and familial conflict (Loeber, Burke,Lahey, Winters & Zera 2000). The relationship between the parents and the child is also significant since parental stress, maternal depression, or lack of warmth and attachment can impact cognitive and emotional features of child development (Lavigne, Dahl, Gouze, LeBailly, & Hopkins 2015). While investigating parental and environmental factors, it is also critical to look into the child's psychological signs that can lead to ODD. Examples of these signs are insecure attachment, sensory regulation difficulties and a low level of effort control (Lavigne et al. 2015). Insecure attachment can lead to difficulties in forging bonds with others. Sensory regulation is critical for child development since it allows them to understand and interact with their environment in a healthy manner. Finally, a low level of effort control is linked to the inability to properly control behaviours that can lead to temperamental problems. The aforementioned factors are directly linked to developmental issues due to a lack of proper parenting skills during the child's early development.

Conduct Disorder

The DSM-V (APA 2013) describes Conduct Disorder as a disruptive, behavioral disorder causing a child or an adolescent to externalize aggressive, destructive, deceitful, and rule violating behaviors. Conduct disorder includes violent symptoms such as physical fights, cruelty towards others, and sexual violence. The symptoms and behavioral patterns in the DSM-V (APA 2013) of CD are more likely to be externalized by an adolescent than a child since they list delinquency, sexual assault, and use of weapons. Conduct disorder can have serious consequences for the child or adolescent's life, since the externalization of these behaviors go against societal norms and laws.

Salvatore & Dick (2018) conducted a meta-analysis on the genetic influences in conduct disorder. They found that multiple types of genes could influence the behaviors that are linked to conduct disorder. One such behavior is substance abuse. A twin study conducted by Kruger et al. (2002) found that substance abuse disorder, conduct disorder, and antisocial disorder were highly heritable. A child born with the genotype predisposing him or her to conduct disorder does not always signify that he/she will, for sure, develop the disorder. Environment is an essential factor to take into account and more importantly, how genes and environment interact. For example, a child living in an urban area with a low level of parental monitoring and peer deviance is more likely to develop conduct disorder (Salvatore & Dick 2018). These are just some of the environmental risk factors that can increase the likelihood of developing conduct disorder.

Conduct and Oppositional Defiant Disorder's Influence on Mental Health

Individuals with CD or ODD are more likely to develop other psychological disorders later in life. Depression and anxiety are the most common mood disorders among children who grow up with ODD (Rowe et al. 2010). Researchers found that children with a childhood-onset type (before the age of 10) of ODD were more prone to develop anxiety and depression. This finding can be explained by the Levigne et al.'s (2015) description of typical predictors of ODD in children. Some of the characteristics the researchers noted were insecure attachment and sensory regulation difficulties, which can play a role in the development of anxiety and depression. Negative family dynamics, such as high parental stress, drug use, or low socioeconomic status can also contribute to the higher likelihood of anxiety in children with ODD. On another note, Loeber et al. (2000) states that children with an anxiety disorder during childhood are considerably less likely to develop a disruptive behavioral disorder while a child with CD has a high risk of developing a comorbid anxiety disorder during adolescence. Antisocial personality disorder (ASPD) and psychopathy can also be developed as a result of CD. The DSM-V (APA 2013) notes that some of the symptoms that can be shown in CD are callousness, lack of remorse or guilt, lack of concern for personal performance, and shallow affect. This list of interpersonal and emotional maladaptive functioning, as stated by the American Psychological Association (2013) can also be a sign of ASPD or psychopathy. Antisocial personality disorder and psychopathy are the most severe psychological outcomes that can be developed as a result of CD, which can have a disastrous impact on an individual's adult life.

The onset type of CD in children and adolescents is also an essential factor to take into account. The DSM-V (APA 2013) states that individuals who exhibit at least one symptom characteristic of conduct disorder before the age of ten, have a childhood-onset form of CD. If the symptoms arise between the ages of ten and eighteen, it is referred to as adolescent-onset. Researchers found that boys were more likely to show symptoms of CD at an earlier stage than girls (Rowe, Costello, Angold, Copeland & Maughan 2010).

Conduct disorder and oppositional defiant disorder are often found in children with attention deficit hyperactivity disorder (ADHD). The relationship between ADHD and disruptive behavior disorders is intriguing since between 40 to 70 percent of children with ADHD had ODD and/or CD (Banaschewski, Brandeis, Heinrich, Albrecht, Brunner, & Rothenberger, A. 2003). This substantial percentage of comorbidity can indicate that hyperactivity influences the development of CD and/or ODD. Researchers are wondering whether ADHD, ODD, and CD should be on the same spectrum of psychopathology (Ghosh&Sinha 2012). Another research study found that 92% of boys with ADHD with comorbid CD were diagnosed at early-onset (Leober, Burke & Lahey et al. 2000). Boys with early-onset CD and ADHD were found to be more prone to become aggressive and violent.

Treatments for Conduct and Oppositional Defiant Disorder

Oppositional defiant disorder and conduct disorder can cause significant psychosocial adversities and can increase the risk of developing other psychopathologies. These difficulties are the reason why treatment should be a priority for parents of children or adolescents with ODD and CD. Parent-Child Interaction Therapy (PCIT), a form of treatment for disruptive behavior disorders, has been shown to be clinically and statistically effective (Schuhmann, Foote, Eyberg, Boggs & Algina, J. 1998). PCIT is a form of family therapy that includes two phases; the first phase is directed towards child interaction, and the second phase is parent-directed. The first stage focuses on different forms of positive interactions with the child, such as playtime. The second stage teaches methods for child compliance, such as praising and time out techniques. Schuhmann et al. (1998) conducted a study investigating PCIT's efficacy through families seeking treatment at a psychiatric hospital for their preschool-aged child. They found that the families who finished full family therapy had a significantly better parent-child relationship and the child presented nearly no symptoms of the behavioural disorder they were diagnosed with at the beginning of the experiment. All of the children in the study had ODD and most of them had comorbid CD and/or ADHD, but the impact on the hyperactive symptoms, were not discussed. While it's effect on ADHD symptoms are not clear, the findings support Parent-Child Interaction Therapy as an effective treatment for disruptive behavioural disorders. However, parents who admit their child with a disruptive behavioral disorder to a psychiatric clinic are more likely to have positive outcomes from therapy, since seeking treatment shows signs of motivation and care for the child (Schuhmann et al. 1998). Therefore, the impressively positive results of the research might be due to the fact the families were already seeking help. By investigating families who are reported by teachers or social services, the findings may show a less effective side of PCIT.

There are other alternatives available for parents with older children who do not qualify for PCIT. Mindfulness, Multisystemic, and Cognitive Behavioral Therapy (CBT) are different options that are effective and can be applied to adolescents. Mindfulness Therapy focuses on learning how to control impulsive behavior through meditation techniques (Bögels, Hoogstad, Van Dun, de Schutter & Restifo 2008). Multisystemic therapy is aimed at adolescents with high levels of delinquency and serious psychopathologies such as CD, ASPD and psychopathy (Henggeler & Sheidow 2012). Finally, CBT is a widely used form of therapy that aims to suppress negative thoughts or behaviors through behavioral exercises and talk therapy (Smeets et al. 2015).

Issues, Controversies, Problems

Informants

A child or adolescent with disruptive behavioral disorders such as opposition defiant disorder and conduct disorder are commonly reported by an authoritative familial figure such as a parent or a teacher. Discrepancies between the various informants' perspectives of the child's mental health are often striking. The teacher or school counsellor has an outsider's point of view and better knowledge of the child's peer relationships (Lavigne, Dahl, Gouze, LeBailly, & Hopkins 2015). Deviant peer relationships, bullying, alienation, and physical fighting are definite signs of CD, which is why teachers are often the informants (APA 2013) (Salvatore & Dick 2018). The researchers found that teachers seem to be informants mostly when there is poor academic performance involved with the maladaptive behavior at school. Parents of children with a disruptive behavioral disorder are usually described as individuals who are stressed, depressed, have a poor parent-child relationship and are from a low socioeconomic status (Lavigne et al. 2015). This list of characteristics can be an explanation for the discrepancy between the teachers' and parents' reports since they might be less aware of their child's behavior. On another note, informant children are a valuable source of information. If a child has covert conduct disorder, it can be difficult for the parents or teachers to notice the maladaptive behaviors. Covert meaning that the behaviors are more discreet such as secretive theft whereas overt is visible such as fighting and confronting others publicly (Loeber et al. 2000). When a child has covert CD, the behaviors can often go unnoticed by teachers or parents, therefore the child is the only possible informant.

Is Oppositional Defiant Disorder a Milder Form of Conduct Disorder?

Some researchers believe that oppositional defiant disorder is a milder version of conduct disorder due to their similar symptoms. Before the DSM-V was published in 2013, researchers believed that ODD should not be separated from CD. All of ODD's symptoms are present in CD's symptomatology (American Psychiatric Association 1994). Rowe et al. (2010) conducted a study to investigate whether ODD should be a separate behavioral disorder from CD in the DSM-V. The researchers noted that some psychologists believe ODD is a "rebellious phase" and should not be treated as a mental illness. Rowe et al. (2010) found some empirical differences between CD and ODD, confirming that they should be classified as different disorders. Conduct disorder is often diagnosed in adolescence rather than during childhood. The symptomatology of CD could explain this finding since it includes violent behavior such as the use of a weapon and sexual violence, behaviors more commonly found in adolescents than in children (American Psychiatric Association 1994). ODD, in contrast, has a more stable onset since it is just as likely to be diagnosed in early childhood as in adolescence (Rowe et al. 2010). Rowe et al. (2010) noted that some researchers found that children with ODD were more likely to develop CD in their adolescence than children who did not have any disorders at all. This is an interesting finding since they also found that there is no continuity of CD to ODD. The continuity between ODD and CD is still in question since not many studies have investigated the subject. However, if this is to be verified in future research, it could reinforce the idea that ODD is a milder form of CD.

Lahey et al. (1994) also investigated this controversial belief that ODD should be considered as a milder form of CD. They found that some of the similarities, especially in the predictors of the disorders such as a low social-economic status, low parenting skills and parents with mental disorders such as antisocial personality disorder, can support the belief that they are the same disorder. However, the researchers also noted that most of the children and adolescents with ODD do not meet enough of the criteria to be diagnosed with CD. As stated earlier, CD is also believed to be a continuity of ODD, however, research shows that many individuals diagnosed with CD with an adolescent-onset never showed signs of ODD in their childhood. ODD and CD cannot be seen on the same spectrum and this distinction is clearly shown in both the DSM-IV and DSM-V since CD is more aggressive and violent.

The serious psychological outcomes of CD and ODD can be used as evidence to argue that they are separate disorders, as well. The prevalence of antisocial personality disorder in adulthood of individuals with either ODD or CD during their childhood years is not identical. Simonoff et al. (2004) investigated the continuity of behavioral disorders in childhood to antisocial disorder in adulthood. They found that individuals who were diagnosed with conduct disorder in their childhood and adolescence were more likely to have ASPD in adulthood. They noted that a child with high levels of CD symptoms as well as hyperactivity was more likely to develop ASPD than a child with moderate symptoms. The research concludes that CD needs to be assessed as a severe mental illness and the changes in symptoms need to be monitored throughout adolescence as a way of avoiding the development of ASPD. This would apply to a lesser extent for ODD.

Gender is a subject widely discussed due to its disparities in CD and ODD. Rowe et al. (2010) noted that males have a higher risk of developing conduct disorder, whereas oppositional disorder seems to affect females and males equally. The increased risk for CD in males could be explained by the physical and aggressive characteristics of the disorder, such as constant fighting. Females with CD have been observed to exhibit less physical aggressiveness, but instead use verbal violence such as defamation and the alienation of others (Loeber et al. 2010). These different forms of aggression have raised questions as to whether CD should have separate diagnostic criteria for females.

While the symptomatology of CD and ODD are similar, the American Psychiatric Association (2013) has concluded that ODD should not be classified as a milder subtype of CD. There are enough signs showing that they are different forms of disruptive behavior disorders. Gender, maladaptive behavioral patterns, and the psychological outcome disparities of CD and ODD confirm that they are not meant to be diagnosed or treated the same way.

Aggressive and Non-Aggressive Conduct Disorder

Conduct disorder is mostly associated with aggressive behaviors. The DSM-V (APA 2013) states that aggression towards others, physical cruelty, use of weapons, and forced sexual activity are some of the most prominent symptoms of CD. Conduct disorder has a non-aggressive subtype, meaning that the client meets the criteria of the disorder without displaying aggressive behaviors. Theft, destruction of property, and severe rule violation such as not respecting curfew (APA 2013) are the other categories of CD's symptomatology that the non-aggressive subtype would fit into. Being diagnosed with this form of CD seems less detrimental in the long-term for the child, since aggressivity is often linked to higher criminal activity (Loeber et al. 2010). Some of the non-aggressive symptoms, like theft, can still be linked to delinquency. Some genetic differences can be found between the two subtypes. Salvatore and Dick (2018) state that there is a higher heritability for the aggressive subtype as compared to the non-aggressive subtype. This finding may hint that aggressivity might be the heritability gene influencing the development of the disorder. The overt and covert forms of conduct disorder can be another way of describing aggressive versus non-aggressive CD. Overt CD includes externalized and apparent maladaptive behavior such as physical fighting whereas covert is the hidden side of CD such as theft and concealing actions (Loeber et al. 2000). Covert and non-aggressive CD is a lot more difficult to notice for the parents and teacher, which is a risk factor of these subtypes.

Social Adversities

Peer rejection and aggression can have detrimental effects on children during their development. Research shows that children who have suffered from rejection, alienation and aggressive behaviors from peers are more likely to develop an externalized disruptive behavior disorder such as CD (Miller-Johnson, Coie, Maumary-Gremaud, & Bierman 2002). Miller-Johnson et al.'s (2002) investigation of the subject found that social rejection was more difficult for a child to cope with than singular aggression. Their study evaluated young children in first grade. The researchers found that there was a link between being rejected by peers at school and the reason that children with CD often socialize in deviant circles. These findings hint that social adversities at a young age can have long-term effects on the mental health of a child. Boys with CD are more likely to socialize with delinquent peers, especially during puberty (Burke, Loeber, & Birmaher 2004). The link seems simple; however; it can show how critical it is to pay attention to early signs of a child's social adversities in a school environment. Peer deviance can lead to severe maladaptive behavioral patterns such as criminal activity during the middle school and high school years. The rejection can also contribute to a general misunderstanding of social norms, which can initiate problematic conduct and early signs of ASPD (Miller-Johnson et al. 2002). The inability to respect others and norms creates evident difficulties for a child to develop healthy peer relationships.

A study investigating parent-child relationships found that there were evident discrepancies concerning their views on their familial environment (Booker, Ollendick, Dunsmore & Greene 2016). One-third of the children in the study perceived their relationship with their parents in a more positive light than did their parents. This is a sign that the children with CD are unaware of how badly their behavior impacts their relationships with their peers and parents. The maladaptive behaviors externalized by the children are a form of self-alienation, which can further silence the positive influences and reinforce the negative. The significant dangers that accompany disruptive behavioral disorders are the psychopathologies that can follow social withdrawal, such as anti-personality disorder and psychopathy (Simonoff et al. 2004).

Familial Environment

The familial environment in which a child grows up, plays a crucial role in a child's likelihood of developing ODD or CD. Throughout children's development, it is essential for them to get the care and parenting they need. Emotional control and a suitable attachment level are crucial for a child to grow up in harmony with others. A lack of emotional effort, emotional control and an insecure attachment is due to poor parenting during the child's early development. While parenting skills are essential, they are a controllable variable since the parents can learn the skill through classes or therapy such as PCIT.

The mental health of the child's parents is important. Researchers have discovered that maternal depression, antisocial personality disorder, and stress (Salvatore & Dick 2018) can profoundly impact the likelihood of developing disruptive behavior disorders. When a parent has psychopathology, it can impact the way he/she raises the child. For example, while investigating the efficacy of parent-child interaction therapy, Schuhmann et al. (2018) found that a parent with a mental health disorder as well as a lower socioeconomic status was less likely to seek therapy for his/her child with a disruptive behavioral disorder. This finding can be explained either as a lack of attention these parents might give towards their child or that the parents are financially unable to seek therapy, which is alarming.

Substance abuse in parents is also often noted as a risk for the child's mental health. Paternal drug use is often discussed in research as a predictor of developing disruptive behaviour disorders (Salvatore & Dick 2018). Addiction-tendencies are highly heritable, which can lead a child to inherit these genes from their parents (Krueger, Hicks, Patrick, Carlson, Iacono, McGue, 2002). The DSM-V does not state that substance abuse is a criterion for the disorder; however; Kruger et al. (2002) state that the addictive genes might increase the risks of conduct disorder. A child with a substance abusing parent has a high chance of having the substance abuse trait which is also a predictor of CD. A parent with substance abuse will also not be able to provide a safe and stable environment for his/her child to grow. Physical, sexual, and verbal abuse towards a child can also increase the chances of developing conduct disorder. The development of an aggressive subtype of CD is also specifically influenced by witnessing and being a victim of domestic abuse (Henggeler, & Sheidow 2012).

Biological Factors

The neurological aspect of ODD and CD has been investigated to understand how the brain of a child diagnosed with a disruptive disorder works and changes. Serotonin is a neurotransmitter that affects mood regulation and aggressive behavior. Levels of serotonin neurotransmitters are different in children with conduct disorder, which can be an explanation for the behavioral patterns of a child with CD (Burke et al. 2004). Findings show that boys who have conduct disorder with an early-onset have a higher level of serotonin in their blood than boys with the adolescent-onset type. This difference in levels of serotonin explains the higher levels of aggressivity of individuals with conduct disorder. On another note, Burke et al. (2004) also found that higher salivatory cortisol levels were found in children with oppositional defiant disorder and early-onset type CD in boys. A low functioning amygdala can also impair the way an individual understands social cues. These impaired understandings of social cues are linked to behavioral disorders since some children with CD find harmful intentions in healthy peer behaviors (Davidson, Putnam, Larson 2000). Antisocial personality disorder is strongly associated with disruptive behavioral disorders. In addition, researchers found that a lower heart rate is widely found in adolescents with ASPD symptoms (Ortiz& Raine 2004). This finding raises the question of whether a low heart rate could be a predictor of a disruptive behavioral disorder developing into ASPD. These findings on low heart rates could relate to the lack of guilt and empathy in individuals with ASPD, which could be an interesting subject for future research to investigate. Miller-Johnson et al. (2002) noted that ODD has not been found to be related to a lower heart rate, in contrast to CD. These heart rate disparities coalesce with conduct disorder's higher risk of developing into ASPD than ODD (Rowe et al. 2010). Oppositional defiant disorder is mostly associated with anxiety and depression (Booker, Ollendick, Dunsmore & Greene 2016) especially in girls, which are both linked to a higher heart rate (Miller-Johnson et al. 2002). Most research investigating the neurological function of CD focuses on the aggressivity aspect of the disorder, however; as aforementioned, conduct disorder can be non-aggressive. In future studies, it would be interesting to investigate the differences between the aggressive and non-aggressive subtypes of CD and see whether the serotonin levels in the blood follow the same patterns for both the aggressive and non-aggressive types. .

Prenatal problems can also affect the child and increase their chances of developing a disruptive, behavioral disorder. Substance abuse during pregnancy, as well as after, has been linked to conduct disorder development (Miller-Johnson et al. 2002). Smoking during pregnancy is a predictor of early-onset conduct disorder in boys, with a particular link to high levels of aggressivity. Epigenetic research found that mothers with psychopathology, such as maternal depression, and those who pursued criminal behavior during their pregnancies, was predictive of higher levels of methylation around the oxytocin receptors (Salvatore & Dick 2018). Methylation can change the activity of a DNA segment. When a woman gives birth, and methylation occurs, findings show that there is a higher chance for the child to have the callous-unemotional trait (Salvatore & Dick, 2018). Callousness is a trait found in disruptive behavioral disorders (APA, 2013) which hints that there is a link between the mother's behavior or psychological state during pregnancy and the development of CD or ODD in the child. Many studies note that maternal depression, substance abuse, and criminal behavior are familial environmental factors that raise a child's chance of developing ODD or CD. However, researchers do not state that negative prenatal factors cause a biological change in the child's genes.

Social Economical Status

Socioeconomic status (SES) is believed by many researchers to affect a child's likelihood of developing a disruptive behavioral disorder. Coming from a high SES background might lower the risk of a child having ODD or CD. Parental stress is shown throughout the research to be a familial environmental factor that affects the likelihood of a child developing CD or ODD (Lavigne et al. 2015). A lack of financial stability can have a substantial impact on a parent's stress levels, which can increase the chances of CD and ODD development (Salvatore & Dick 2018). On another note, families from low SES backgrounds are more likely to live in neighbourhoods with high crime rates (Loeber et. 2000) which can influence children to take part in criminal behavior as they grow up. Loeber et al, (2000) showed that high crime areas are linked to higher levels of peer deviance, an influential factor in the development of CD and ODD (Salvatore & Dick). A lower socio-economic status can also lead to a lower chance of seeking treatment due to financial restrictions. Schuhmann et al. (1998) found that the cost of public service interventions is three times more expensive for children that meet the criteria of CD, which leads to a lack of affordable solutions for families seeking therapy. Researchers note that children who have early-onset CD or ODD have a high chance of continuity into adolescence (Murray & Farrington 2010). Early intervention through therapy could help avoid this continuity. While a low socioeconomic status seems to be an influential factor, children with a favorable genotype to ODD and CD, who grow up in a high SES home are believed to be just as likely to develop a disruptive behavior disorder (Salvatore & Dick 2008). The high cost of therapy is one of many reasons that prevention programs in communities and schools need to be widely set up to raise awareness of conduct and oppositional defiant disorder. Government or association funded parenting skill training for young parents and counselling options at schools for diagnosed children can be a good option to limit costs for families. While these exist today, they need to be widespread to be effective on a larger scale.

Delinquency

Delinquency in children and adolescents with disruptive behavior disorders such as CD is one of the most concerning outcomes of their symptomatology. Delinquency can lead to life-long consequences, such as having a criminal record and imprisonment. While adolescents diagnosed with CD are often delinquents, they are found to rarely follow a criminal path in their adult years (Henggeler, & Sheidow 2012). Murray & Farrington (2010) found that the average age for delinquent behavior was between thirteen and sixteen years of age. Delinquency takes into account violent offenses such as burglary, theft, vandalism, drug use, and more.

Past research has found that there are gender disparities in CD criminal behavior since only thirty percent of the juvenile violent offenses were conducted by females in 2008 (Henggeler, & Sheidow 2012). This gender difference reflects the generally higher rate of disruptive behavior disorders in males as well as their prevalent tendencies toward violence. The researchers also found that children and adolescents who grow up in a disadvantaged and a low academic-focused environment were more likely to take part in delinquency. Henggeler & Sheidow (2012) state that being part of a lower SES can have an impact on the likelihood of developing a delinquent form of a disruptive behavior disorder. Some other risk factors are impulsivity, restlessness, and hyperactivity, which are all symptoms of ADHD (Murray & Farrington 2010). This directly links ADHD's substantial prevalence in children with CD and ODD and their criminal behavior. Henggeler & Sheidow (2012) also found that a child or adolescent who has an incarcerated parent has a higher chance of being delinquent and arrested, as well.

A low intellectual quotient (IQ) can also predict a higher likelihood of conducting offenses and crimes. Individuals with a lower IQ are found to spend less time in school settings as well as to not understand the consequences of their actions (Murray & Farrington 2010). Burke et al. (2004) state that a higher level of verbal IQ decreases the likelihood of developing CD which coincides with Murray &Farrington (2010)'s findings, that adolescents with a lower verbal IQ had a higher chance of being delinquents. While Burke et al. (2004) do note that IQ and conduct disorder development have a nearly non-significant relationship, there are some signs that verbal IQ might play a role in criminal behavior for children and adolescents with CD. The researchers note that this link could be due to the need for strong verbal intellectual capacities for schoolwork. A weakness in verbal intellectual abilities can lead to stepping out of the school system and turning to delinquent behaviors (Murray & Farrington 2010).

Child abuse and witnessing violent behavior can be a risk factor for delinquent behavior, as well. The link between a weak familial dynamic and the development of disruptive behavior disorder is clear (Salvatore & Dick 2018). In addition to that link, previous research has found that being a witness to domestic violence and substance abuse are factors that contribute to an increased risk of delinquent behavior (Murray & Farrington 2010). On the other hand, comfortable housing, a positive interparental relationship as well as high academic performance are linked to lowering the likelihood of delinquency in children with disruptive behavior disorders (Henggeler, & Sheidow 2012). The importance of the environment in a child's life is critical since it can trigger a criminal behavioral pattern in a child with ODD or CD. This is why teacher informants can be of great help since they can be useful from an outsider's perspective such as alarming social services and providing tools to help the child through dysfunctional family situations.

Attention Deficit Hyperactivity Disorder

Attention-deficit-hyperactivity disorder (ADHD) is linked to disruptive behavior disorders such as CD and ODD. ADHD is described by the DSM-V 5 (APA 2013) as "a persistent pattern of inattention and/or hyperactivity-impulsivity that interferes with functioning or development." A study found that forty to sixty percent of children with ODD or CD also have ADHD (Banaschewski, Brandeis, Heinrich, Albrecht, Brunner, & Rothenberger 2003). These results show that there is a high rate of comorbidity between ADHD and CD or ODD. The researchers hypothesize that ODD and CD could be a complication of the hyperactivity in ADHD's symptoms. ADHD, conduct disorder, and oppositional defiant disorder all generate a lack of inhibition. This raises the question as to whether hyperactivity or the lack of inhibition might be the reason why ADHD is so often comorbid with CD and ODD. Some researchers believe that ADHD could have a particular subtype that is comorbid with disruptive behavioural disorders (Banaschewski et al 2003). While the DSM-V (APA 2013) has not yet created this sub-classification, the high prevalence of comorbid ADHD and CD and/or ODD could support this proposition by Banaschewski et al (2003).

There are some gender differences concerning ADHD, CD, and ODD development. Boys with ADHD are more likely to develop conduct disorder at early-onset and to externalize aggressive behavior (Loeber et. 2000). There are few findings on females with CD and ADHD due to the higher prevalence in males. A four year follow up study on children with CD and ODD investigated the numerous ways ADHD affects disruptive behaviour disorders (Biederman, Faraone, Milberger, Jetton, Chen, Mick, ... & Russell 1996). The researchers found that ADHD with comorbid ODD and CD could be a predictor of antisocial personality disorder. This can support Lahey and Loeber's hypothetical model (Loeber et. 2000) that suggests that ASPD needs to be preceded by a continuity of ADHD, ODD, and CD to be developed. The link between ADHD and the higher severity of CD's symptoms is clear. It is essential to be vigilant about any evident signs of conduct and oppositional defiant disorder in children with ADHD since they are more vulnerable to developing them.

SOLUTIONS AND RECOMMENDATIONS

Conduct disorder and oppositional defiant disorder are both prominent in children today. These disruptive behavior disorders are shown to have detrimental effects on the individual's social life, education, and sometimes with the law. This is the reason that it is so important for parents to act rapidly and seek treatment for their child. Therapies such as parent-child interaction therapy, cognitive behavioral therapy, and mindfulness are great tools to help with maladaptive externalizing behaviors, such as aggression, hostility, and impulsivity.

Parent-Child Interaction Therapy (PCIT)

PCIT is a therapy for children with disruptive behavior disorder which includes conduct disorder, oppositional defiant disorder, and attention deficit hyperactivity disorder. PCIT is directed towards children ranging from the age of two to seven, which uses social learning and attachment theory (Ward, Theule, & Cheung 2016). Parents play a crucial role in PCIT since the therapy focuses on helping them with parenting skills, child-play, and more importantly creating a healthy parent-child relationship.

PCIT includes nine to twelve weekly one-hour sessions with a therapist. There are two parts to it; the child-directed interaction phase (CDI) and the parent-directed interaction phase (PDI) (Ward, Theule, & Cheung 2016). The first part aims at helping parents have friendly interactions with their child during therapy sessions. CDI includes strategies that will help the parent create a bond with their children as well as suppress any negative remarks or behaviors they might ordinarily have towards them. Parents will learn how to give positive feedback, praise, and play with their child. CDI gives the child the ability to be autonomous during the session, since the parents are not supposed to control any part; this offers great insight into the familial situation and relationship to the therapist. PDI is the second part, where the parents learn and put into action various parenting techniques. The parents will learn how to engage with their child during playtimes or activities while following CDI's parenting strategies. PCIT focuses on giving parents new ways of interacting with their child through reinforcing good behavior and appropriately suppressing maladaptive behavior (Schuhmann et al. 1998). The parenting strategies will help the parent create boundaries and enforce rules. This form of therapy can be very efficient since it is directed towards younger children and can improve the relationship between the parent and the child rather than trying to fix the problematic behavior itself. As research has shown, parents are a leading influence on the development of conduct disorder and oppositional defiant disorder through a lack of parenting skills and hostility (Lavigne et al. 2015). PCIT is a way to address the problem at its source, early on.

Schuman et al. (1998) conducted a follow-up study investigating the efficacy of PCIT. Sixty-four families seeking treatment for their child's conduct problems participated in the study. While the sample was not quantitative, the results were striking. Most of the parents who finished all of the PCIT sessions reported, four months later, that their child was showing no signs of any disruptive behavior disorder. The results were impressive since the control families who did not complete or partake in PCIT reported that their child was still having behavioral issues. The study does have some limitations: eighty-one percent of the participants were boys and the participating families were actively seeking treatment, which shows concern for their child's mental health. Parents of children with disruptive behavioral disorders are often from a lower socio-economic status and may be more likely to have mental health disorders, which may mean they are less likely to seek out treatment for their child (Loeber et al 2000). Randomly selecting families within their communities could have provided more useful data into the efficacy of PCIT rather than directly examining its efficacy at the clinic. Parents, who seek treatment for their children, show a signs of care and attachment to their child, which is a definite starting point for PCIT.

On another note, a study following children through school assessments after PCIT, found mixed results concerning the therapy's efficacy (Funderburk, Eyberg, Newcomb, McNeil, Hembree-Kigin, & Capage 1998). The results showed that after a twelve-month follow-up, the signs of disruptive behavioral disorders were less severe. However, the researchers found that the symptoms of CD, ODD, or ADHD were coming back after eighteen months. This raises the question as to whether PCIT needs to include follow-up sessions after a year to make sure the symptoms will not recur. Efficacy studies can sometimes show stronger results in favour of therapy since many variables are controlled, such as the therapists, the clinical environment and the structure of the therapy session (Schuman et al. 1998). Funderburk et al.'s (1998) study gives us a more realistic insight into the long-term effect of PCIT on children. Parent-child interaction therapy could possibly include follow up sessions after a year to make sure that no problematic behavioural patterns will recur. The results are mixed, however; both Funderburk et al. (1998) and Schuman et al. (1998) support PCIT as an effective form of therapy for preschool-aged children with disruptive behavior disorders.

Cognitive Behavioral Therapy (CBT)

CBT is used for a wide range of psychological disorders such as anxiety, depression, post-traumatic stress disorder, or anger management issues. CBT targets cognitive processes such as a patient's thoughts, fears, or beliefs and relating them to the patient's behavior. Once the relationship between the cognitive and the behavioral is made, problem-focused strategies are set up. Children and adolescents with conduct and oppositional defiant disorder can have problems controlling their anger and aggressivity (APA 2013). CD and ODD with high aggressivity can lead to severe outcomes such as problems with the law, social adversities and a higher risk of developing severe psychopathologies (ASPD or psychopathy) (Loeber et al. 2000). CBT can be an effective way of calming the aggressive symptoms of disruptive behavior disorders.

Anger management, social skills training, and assertiveness training CBT are most commonly used to treat the symptoms of conduct disorder and oppositional defiant disorder (Smeets et al. 2015). CBT therapists coach and provide strategies for patients to improve their problematic behaviors. Through new skills and strategies, the patients can slowly change their dysfunctional behaviors or thinking patterns. CBT can be offered in a clinical or school-based environment. School CBT interventions can be more comfortable and less expensive; this is its positive aspect. Smeets et al. (2015)'s meta-analysis of CBT's effectiveness on conduct and oppositional defiant disorder found that the results were not affected by the environment (school or clinical) nor were they impacted by the length of the intervention. Both of these findings are surprising and positive since they show that school-based CBT interventions can be as effective as those in a clinical environment.

Multisystemic Therapy

Multisystemic therapy aims at treating children and adolescents with disruptive behavior disorders with strong delinquent tendencies. This form of therapy is not singularly restricted to these disorders since any juvenile committing severe offenses, and with severe clinical problems can seek this form of intervention (Henggeler & Sheidow 2012). The DSM-V criteria for conduct disorder involve vs. state that theft, sexual offenses, burglary, and violent crimes as some of its symptomatology. Multisystemic therapy includes highly trained psychologists or psychiatrists who are on call at any time of the day in case of a crisis. While some other forms of therapy are focused on solving one specific problem, Multisystemic Therapy takes into account all of the influential factors of maladaptive behavior and tries to solve them. The therapist will also help with parental problems such as substance use and poor parenting skills, which are a leading cause of ODD and CD development

(Loeber et al. 2000). Henggeler & Sheidow (2012) investigated the efficacy of this form of therapy and noted that a poor familial relationship, peer deviance, and poor grades were some of the most problematic areas in patient's lives. They also noted that Multisystemic Therapy incorporates CBT techniques when anger management problems and substance abuse are present in patient behavior. The research showed that Multisystemic Therapy leads to a lowering of delinquent behavior and a better familial relationship. This is a good option for adolescent-onset CD and ODD with strong maladaptive behavior, since there are few practical alternatives for them. Multisystemic Therapy is found to be one of the most effective forms of treatment for adolescents with a high level of delinquency.

Mindfulness

Mindfulness is a therapy that is based on meditation training; it is useful for adults with depression, anxiety, and eating disorders (Bögels, Hoogstad, Van Dun, de Schutter & Restifo 2008). Bögel et al. (2008) researched the effectiveness of mindfulness for children and adolescents with a disruptive behavior disorder. The researchers describe mindfulness as a relatively new form of therapy that treats problematic behaviors and thoughts through focusing on the "here and now" with the purpose of learning how to cope with negative feelings through meditation. The "here and now" technique is a way to calm the hyperactive and impulsive side of disruptive behavior disorders since it teaches the patient to focus only on specific tasks in a non-judgmental way. This new form of therapy is a way of helping the problematic externalizing behaviors at their base, while using a holistic method. Mindfulness can also be an effective method for people against medication, such as Methylphenidate, which is a medication used for treating impulsive behaviors found in disruptive behavior disorders. While Bögel et al. (2008) noted that Methylphenidate is effective; it can have side effects and can be unendorsed by some parents. Some of the meditation exercises stated were mindful eating, speaking, walking, and yoga practice. Body scans and breathing exercises are planned for the patient to follow at home (Bögel et al. 2008). The ability to practice the therapy alone and at home can create a sense of security and comfort for the client. These activities are a way to teach children and adolescents how to entirely focus on one activity and to control their impulsiveness through relaxation.

Interestingly enough, Mindfulness Therapy included a delayed gratification exercise. The exercise asked the children to wait for an extended period of time in front of half a chocolate bar for the clinician to come back with the other half (Biederman et al. 1995). While it is generally a difficult task for children and adolescents with disruptive behaviour disorders, through numerous trials the exercise is successful at enhancing delay. Child reports state that they were satisfied with the outcome of their delayed gratification task and felt that they learned something. This is a way of teaching the clients how to control their impulsivity as well as understanding the gratification that can result (Biederman et al. 1995). Not a lot of research focuses on mindfulness for children with ODD or CD since it primarily relates to children with ADHD. However, many studies have found that ODD and CD are often comorbid with ADHD (Biederman et al. 1995). Mindfulness can help with some of the impulsivity and can offer techniques for the children to calm down when they feel frustrated. While this new form of therapy does not tackle the problematic externalizing behaviors correctly, it offers the tools to the client to control his/her emotions and actions.

FUTURE RESEARCH DIRECTIONS

Today's knowledge on Conduct Disorder and Oppositional Defiant Disorder is vast. Many researchers are still investigating these disorders since there are still some unanswered questions on the subject. Some biological aspects still remain uninvestigated and unknown, such as the neurological differences between aggressive and non-aggressive CD. Most of the neurological and biological studies on CD and ODD focus on the aggressivity aspect of the disorder rather than its non-aggressive subtype. It would be interesting to see if there are some other signs of behavioral disorders that are unknown today.

There are some studies looking into the lives of incarcerated juveniles with CD such as Boduszek, Belsher, Dhingra & Ioannou (2014), who investigated the prevalence of alcohol abuse and imprisonment. It would be interesting to create intervention programs in juvenile prison facilities for disruptive behavior disorders or to test their efficacy and prevalence if they are already in place. They might lower the risk of recidivism and of developing more serious psychopathologies linked to delinquency such as ASPD.

While there is awareness of gender disparities in CD, since boys are more likely to develop it, most studies have a larger percentage of male participants. It would be interesting to conduct studies specifically investigating females with conduct disorder since some findings have shown they do not externalize the same maladaptive behavior as boys (Loeber et al 2000). The neurological and biological differences due to these behavioral disparities could also become a new direction for further investigation

Raising awareness about conduct and oppositional defiant disorder is critical since some parents may not be aware of its prevalence in today's child population. While some might believe it is simply a rebellious phase, schools can inform parents of the early signs of CD and ODD to help prevent and treat the problematic behaviors in time.

CONCLUSION

Conduct and Oppositional Defiant Disorders are both disruptive behavior disorders. These psychopathologies affect children and adolescents during their development and are prone to developing serious mood disorders as well as antisocial personality disorder and psychopathy. CD and ODD can also increase the likelihood of mood disorders such as depression and anxiety. It is now known that CD and ODD also negatively affect a child's social life and academic work leading to long-term consequences. Having deviant peers and stepping out of the school system are linked to delinquency. Due to these serious outcomes, noticing the symptoms early, and seeking therapy as early as possible is the best way to help children with disruptive behavior disorder and give them the tools to experience healthy development.

A major controversy that is widely discussed in studies is whether ODD is a milder form of CD and whether it should be reclassified in the DSM-V (APA 2013). ODD's symptomatology is part of CD's which can lead to misdiagnosis and can support the belief that the two disorders should be the same disorder. While there are commonalities among the disorders, this chapter investigates numerous differences that separate ODD and CD. There are gender, long-term psychological outcomes and biological disparities for both CD and ODD, which lead us to believe that they are not to be classified as the same disorder.

The impact of CD and ODD on a child's social life and ability to function in society can be severe due to their maladaptive externalized behaviors. The risks linked to these social adversities can lead to alienation from positive social circles and can cause those affected to gravitate towards socializing with deviant peers. For some of them, the social influences can lead to poor choices and to following a delinquent path of CD. It is therefore crucial to carefully monitor a child or adolescent's social well-being in the school setting. Academic performance is also a strong indicator of conduct problems, while poor grades are not a criterion for CD or ODD, they can be risk factors for developing the disorders.

The biological and environmental factors interact in the development of CD and ODD. If there are some heritable traits in the family such as, substance abuse, aggressivity or ASPD, it is important to keep an eye on environmental factors to prevent the development of the disorders. The concerning aspect of these factors is that often a negative environment and genes go hand–in-hand which is a reason that preventing CD and ODD can be difficult. Community prevention programs funded by the government or associations can be helpful in providing support for children with familial problems.

The awareness of conduct and oppositional defiant disorder in children and adolescents has allowed for the creation of therapies aimed at children with disruptive behavior disorders. PCIT is known for being very effective in young children through parenting training and creating a healthier familial environment. Multisystemic therapy can also be very helpful for older children and adolescents with CD and delinquency. CBT has shown its effectiveness in suppressing the maladaptive behaviors through anger management. Finally, mindfulness therapy is another option for lack of impulsivity control through teaching meditation techniques and focusing on the present moment. Conduct and oppositional defiant disorder need to be taken seriously, and parents should seek therapy to help their children develop healthfully.

ACKNOWLEDGMENT

This research received no specific grant from any funding agency in the public, commercial, or not-for-profit sectors.

REFERENCES

Banaschewski, T., Brandeis, D., Heinrich, H., Albrecht, B., Brunner, E., & Rothenberger, A. (2003). Association of ADHD and conduct disorder–brain electrical evidence for the existence of a distinct subtype. *Journal of Child Psychology and Psychiatry, and Allied Disciplines*, *44*(3), 356–376. doi:10.1111/1469-7610.00127 PMID:12635966

Biederman, J., Faraone, S. V., Milberger, S., Jetton, J. G., Chen, L., Mick, E., ... Russell, R. L. (1996). Is childhood oppositional defiant disorder a precursor to adolescent conduct disorder? Findings from a four-year follow-up study of children with ADHD. *Journal of the American Academy of Child and Adolescent Psychiatry*, *35*(9), 1193–1204. doi:10.1097/00004583-199609000-00017 PMID:8824063

Boduszek, D., Belsher, R., Dhingra, K., & Ioannou, M. (2014). Psychosocial correlates of recidivism in a sample of ex-prisoners: The role of oppositional defiant disorder and conduct disorder. *Journal of Forensic Psychiatry & Psychology*, *25*(1), 61–76. doi:10.1080/14789949.2013.862293

Bögels, S., Hoogstad, B., van Dun, L., de Schutter, S., & Restifo, K. (2008). Mindfulness training for adolescents with externalizing disorders and their parents. *Behavioural and Cognitive Psychotherapy*, *36*(2), 193–209. doi:10.1017/S1352465808004190

Booker, J. A., Ollendick, T. H., Dunsmore, J. C., & Greene, R. W. (2016). Perceived parent–child relations, conduct problems, and clinical improvement following the treatment of Oppositional Defiant Disorder. *Journal of Child and Family Studies*, *25*(5), 1623–1633. doi:10.100710826-015-0323-3 PMID:27284234

Burke, J. D., Loeber, R., & Birmaher, B. (2004). Oppositional defiant disorder and conduct disorder: A review of the past 10 years, part II. *Focus (San Francisco, Calif.)*, *41*(4), 1275–1576. PMID:12410070

Funderburk, B. W., Eyberg, S. M., Newcomb, K., McNeil, C. B., Hembree-Kigin, T., & Capage, L. (1998). Parent-child interaction therapy with behavior problem children: Maintenance of treatment effects in the school setting. *Child & Family Behavior Therapy*, *20*(2), 17–38. doi:10.1300/J019v20n02_02

Henggeler, S. W., & Sheidow, A. J. (2012). Empirically supported family-based treatments for conduct disorder and delinquency in adolescents. *Journal of Marital and Family Therapy*, *38*(1), 30–58. doi:10.1111/j.1752-0606.2011.00244.x PMID:22283380

Krueger, R. F., Hicks, B. M., Patrick, C. J., Carlson, S. R., Iacono, W. G., & McGue, M. (2002). Etiologic connections among substance dependence, antisocial behavior and personality: Modeling the externalizing spectrum. *Journal of Abnormal Psychology*, *111*(3), 411–424. doi:10.1037/0021-843X.111.3.411 PMID:12150417

Lahey, B. B., Applegate, B., Barkley, R. A., Garfinkel, B., McBurnett, K., Kerdyk, L., ... Biederman, J. (1994). DSM-IV field trials for oppositional defiant disorder and conduct disorder in children and adolescents. *The American Journal of Psychiatry*, *151*(8), 1163–1171. doi:10.1176/ajp.151.8.1163 PMID:8037251

Lavigne, J. V., Dahl, K. P., Gouze, K. R., LeBailly, S. A., & Hopkins, J. (2015). Multi-domain predictors of oppositional defiant disorder symptoms in preschool children: Cross-informant differences. *Child Psychiatry and Human Development*, *46*(2), 308–319. doi:10.100710578-014-0472-4 PMID:24997089

Loeber, R., Burke, J. D., Lahey, B. B., Winters, A., & Zera, M. (2000). Oppositional defiant and conduct disorder: A review of the past 10 years, part I. *Journal of the American Academy of Child and Adolescent Psychiatry*, *39*(12), 1468–1484. doi:10.1097/00004583-200012000-00007 PMID:11128323

Miller-Johnson, S., Coie, J. D., Maumary-Gremaud, A., & Bierman, K. (2002). Peer rejection and aggression and early starter models of conduct disorder. *Journal of Abnormal Child Psychology*, *30*(3), 217–230. doi:10.1023/A:1015198612049 PMID:12041708

Murray, J., & Farrington, D. P. (2010). Risk factors for conduct disorder and delinquency: Key findings from longitudinal studies. *Canadian Journal of Psychiatry*, *55*(10), 633–642. doi:10.1177/070674371005501003 PMID:20964942

Ortiz, J., & Raine, A. (2004). Heart rate level and antisocial behavior in children and adolescents: A meta-analysis. *Journal of the American Academy of Child and Adolescent Psychiatry*, *43*(2), 154–162. doi:10.1097/00004583-200402000-00010 PMID:14726721

Rowe, R., Costello, E. J., Angold, A., Copeland, W. E., & Maughan, B. (2010, November). Developmental pathways in oppositional defiant disorder and conduct disorder. *Journal of Abnormal Psychology*, *119*(4), 726–738. doi:10.1037/a0020798 PMID:21090876

Salvatore, J. E., & Dick, D. M. (2018). Genetic influences on conduct disorder. *Neuroscience and Biobehavioral Reviews*, *91*, 91–101. doi:10.1016/j.neubiorev.2016.06.034 PMID:27350097

Schuhmann, E. M., Foote, R. C., Eyberg, S. M., Boggs, S. R., & Algina, J. (1998). Efficacy of parent-child interaction therapy: Interim report of a randomized trial with short-term maintenance. *Journal of Clinical Child Psychology*, *27*(1), 34–45. doi:10.120715374424jccp2701_4 PMID:9561935

Simonoff, E., Elander, J., Holmshaw, J., Pickles, A., Murray, R., & Rutter, M. (2004). Predictors of antisocial personality: Continuities from childhood to adult life. *The British Journal of Psychiatry*, *184*(2), 118–127. doi:10.1192/bjp.184.2.118 PMID:14754823

Smeets, K. C., Leeijen, A. A., van der Molen, M. J., Scheepers, F. E., Buitelaar, J. K., & Rommelse, N. N. (2015). Treatment moderators of cognitive behavior therapy to reduce aggressive behavior: A meta-analysis. *European Child & Adolescent Psychiatry*, *24*(3), 255–264. doi:10.100700787-014-0592-1 PMID:25138144

Ward, M. A., Theule, J., & Cheung, K. (2016, October). Parent–child interaction therapy for child disruptive behaviour disorders: A meta-analysis. In *Child & Youth Care Forum* (Vol. 45, No. 5, pp. 675-690). Springer US.

ADDITIONAL READING

Burke, J. D., Loeber, R., & Birmaher, B. (2004). Oppositional defiant disorder and conduct disorder: A review of the past 10 years, part II. *Focus (San Francisco, Calif.)*, *41*(4), 1275–1576. PMID:12410070

Ford, J. D., Racusin, R., Ellis, C. G., Daviss, W. B., Reiser, J., Fleischer, A., & Thomas, J. (2000). Child maltreatment, other trauma exposure, and posttraumatic symptomatology among children with oppositional defiant and attention deficit hyperactivity disorders. *Child Maltreatment*, *5*(3), 205–217. doi:10.1177/1077559500005003001 PMID:11232267

Hutchings, J., Bywater, T., Daley, D., Gardner, F., Whitaker, C., Jones, K., ... Edwards, R. T. (2007). Parenting intervention in Sure Start services for children at risk of developing conduct disorder: Pragmatic randomised controlled trial. *BMJ (Clinical Research Ed.)*, *334*(7595), 678. doi:10.1136/bmj.39126.620799.55 PMID:17350966

Loeber, R., Burke, J. D., Lahey, B. B., Winters, A., & Zera, M. (2000). Oppositional defiant and conduct disorder: A review of the past 10 years, part I. *Journal of the American Academy of Child and Adolescent Psychiatry*, *39*(12), 1468–1484. doi:10.1097/00004583-200012000-00007 PMID:11128323

Maughan, B., Rowe, R., Messer, J., Goodman, R., & Meltzer, H. (2004). Conduct disorder and oppositional defiant disorder in a national sample: Developmental epidemiology. *Journal of Child Psychology and Psychiatry, and Allied Disciplines*, *45*(3), 609–621. doi:10.1111/j.1469-7610.2004.00250.x PMID:15055379

Puig-Antich, J. (1982). Major depression and conduct disorder in prepuberty. *Journal of the American Academy of Child Psychiatry*, *21*(2), 118–128. doi:10.1016/S0002-7138(09)60910-9 PMID:7069078

Rowe, R., Costello, E. J., Angold, A., Copeland, W. E., & Maughan, B. (2010). Developmental pathways in oppositional defiant disorder and conduct disorder. *Journal of Abnormal Psychology*, *119*(4), 726–738. doi:10.1037/a0020798 PMID:21090876

Salvatore, J. E., & Dick, D. M. (2018). Genetic influences on conduct disorder. *Neuroscience and Biobehavioral Reviews*, *91*, 91–101. doi:10.1016/j.neubiorev.2016.06.034 PMID:27350097

Schuhmann, E. M., Foote, R. C., Eyberg, S. M., Boggs, S. R., & Algina, J. (1998). Efficacy of parent-child interaction therapy: Interim report of a randomized trial with short-term maintenance. *Journal of Clinical Child Psychology*, *27*(1), 34–45. doi:10.120715374424jccp2701_4 PMID:9561935

Tremblay, R. E., LeMarquand, D., & Vitaro, F. (1999). The prevention of oppositional defiant disorder and conduct disorder. In *Handbook of disruptive behavior disorders* (pp. 525–555). Boston, MA: Springer. doi:10.1007/978-1-4615-4881-2_25

Zoccolillo, M., Pickles, A., Quinton, D., & Rutter, M. (1992). The outcome of childhood conduct disorder: Implications for defining adult personality disorder and conduct disorder. *Psychological Medicine*, *22*(4), 971–986. doi:10.1017/S003329170003854X PMID:1488492

KEY TERMS AND DEFINITIONS

Aggression: Behavior that leads to the harm of others and objects with a purpose.

Delinquency: Committing crimes at a young age, such as property theft or violent crimes with weapons.

Disruptive Behavior Disorders: A group of disorders that includes Conduct Disorder and Oppositional Defiant Disorder.

Epigenetic: The study of phenotype changes that are not genetically influenced.

Genotype: The genetic constitution of one's organism.

Informants: The individual or group that will inform when there is a problematic situation.

Maladaptive Behavior: In children, maladaptive behavior is shown through tantrums, the inability to adjust to situations and through externalizing behaviors that do not fit societal norms.

Methylation: When methyl groups are added to one's DNA. Methylation can alter the DNA and therefore change one's genotype.

Phenotype: The externalization of a gene's characteristic through observable behavior.

Chapter 9
Parenting in Dyads With an ASD-Child:
An Overview of the Challenges and Intervention Perspectives Through Attachment Theoretical Framework

Giulia Perasso
https://orcid.org/0000-0003-3265-3869
University of Pavia, Italy

Nava R. Silton
Marymount Manhattan College, USA

Jacopo De Angelis
University of Milano-Bicocca, Italy

ABSTRACT

This chapter provides an overview of the complex experience of parenting children with Autism Spectrum Disorders (ASDs) from an attachment-based perspective. The role of parental sensitivity, intrusiveness, and self-efficacy will be discussed in detail. These parental characteristics were indeed found to positively affect the parent-ASD-child bond and, in turn, to modulate the developmental course of ASDs. Likewise, the nature of symptomatology pertaining to autism (i.e., strong impairment in social and communication skills) represents an obstacle for parents to effectively attune to their children's needs or emotions. A number of interventions aimed at improving the quality and the attunement level in the parent-ASD-child dyad are presented. A specific focus is dedicated to attachment-based interventions such as the video feedback intervention to promote positive parenting – AUTI (VIPP-AUTI).

DOI: 10.4018/978-1-7998-2940-9.ch009

INTRODUCTION

Caring for a child with a disability can be very stressful, but it can also be an opportunity to discover new psychological resources that can be useful for the situation. One of the main challenges of parenting a child with a disability is to seek behavioral and emotional strategies to effectively meet the child's emotional needs. This process proves even more difficult in families with a child with autism since social communication impairments associated with autism represent a more complex obstacle to overcome for parents. However, research is providing families with new intervention perspectives to facilitate everyday life interactions.

The present chapter intends to show the complexity of parenting a child with ASD and to review some of the interventions that are designed to improve the quality of parent-ASD-child interactions. Specifically, it will be structured in the following manner. The first paragraph will provide a brief overview of Autism Spectrum Disorders by reporting diagnostic criteria, prevalence data, and debates on their etiology. The second paragraph will focus on the principal challenges of parenting children with ASD through the lens of a theoretical attachment perspective (Bowlby, 1969; Ainsworth & Bowlby, 1991). Three constructs will be analyzed in detail: parental sensitivity, parental intrusiveness, and parental self-efficacy. The third paragraph will review the main interventions targeted at improving the quality of parent-ASD-child interactions by boosting parental competencies and reducing parental intrusiveness. The chapter will also focus on the Video Feedback Intervention to Promote Positive Parenting – AUTI (VIPP-AUTI; Poslawsky, Naber, Bakermans-Kranenburg, De Jonge, Van Engeland, Van IJzendoorn, 2014). Finally, clinical and experimental limitations, as well as future directions of research in this field, will be discussed. Therefore, the current chapter is targeted at examining the parent-ASD-child dyad's bonding in light of recent intervention perspectives.

AN OVERVIEW OF AUTISM SPECTRUM DISORDERS

Diagnostic Features and Epidemiology

Autism Spectrum Disorders constitute a multi-faceted and pervasive neurodevelopmental syndrome characterized by both social and non-social impairments. Specifically, the *Diagnostic Statistical Manual of Mental Disorders* (*DSM-5*) focuses on impairments in social interaction and communication, and restricted, repetitive patterns of behaviors, interests, or activities as key criteria for ASD diagnoses (APA, 2013). The severity of the disorder varies as a function of the general cognitive profile and the behavior of the individual. Accordingly, there are three levels to describe the severity of impairment that needs to be reported when diagnosing ASDs. Level 1 includes those cases requiring limited support, whereas Level 2 and 3 respectively refer to cases requiring substantial and very substantial support (APA, 2013). An ASD diagnosis is mainly based on behavioral indicators due to the lack of clear and validated early biological markers, although some promising objective diagnostic tools have been validated and are expected to be used in clinical settings (e.g. Eye-tracking based tools; Frazier, Klingemier, Beukemann, Speer, Markowitz et al., 2016). In addition, early diagnoses (< 3 years old) are very rare (Fountain, King & Baerman, 2011) because of the difficulty of effectively quantifying non-social symptoms such as stereotypic and repetitive behaviors. Therefore, young children (< 3 years old) who present early symptomatology are typically classified as "at-risk" and their neuropsychological development is monitored until the age of diagnosis. A possible factor that was demonstrated to predict the age of diagnosis is parental education since children of highly educated parents seem to be likely to receive a diagnosis earlier than children with less-educated parents (Fountain et al., 2011). Specifically, this discrepancy reflects a gap between high and low family socioeconomic status impacting the age of diagnosis.

The prevalence rate of ASD is currently estimated at 1-2% (Kim, Leventhal, Koh, Fombonne, Laska, Lim, et al., 2011) and, as reported by Fisch (2012), prevalence rates have dramatically increased in the past twenty years. The increase of diagnoses can be in part explained by the changing diagnostic features resulting in more strict criteria (Fisch, 2012). Among individuals with autism, no cross-cultural differences in ASD rates were found (Fombonne, 2009), while a higher prevalence rate of men with ASD has typically been observed with a commonly referenced male: female consensus ratio of 4:1 (Werling & Geschwind, 2013). However, this male bias has been questioned for two reasons. First, the specific factors responsible for the higher prevalence rates of men diagnosed with ASD are still partially unclear (Baron-Cohen, Lombardo, Auyeung, Ashwin, Chakrabati & Knickmeyer, 2011). Secondly, this bias likely reflects the difficulty in diagnosing autism in females (Baron-Cohen et al., 2011). According to Holliday-Willey (1999), the under-diagnosis of ASD in females could be explained by the fact that females may be more motivated to conform socially and to adapt their behaviors to the external social context.

Etiology

The etiology of ASD includes a combination of genetic variants interacting with environmental factors (Chaste & Leboyer 2012; Newschaffer Croen, Daniels, Giarelli, Grether, Levy, et al. 2007). Approximately, 400-1000 genes are likely to be related to a susceptibility to autism (He, Sanders, Liu, Rubeis, Lim, Sutcliffe, & Devlin, 2013) that, in turn, seem to explain abnormalities in the developmental stages of the brain (Krishnan, Zhang, Yao, Theesfeld, Wong, Tadych, et al., 2016; Masi, De Mayo, Glozier, & Guastella, 2017). Recently, researchers have mapped a specific set of alleles that explain a consistent number of variants (Lord, Elsabbagh, Baird, & Veenstra-Vanderweele, 2018). However, the genes-based explanation was unable to explain at least 70% of cases of autism (Schaaf & Zoghbi, 2011; Masi, Quintana, Glozier, Lloyd, Hickie., & Guastella, 2015). This discrepancy is probably due to the existence of concurrent environmental factors that emerge during prenatal growth and/or postnatal development. For instance, maternal infection has been hypothesized as a possible prenatal environmental risk factor for ASDs (Malkova, Collin, Hsiao, Moore, & Patterson, 2012), as well as the use of valproate (a medication primarily used for the treatment of epilepsy and migraine) (Gardener, Spiegelman, & Buka, 2011). On the other hand, the susceptibility to some organic pollutants was reported to be a possible predictor of ASD symptomatology severity during the postnatal period (Boggess, Rahman, Pamukcu, Faber, & Kingston, 2014). Furthermore, a 2014 meta-analytic study completely discarded any possible link between vaccines and autism (Taylor, Swerdfeger, & Eslick, 2014).

Broader Autism Phenotype

The genetic susceptibility for ASDs was demonstrated to have a phenotypic expression in the so-called Broader Autism Phenotype (BAP; Baron-Cohen & Hammer, 1997; Gerdts & Bernier, 2011). The BAP refers to a substantial number of parents and siblings of children with ASD exhibiting behavioral features that are similar to some of the symptoms of ASDs, although in a milder form (Baron-Cohen & Hammer, 1997; Gerdts & Bernier, 2011; Sasson, Lam, Parlier, Daniels, & Piven, J, 2013). There is consistent evidence showing mild problems in some social cognitive abilities in parents of children with ASDs (Sucksmith, Roth, & Hoekstra, 2011; Sasson et al., 2013) that are usually reported to be substantial predictors of effective parent-child interactions (e.g., eye-contact and joint attention, Vernetti, Senju, Charman, Johnson, Gliga et al.,2018). Interestingly, it seems that the presence of a single parent with BAP is more common than both parents with BAP in families with children on the spectrum (Sasson et al., 2013). The presence of BAP predicts the severity of children's autistic symptomatology (Sasson et al., 2013). Specifically, children with BAP parents were reported to exhibit a more severe profile than other groups of children (Sasson et al., 2013). It is not completely clear if the BAP is the behavioral expression of a genetic pattern or the consequence of strategies that parents of children with ASD adopt to feel more attuned to their children. Indeed, as shown in the next paragraph, difficulty adapting to child interactions, communication styles, and the emotional world represent some of the main challenges of parenting in families with an ASD-child. Regardless of the nature of BAP, the existence of this behavioral phenotype further highlights the importance of better understanding the role of parenting in ASDs as a mediator of children's socio-emotional skills development and treatment effectiveness.

THE CHALLENGES OF PARENTING IN DYADS WITH AN ASD-CHILD

Social communication impairment characterizing ASDs represents one of the main obstacles to effective parenting strategies. Children with autism exhibit a constellation of early symptoms that put a strain on the relationship with their caregivers. These include issues in reciprocal social interaction (e.g. aversion to social touch, lack of eye contact, lack of response to social cues, lack of joint attention) and emotion regulation (e.g. difficulty in calming when distressed) (Wheterby, Woods, Allen, Cleary, Dickinson, & Lord, 2004). Many parents report great difficulties in attuning to their child due to feelings of disappointment, rejection, and anger (Benson & Karlof, 2009). Accordingly, these feelings affect the parenting style in a way that the parent is described as "cold" (Crowell, Keluskar, & Gorecki, 2019). Unlike disconfirmed theories presented in the 1960s (Bettelheim, 1967) intending "parental coldness" as an ASD etiologic factor, nowadays this cold parenting is seen as the reaction to the stress related to parenting a child with autism (Crowell et al., 2019). Other factors were demonstrated to determine this sense of frustration such as social isolation and maladaptive coping strategies (e.g. avoidant strategies; Dunn, 2001) causing a "closed" attitude toward social relationships in general.

This evidence stresses the importance of deeply understanding parental behavior in parents-ASD-child dyads since it plays a significant role in child development as in neurotypical children. In the next section, the parental characteristics impacting the relationship in these dyads will be presented from an attachment-based theory perspective. This approach constitutes a new angle to study parents-ASD child interactions, where the focus is on the dyadic bond rather than on the child's atypicality. Accordingly, the next section will focus on parental sensitivity, parental intrusiveness, and parental self-efficacy.

Parental Sensitivity

Parental sensitivity is defined as the parent's capacity to detect and interpret children's attachment signals, and the ability to adequately provide answers (Ainsworth, Blehar, Waters, & Wall, 1978). Attachment signals are the infants' contributions to help caregivers protect them by activating the attachment system (Crittenden, 2005). Parental sensitivity represents one of the main issues of parenting in families with children on the spectrum. It is intrinsically challenged by autistic symptomatology (Dawson, Hill, Spencer, Galpert, & Watson 1990) since -infants with ASD present issues in many social domains (Gervais, Belin, Boddaert, Leboyer, Coez, Sfaello, et al. 2004; Jermann, Basilio, Ansermet, Hentsch, Nadel, & Billard, 2013; Ploog, 2010). These domains include deficits in joint attention processes (Mundy, Sigman, Ungerer, & Sherman, 1986), pointing and showing behavior, eye contact, and other social behaviors (Mundy et al. 1986; McEvoy, Rogers, & Pennington. 1993). In the context of the parent-child relationship, children with autism do not show the same reciprocal affection or communication as neurotypical children. This behavior implies that parents of children with ASD have to adjust their verbal and non-verbal communication processes to effectively interact with their children (Doussard-Roosevelt, Joe, Bazhenova, & Porges, 2003). In other words, parents of children with ASD are required to learn new communication channels to attune to the emotional world of their child. For instance, mothers of preschoolers with ASD present more physical contact and fewer verbal approaches during play sessions as compared to mothers of preschoolers without ASD (Doussard-Roosevelt et al., 2003).

Parental sensitivity is an indicator typically used to describe the attachment bond between a parent and his/her child (Ainsworth et al., 1978). Indeed, parental sensitivity was reported to be associated with secure attachment (Prior & Glaiser, 2006). The secure child-parent bond represents a precursor of many human beings' socio-emotional capacities such as the ability to control negative and stressful emotions or to develop stable and long-term relationships (De Wolff & Van IJzendoorn, 1997). This also applies to families of children with disabilities as in the case of parents of children with ASD (Crowell et al., 2019). In a recent study by Rozga and colleagues (2018) 30 preschool children with ASD participated in a Strange Situation Procedure (Ainsworth et al., 1978), and they were also observed while interacting with the primary caregiver at home. One year later, the same group of children were assessed with a battery of tests evaluating their cognitive and emotional functioning. Interestingly, about forty-five percent (45%) of the children with ASD were found to be securely attached. Securely attached children showed better language, emotional and social skills than insecure and disorganized children. Furthermore, parents of children with secure attachment were rated as more sensitive than parents of insecurely attached children. These findings are consistent with other pioneering studies in the field (e.g., Sigman & Ungerer, 1984) and presented – and partially answered – two important research questions: 1) Do children with ASD exhibit a similar sequela of attachment security to those observed in typically developing children? 2) Does attachment have an impact on the development of children with ASD to the same extent as typically developing children?

In reference to the first question, the evidence above clearly demonstrates that attachment security in children with ASD emerges with the same frequency as in typically developing children. With regard to the second question, the reported evidence stressed how secure attachment can modulate the expression of autistic symptomatology severity since children with ASD who manifest secure attachment seem to have superior cognitive and emotional functioning. This connection was replicated by several studies. For instance, Sigman & Ungerer (1984) found that securely attached children with ASD had better linguistic skills and engaged in more symbolic play and joint attention, while Naber and colleagues (2008) found that increased fictional play seems to be positively associated with secure attachment in children with ASD. These data are in line with Losh and colleagues' study (2017), showing that social interaction and communication difficulties in parents represent substantial predictors of ASD severity in children.

Taken together, these results demonstrate the positive impact of effective ASD-child-parent relationships on the development of social, cognitive and emotional skills in children with autism. Likewise, they give an overview of how challenging parenting in a family with a child on the spectrum can be. The degree of effort exercised by parents of children with autism was quantified by Ostfeld-Etzion and colleagues' (2015) research-in which the authors used a Still Face paradigm (Tronick, 1975) to assess the emotion regulation and synchronization in the parent-ASD-child dyad. Still Face paradigm consists of the caregiver's sudden disconnection from the dyadic communication with the child, by interrupting her/his emotional responsiveness toward the child for several seconds. Results showed that both mothers and fathers of children with ASD were more attuned to their children after the Still Face episode and experienced more positive emotions. Interestingly, this was interpreted as an indicator of great parental regulatory effort by parents of children with ASD who need many psychological resources to cope with parenting challenges.

Parental Intrusiveness

Previous literature indicated that parents of children with socio-emotional difficulties tend to be more intrusive than parents of typically developing children (Dollberg, Feldman & Keren, 2010). Intrusive behavior enhances the parent's sense of control since parents report experiencing more self-efficacy when asked to manage their children's difficulties. However, intrusiveness undermines the child's autonomy, as well as his/her capacity to independently explore the environment (Biringen, 2000).

Many caregivers of children with ASD tend to act excessively as teachers guiding children with ASD (Safe, Joosten & Molineux, 2012) by becoming too intrusive and less attuned to children's needs. These behaviors impact children's capacity to play and learn at their own tempo (Jordan, 2003; Pajareya & Nopmaneejumruslers, 2011) and, at the same time, they also have an impact on parental psychological wellbeing. An interesting and recent study by McAuliffe and colleagues (2019), conducted on an Australian sample of mothers with children with ASD, showed how "hyper-performing" parenting can seriously undermine the development of several personal-psychological domains in children. In addition, this study indicated that renouncing "me-time" to assume an exclusive role in caregiving children with disabilities may negatively impact a mother's health and psychological wellbeing (McAuliffe, Thomas, Vaz, Falkmer, & Cordier, 2019). Becoming completely involved in the mother-child relationship may often result in a loss of psychological and social resources that necessarily lead mothers to that sense of desperation and frustration described earlier. Therefore, this evidence highlights the importance of developing interventions targeted at encouraging mothers to participate in "me-time" activities to reduce their sense of isolation and to enhance their coping strategies (McAuliffe et al., 2019).

This parental tendency toward intrusiveness has also been reported in fathers of children with ASD. Konstantareas (2008) analyzed language patterns employed by fathers and mothers of children with ASD. Children were videotaped while interacting with their mothers and fathers. It was found that mothers were more inclined to suggest prompts whereas fathers were reported to give more explicit suggestions and to be more directive. Moreover, this greater paternal directiveness is often accompanied by less social engagement with children with ASD as reported by Flippin and Watson's (2015) study. These findings suggest how working on parent-child boundaries is critical to the health of both of the dyad members. In other words, it is evident how important it is to reinforce mothers' and fathers' identities outside of their parental roles.

Parental Self-Efficacy

Another conclusion emerging from previous studies on the topic is that the quality of parent-child interactions is influenced by parental self-efficacy (Kuhn & Carter, 2006). Self-efficacy can be defined as how well a person perceives him/herself as able to execute courses of action to address prospective situations (Bandura, 1982). Kuhn & Carter's study (2006) clearly showed that self-efficacy is a substantial predictor of well-being and agency in mothers of children with autism. Importantly, experiencing self-efficacy is not explained by the acquired technical knowledge of autism. In clinical practice, clinicians often report that parents of children with ASD tend to accumulate technical knowledge of the syndrome that, in turn, seems to guarantee a better sense of control. This attitude can be better identified as the defense mechanism called "Intellectualization:" that is a strategy used by the person to manage and block unconscious conflicts or emotional suffering (Vaillant, 1992). Conversely, self-efficacy refers to the ability to manage situations and face different obstacles. It strongly relies on coping strategies that enable the individual to contend with all of the emotional and practical stressors implied in the situation, without avoiding difficulties or negative emotions.

There is also evidence of a negative association between parental self-efficacy and parental distress (Giallo, Rose & Vittorino, 2011; Bekhet, Johnson, & Zauszniewski, 2012), stating that self-efficacy is a powerful and critical protective factor preventing parental desperation and stressful, negative experiences. Accordingly, parental self-efficacy is considered to be one of the most important predictors of parent-child relationship effectiveness both in families of typically developing children and in those with children with neurodevelopmental disorders.

What Should Be the Aims of an Intervention Targeting the Parents-ASD-Child Dyad?

This paragraph outlines the main challenges parents of children with ASD have to endure. Additionally, what clearly emerges from the presented findings is the role played by the environment in modulating the course of the disorder. In other words, even though autism has a strong genetic component, the environment can actively intervene in the development of psychological skills as is the case in typically developing children. Therefore, literature suggests to clinicians and researchers the importance of developing intervention tools to boost parental sensitivity to increase the attunement level between members of the dyads. Secondly, another aim of the interventions is to make parents more sensitive to the needs of their children without being too intrusive. Obviously, each family has its own history and background, meaning that the interventions have to consistently be targeted to the specific situation of each family. These aims can be achieved if parents have the sense to effectively manage critical situations without being overwhelmed. Every intervention should work to enhance parental self-efficacy since it strongly modulates the parent-child relationship quality by affecting parents' well-being. Some recent and innovative interventions addressing these competencies will be presented in the next paragraph of this chapter.

INTERVENTIONS WORKING ON PARENT ASD-CHILD DYADS: A FOCUS ON VIDEO-FEEDBACK INTERVENTIONS

Video-Feedback Intervention: A Tool for Therapeutic Intervention

The portability of video-recording devices extends the observation potential of new techniques that can feasibly apply in different contexts (i.e. ecological and clinical). Video-recording represents a powerful tool for clinicians, since it provides the possibility of code sequences by the delayed re-watching of the clip. Coding is targeted at creating feedback directed to participants of the intervention. Video-feedback (VF) is commonly used with typically developing individuals in education, coaching, supervision, and mental health treatment to enhance skills development and critical thinking stimulation.

In addition, Video-feedback (VF) has been used with parent-ASD-child dyads that represent one of the most challenging contexts for this intervention. As in non-clinical dyads, VF consists of commenting on recorded clips following a protocol, the guidelines of which differ in each evidence-based manualized intervention (i.e. Preschool Autism Communication Therapy, PACT; Parent Mediated Intervention for Autism Spectrum Disorders in South Asia, PASS; Video-feedback to promote Positive Parenting for Children with Autism, VIPP-AUTI). Video clips are usually recorded at home to guarantee an ecological approach to the dyad's everyday routine. The recorded sequences address caregiving interactions, such as meals or play sessions – dyadic playing or child playing alone- with different types of toys.

Regarding every context of parent-child intervention, VF represents a "catalyst for change" to reconsider the established connection with the infant (Adamson, Bakeman, Deckner, & Nelson, 2012; Steele, Steele, Bate, Knafo, Kinsey, Bonuck, et al., 2014). As stressed by Aldred, Taylor, Wan, and Green (2018), it is critical to distinguish VF in psychoeducation from its use in therapeutic interventions. Psychoeducational programs for parents and children with ASD are solely focused on teaching parents the correct techniques to interact with their infants (Steiner, Koegel, Koegel, & Ence, 2012). They can also be practiced along with a therapist who is separately working with the child (Oono, Honey, & McConachie, 2013). In the therapeutic context, as pointed out by a recent literature review (Factor, Ollendick, Cooper, Dunsmore, Rea, & Scarpa, 2019), VF is intended as a technique to promote a "parent-mediated" intervention for the child (Aldred, Taylor, Wan, & Green, 2018). VF has a twofold benefit: 1) to enhance parental skills in the interaction with the child with ASD; and 2) to improve the child's social communication skills by refining parental observation, behaviors, cognitions, morale and confidence within the relationship.

Parents as "Co-Therapists"

A proper premise needs to be drawn. VF interventions are not utilized for parents who present poor parenting skills, but, contrarily, they are aimed at invigorating the already present skills to make parents "co-therapists." A great body of scientific evidence has supported long-term VF benefits in infants (Pickles, Le Couteur, Leadbitter, Salomone, Cole-Fletcher, Tobin et al.,2016; Aldred, Taylor, Wan, & Green, 2018) across a wide range of parents' social classes, cultures, and educational levels. VF methods should be used both in family contexts with typically developing children and with other children suffering from neurodevelopmental disorders such as ASDs (Juffer, Bakermans-Kranenburg & Van Ijzendoorn, 2008; Poslawsky, Naber, Bakermans-Kranenburg, van Daalen, van Engeland, & van IJzendoorn, 2015).

As reported in the previous paragraph, research showed no consistent differences in parental sensitivity (Van Ijzendoorn, Rutgers, Bakermans-Kranenburg, Swinkels, Van Daalen, Dietz, et al., 2007) and in perceived caregiving burden (Rutgers, Van Ijzendoorn, Bakermans-Kranenburg, Swinkels, Van Daalen, Dietz, et al. 2007) among parents of children with ASD and in parents of children with other clinical and non-clinical diagnoses. However, it was already reported how the attachment needs and signals of children with ASD may be too complex for parents to decode (Rutgers et al., 2007). Decoding signals of children with autism is strongly associated with parental stress, as indicated by studies comparing the level of stress of parents of children with ASD with the levels of stress in parents of children with mental retardation and/or typically developing children (Benjak, Vuletić Mavrinac, & Pavić Šimetin, 2009; Higgins, Bailey, & Pearce, 2005; Eisenhower, Baker, & Blacher, 2005). According to these studies, parents of children with ASD report experiencing higher levels of anxiety, burnout, psychosomatic symptoms, depressive symptoms, somatic complaints, and perceived family dysfunction.

As aforementioned, this does not mean that parents of children with ASD are not "good enough," but it underlines the critical importance of early support for the dyads. Early intervention can be a source of support for the family system by promoting its positive functioning as pointed out by Oosterling and colleagues (2010). Therefore, this type of intervention is highly recommended since it constitutes a mitigating factor capable of moderating the severity of ASD symptomatology and problematic behaviors.

Parent-Mediated Interventions in ASD-Child Dyads

In recent decades, a variety of interventions have been implemented in the pharmacological and psychological field, but only a few have been empirically validated by randomized control studies (Green, Pituch, Itchon, Choi, O'Reilly, & Sigafoos, 2006; Ospina, Seida, Clark, Karkhaneh, Hartling, Tjosvold, et al., 2008; Rogers & Vismara, 2008). As stated by the New York State Department of Health Clinical Practice Guideline (1999), the most pioneering intervention approaches were based on the development of several distinguished trainings addressing the specific components typically impaired in autism (e.g., language, autonomy, social skills, etc.). Subsequently, more holistic approaches were structured. For example, the Wieder and Greenspan "Floor time" Approach (2003) constitutes one of the main early interventions used to increase social functioning in children with ASD. The intervention is focused on play sessions where the child is leading the interaction with adults. The final aim is to encourage the development of communication and symbolic abilities in the infant (Wieder & Greenspan, 2003).

To date, researchers suggest how important it is to structure interventions that reflect as best as possible real-life situations by analyzing the child's behavior. Within this approach, Applied Behavioral Analysis (ABA) (Lovaas, 1970) proved to be the most effective methodology used to diminish the impact of ASD symptoms in childhood (Makrygianni & Reed, 2010; Peters-Scheffer, Didden, Korzilius, & Sturmey, 2011). ABA interventions apply operant conditioning to facilitate child behavioral change through reinforcement of some actions and ignoring others (Erba, 2000). Intervention outcomes include the improvement of cognitive functions, adaptation and language skills in children undertaking the ABA Approach compared to controls. These treatment goals are achieved through the use of four behavioral techniques: prompting, shaping, fading, and chaining of the child's actions. *Prompting* involves the use of prompts that are introduced to increase the likelihood that the child will provide the desired response (e.g., teaching pointing behavior by supporting the child's arm). *Fading* aims at increasing the child's autonomy level, by progressively reducing prompts. *Shaping* consists of reinforcing behaviors that are closer to the target behavior (e.g., reinforcing the child whenever he/she orients visual attention to the target object). *Chaining* relies on Task Analysis, that is, disentangling a task in sub-components and teaching them to the child until the entire task is complete. ABA principles and intervention strategies are also partially shared by other validated interventions. Among these, the Early Start Denver Model (ESDM) has been shown to improve adaptive behaviors in toddlers with ASD (Dawson, Rogers, Munson, Smith, Winter, Greenson, et al., 2010). The ESDM model integrates Applied Behavioral Analysis principles with relationship-based and developmental principles. The ESDM was shown to determine normalized brain activity in children with ASD after exposure to the training (Dawson Jones, Merkle, Venema, Lowy, Faja, et al., 2012).

Despite the proven benefits of ABA-based models, some limitations in these programs have emerged. For instance, there is an evident increase in family stress due to the great effort parents need to put forth to learn and reproduce ABA techniques in everyday life (Schwichtenberg & Poehlmann, 2007). Similarly, other interventions are more focused on the development of facilitating environments for children with ASD (i.e. TEACCH by Schopler, 1994) and carry the risk of being unbalanced by underestimating the relationship. The TEACCH (Treatment and Education of Autistic and related Communication Handicapped Children) is intended to create structured learning environments in which the child is continuously stimulated to learn and communicate through the use of visual aids. The development of facilitating environments includes the physical organization (e.g. neither too hyper nor hypo-stimulating) of individualized schedules and the use of materials with a visual structure (e.g. colored cards containing indications on how to perform a task such as brushing teeth).

In the field of ASD treatments, parent-mediation might represent one of the key factors of a powerful intervention in childhood. According to Green and colleagues (2010), parent-mediated communication enhances synchronous responses and improves the likelihood of communication initiation by the child, especially with the support of video-recording of parent-child dyadic interactions. However, parent-mediated communication, behavioral analysis, and environment-based interventions are not meant to be mutually exclusive. Conversely, they can be well-integrated with parent-mediated approaches to work from a 360-degree perspective on parent-child interactions (Oono, Honey, & McConachie, 2013).

Video-Feedback to Address the Challenges of Parenting ASD-Children

VF represents a chance for parents to observe their own behaviors and to actively structure their own feedback in first person, rather than to passively receive evaluations and advice from experts (Vik & Rohde, 2014). However, it does not mean that VF interventions attribute a marginal role to the therapist since the level of collaboration with the parent depends on the underlying intervention guidelines and the related techniques (Benzies, Magill-Evans, Hayden, & Ballantyne, 2013; Buggey & Ogle, 2012). VF methods create awareness and emotional arousal in the parent, allowing for a self-regulated and accelerated learning process, which is more effective than seeing a video-training with neutral examples (Dowrick, 1991). Longitudinal evidence on non-clinical dyads shows that VF increases mentalization – in terms of awareness of own and others' thoughts and feelings (Fonagy & Target, 1998) -thus improving parental empathy and responsiveness, and decreasing the likelihood of a child later developing emotional and behavioral problems (Fonagy & Target, 1997; Wolff & van IJzendoorn, 1997). This feature is particularly interesting when it comes to parent-ASD-child dyads because VF facilitates mentalization in terms of interpretation of the child with ASD's state of mind (Beebe, 2010). This interpretation occurs without the urgency of face-to-face interactions with the child, giving the parent the time to understand and think about her/his infant communication.

To date, as reviewed by Aldred et al., (2018), there are three main VF interventions in the field of parent ASD-child dyads:

- The Preschool Autism Communication Therapy (PACT) (Green et al., 2010) is an 18-session intervention that offers six stages with specific goals and strategies. In each session, dyadic interactions are videotaped and then discussed in the following encounter by the therapist and the parent together.

The order of the stages is preparatory and determined by the child's level of development and ASD deficit severity. PACT has been demonstrated to be effective in increasing parental interactive synchrony and in diminishing ASD-child symptoms' severity in both the social-affective and repetitive interest domains (Green et al., 2010).

- The Parent Mediated Intervention for Autism Spectrum Disorders in South Asia (PASS), a remote training supervision adaptation (Divan et al., 2015; Green, Rahman, Divan, Handani, Vajaratkar, Taylor, et al., 2015) of PASS, was implemented in South Asia with positive results. In detail, findings obtained through the implementation of the UK PACT have been replicated in terms of increased parental synchronicity and enhanced child communication initiations.
- Video-Feedback to promote Positive Parenting for Children with Autism (VIPP-AUTI) (Poslawsky, Naber, Bakermans-Kranenburg, De Jonge, Van Engeland, Van IJzendoorn, 2014), which will be presented in the subsequent paragraphs, is an attachment-based and evidence-based intervention particularly effective to enhance parent-ASD-child dyads' socioemotional interactions.

Video-Feedback to Promote Positive Parenting for Children with Autism

Video-feedback to promote Positive Parenting for Children with Autism (VIPP-AUTI) (Poslawsky et al., 2014) is of particular interest due to its positive socio-emotional outcomes. VIPP-AUTI is an intervention that encompasses video recording, behavioral coding, and feedback of parent-ASD-child dyads. The main aim of VIPP-AUTI is to improve parental sensitivity in understanding and responding to the signals of the child with ASD. Secondly, as a parent-mediated intervention, VIPP-AUTI is targeted at reducing the child's symptomatology as an indirect effect of enhanced parental sensitivity. Findings from Randomized Control Trial (RCT) (Poslawsky et al., 2014; 2015) highlighted that parents undertaking VIPP-AUTI presented reduced intrusiveness on child's exploration and play patterns, measured by Emotional Availability Scales (EAS, Biringen, Robinson, & Emde, 2000). Moreover, VIPP-AUTI resulted in improved parental efficacy at the Parental Efficacy Questionnaire (Rutgers et al., 2007; Yaman, Mesman, Van IJzendoorn, & Bakermans-Kranenburg, 2010). This construct describes the level of personal efficacy (driven by Bandura's Social Cognitive Theory, 1997) perceived in parenting. VIPP has also been adapted for use in the prodromal phase of ASD with the Intervention in the British Autism Study of Infant Siblings (iBASIS-VIPP, Green, Pickles, Pasco, Bedford, Wan, Elsabbagh et al, 2017; Wan, Green, Elsabbagh, Johnson, Charman, Plummer et al.,2012). The ARCT study on iBASIS-VIPP effectiveness showed a significant increase in parental non-directedness, parent-rated adaptive functioning and infant's attentiveness to parents. A reduction of autism prodromes and major attentional flexibility in the child was likewise reported.

VIPP-AUTI has been designed via the collaboration between Leiden University (Center for Child and Family Studies) and University Medical Center Utrecht (Poslawsky, et al. 2014). The intervention arose from the VIPP-Sensitive Discipline (SD) (Juffer, Bakermans-Kranenburg, & van IJzendoorn, 2008) version, which is tailored to dyads with a typically developing child. The adaptation of VIPP-SD has been conducted by the authors to meet specific characteristics of parent ASD-child dyads, by applying clinical knowledge about autism symptomatology to the intervention. This attachment-based and home-based intervention has been revised to be targeted to impairments in communication, altered play patterns and stereotypical behaviors of children with ASD. Like the VIPP-SD, each VIPP-AUTI session involves: 1) parent-child interactive situations (e.g. playing, or mealtime) that are video-recorded by the intervener; and 2) a feedback moment in which the intervener and the parent watch the previous session's video-recordings. This part is particularly significant since the video enables the parent to think about aspects of the child's behavior that would be otherwise difficult to verbally describe. As stated by the intervention's guidelines, the intervener has to remain neutral during the video-recording to allow parent-child interactions to be as natural as possible. This neutrality principle is shared by many observation techniques (e.g. infant observation) taking place in ecological settings but it becomes even more critical for parent ASD-child dyads (Wallace & Rogers, 2010). A natural environment is fundamental to capture the whole behavioral repertoire of children with autism (McConnell, 2002). Professionals working with children with ASD (e.g. psychologists, social workers, nurses, etc.) can become VIPP-AUTI interveners by attending a specific training and a certain number of supervisions.

VIPP-AUTI, like the VIPP-SD, is targeted at the dyad constituted by the child and one caregiver (commonly the mother or the father). This means that the intervention has to be directed with continuity to the child and the mother or father from the first to the last session. The interchange between parents is not allowed within VIPP interventions, but the two parents can both undertake the VIPP intervention separately by constituting two different dyads with the same child.

The VIPP-AUTI protocol is divided into five sessions. Similarities with VIPP-SD (Juffer et al., 2008) can be found in recurrent themes (i.e. Attachment and Exploration, Sharing Emotions, etc.), or techniques (i.e. Speaking for the child, Sensitivity chain, Sensitive time-out, etc.). Specific themes for parent ASD-child dyads have been included (i.e. mastery motivation and play, joint attention, daily problems and routine, emotions and stereotypical behavior). VIPP-AUTI sessions are structured as follows:

- *Session 1*: The first session of VIPP-AUTI, as in the original version of VIPP, deepens the theme of Attachment and Exploration. Distinguishing proximity-seeking behavior and the need to explore the environment is one of the crucial steps toward improved parental sensitivity. This session can help the parent learn how to respond to a child's signals, both when he/she is eager to get close to the caregiver for comfort, and when he/she prefers playing alone. The restricted play repertoire of individuals with ASD makes it more complex for the parents to recognize proximity-seeking and exploration signals. Indeed, VIPP-AUTI's first session is targeted toward enhancing parental support and the acceptance of child's play.
- *Session 2*: In the second session of VIPP-AUTI, the intervener introduces the "speaking for the child" technique, consisting of verbally expressing the child's signals (e.g. what he/she is thinking, what he/she wants to communicate to the caregiver, what he/she is trying to do). Since this technique implies the intervener commenting and interpreting the child's state of mind and his/her actions, it is similar to dubbing a movie as the intervener's comments are giving voice to the child's behaviors, emotions, and cognitions. In particular, the technique is applied to three play-situations (a child playing alone with a toy, a child and parent playing together, and a child and parent playing together interrupted by an unexpected event) after the accurate coding of the video by the intervener, who is trained at interpreting the child's facial expression and non-verbal signals. In dyads with an ASD-child, the intervener discusses alternative communication strategies with the parents (e.g. the use of a glove puppet) to overcome the child's limited eye contact. Additionally, the intervener emphasizes the importance of verbally guiding the child's behavior (e.g. using compliments, describing what he/she is doing), even when the child does not respond through the same communicative channel.
- *Session 3*: In VIPP-AUTI's third session, the intervener introduces "sensitivity chains." Sensitivity chains stress the importance of parental sensitivity since this type of interaction is characterized by three components: 1) A signal from the child (e.g. crying), 2) the corresponding adequate and on-time response by the parent (e.g. consoling), and 3) a subsequent reaction from the child (e.g. stopping crying and/or smiling). Autism social and communication symptoms complicate the chain-of-events of parent-child interactions in everyday life. Managing challenging behaviors, sleep problems and eating problems is one of the goals of VIPP-AUTI, by combining procedures of VIPP (e.g. sensitive chains, sensitive time out, reinforcement) with new elements. In fact, VIPP-

AUTI includes feedback on the organization of a predictive daily routine, and the use of pictograms (texts or photographs) to improve communication exchange in daily interactions.

- *Session 4:* VIPP's fourth session is centered on emotion recognition, affective attunement and emotion sharing between parent and child. Given ASD problems in emotion regulation and stereotypical behaviors (tics, manipulation of the object, repeated movements or repetitive language), affective attunement in the dyad could be difficult to reach. In this session of VIPP-AUTI, the video-recorded situations are making music together by using a xylophone, singing and producing gestures to trigger imitation, and blowing soap bubbles. These clips have been thought to be particularly stimulating for the emotional processes and communication skills of children with ASD. In the feedback part, the intervener emphasizes the importance of labeling the child's emotional states and the context-related factor triggering emotional activation, by distinguishing emotional excitement from stereotypical behaviors.
- Session 5: In the final VIPP-AUTI home-visit, the precedent topics are revised by watching three previously filmed situations (child and parent playing together with a fruit set, reading a book together, playing with a marble run). The intervener invites parents to use the technique of "*speaking for the child*" and sensitivity chains. The other parent is also invited to participate in the session to discuss together positively- achieved parent-child interactions and how they can be implemented in everyday routines. In the final session, the VIPP-AUTI intervener can leave a written summary for the parents to describe the child's competencies and the main issues faced by the dyad as a reminder of the achieved strengths and weaknesses to consider when encountering parenting challenges.

LIMITATIONS AND FUTURE DIRECTIONS

Clinical Limitations

The main concern related to Video Feedback techniques relates to the intervener's level of adherence to manualized protocol guidelines as a possible source of distortion and misinterpretation. Once one completes the training and obtains the VIPP-AUTI certification, it is fundamental that clinicians follow the manual's instruction to guarantee a gold standard in treatment administration. A second potential issue is given by parents' expectations about the treatment – as stated by Aldred et al. (2018). Parents tend to exhibit different responses toward the treatment that requires the therapist to adapt to different parenting attitudes (i.e. encouraging motivation in non-compliant parents). Additionally, parents' adherence to the principles of the Video Feedback-based interventions can substantially impact its effectiveness.

Experimental Limitations

Several post-intervention outcomes used by the aforementioned studies come from measures such as self-reports and observation techniques. However, it is well known how these measures can be affected by confounding variables impacting assessment reliability. These confounders can concern the characteristics of the rater (clinician or researcher). Specifically, rater biases include both personal characteristics of the rater that might systemically influence the evaluation (e.g. mood, personality traits) and problems related to the arbitrariness of the subjective rating (e.g. prejudices, a-priori knowledge). Although clinicians' trainings are structured to prevent these sources of error, they cannot be totally limited. In light of these issues, future lines of research should work on developing more objective standards of evaluation and automatized coding procedures. For instance, the use of mobile eye-tracking technology might be introduced in clinical settings to objectively measures social cognitive processes, such as joint attention, mutual eye contact, and responsiveness to social cues, when the child is involved in the interaction with his/her parents. It would also be interesting to look at the physiological reactions of the child to monitor the anxiety level experienced in parent-child dynamics. Possibly, Galvanic Skin Response (GSR) or Heartbeat (HB) measurement tools might become critical to assess the VF interventions' outcome. In other words, this combination of techniques would open a dialogue between parenting psychology and social neuroscience methods by laying the foundation of a "neurocognitive approach to parenting."

CONCLUSION

This chapter has shown the main challenges that parents of children with ASD experience and focuses on evidence-based intervention strategies to boost parental skills through the use of Video-Feedback. Particular attention is paid to the description of VIPP-AUTI since it enables families and professionals to look at parent ASD-child dyads through the lens of Attachment Theory (Bowlby, 1969). The reported evidence suggests to parents and to a wide range of professionals (e.g., counselors, educators, psychologists, and social workers) that empowering attunement in the dyad might help parents to trust themselves and to positively modulate ASD-child social and emotional skills development.

REFERENCES

Adamson, L. B., Bakeman, R., Deckner, D. F., & Nelson, P. B. (2012). Rating parent–child interactions: Joint engagement, communication dynamics, and shared topics in autism, Down syndrome, and typical development. *Journal of Autism and Developmental Disorders*, *42*(12), 2622–2635. doi:10.100710803-012-1520-1 PMID:22466689

Ainsworth, M. D. S., Blehar, M., Waters, E., & Wall, S. (1978). Patterns of attachment: Observations in the Strange Situation and at home. Hillsdale, NJ: Erlbaum.

Ainsworth, M. S., & Bowlby, J. (1991). An ethological approach to personality development. *The American Psychologist*, *46*(4), 333–341. doi:10.1037/0003-066X.46.4.333

Aldred, C., Taylor, C., Wan, M. W., & Green, J. (2018). Using video feedback strategies in parent-mediated early autism intervention. In *Handbook of Parent-Implemented Interventions for Very Young Children with Autism* (pp. 221–239). Cham: Springer. doi:10.1007/978-3-319-90994-3_14

American Psychiatric Association. (2013). *Diagnostic and statistical manual of mental disorders* (5th ed.). Washington, DC: Author.

Bandura, A. (1982). Self-efficacy mechanism in human agency. *The American Psychologist*, *37*(2), 122–147. doi:10.1037/0003-066X.37.2.122

Baron-Cohen, S., & Hammer, J. (1997). Parents of children with Asperger syndrome: What is the cognitive phenotype? *Journal of Cognitive Neuroscience*, *9*(4), 548–554. doi:10.1162/jocn.1997.9.4.548 PMID:23968217

Baron-Cohen, S., Lombardo, M. V., Auyeung, B., Ashwin, E., Chakrabarti, B., & Knickmeyer, R. (2011). Why are autism spectrum conditions more prevalent in males? *PLoS Biology*, *9*(6), e1001081. doi:10.1371/journal.pbio.1001081 PMID:21695109

Beebe, B. (2010). Mother–infant research informs mother–infant treatment. *Clinical Social Work Journal*, *38*(1), 17–36. doi:10.100710615-009-0256-7

Bekhet, A. K., Johnson, N. L., & Zauszniewski, J. A. (2012). Resilience in family members of persons with autism spectrum disorder: A review of the literature. *Issues in Mental Health Nursing*, *33*(10), 650–656. doi:10.3109/01612840.2012.671441 PMID:23017040

Benjak, T., Vuletić Mavrinac, G., & Pavić Šimetin, I. (2009). Comparative study on selfperceived health of parents of children with autism spectrum disorders and parents of nondisabled children in croatia. *Croatian Medical Journal*, *50*(4), 403–409. doi:10.3325/cmj.2009.50.403 PMID:19673041

Benson, P. R., & Karlof, K. L. (2009). Anger, stress proliferation, and depressed mood among parents of children with ASD: A longitudinal replication. *Journal of Autism and Developmental Disorders*, *39*(2), 350–362. doi:10.100710803-008-0632-0 PMID:18709548

Benzies, K. M., Magill-Evans, J. E., Hayden, K. A., & Ballantyne, M. (2013). Key components of early intervention programs for preterm infants and their parents: A systematic review and meta-analysis. *BMC Pregnancy and Childbirth*, *13*(1Suppl 1), S10. doi:10.1186/1471-2393-13-S1-S10 PMID:23445560

Bettelheim, B. (1967). *The empty fortress*. New York: Free Press.

Biringen, Z. (2000). Emotional availability: Conceptualization and research findings. *The American Journal of Orthopsychiatry*, *70*(1), 104–114. doi:10.1037/h0087711 PMID:10702855

Biringen, Z., Robinson, J. L., & Emde, R. N. (2000). Appendix B: The emotional availability scales; an abridged infancy/early childhood version). *Attachment & Human Development*, *2*(2), 256–270. doi:10.1080/14616730050085626

Boggess, A. J., Rahman, G. M., Pamukcu, M., Faber, S., & Kingston, H. S. (2014). An accurate and transferable protocol for reproducible quantification of organic pollutants in human serum using direct isotope dilution mass spectrometry. *Analyst (London)*, *139*(23), 6223–6231. doi:10.1039/C4AN00851K PMID:25302342

Bowlby, J. (1969). Attachment and loss: Vol. 1. *Attachment*. London: Hogarth.

Buggey, T., & Ogle, L. (2012). Video self-modeling. *Psychology in the Schools*, *49*(1), 52–70. doi:10.1002/pits.20618

Chaste, P., & Leboyer, M. (2012). Autism risk factors: Genes, environment, and gene-environment interactions. *Dialogues in Clinical Neuroscience*, *14*(3), 281. PMID:23226953

Crittenden, P. M. (2005). Attachment theory, psychopathology and psychotherapy: The dynamic-maturational approach. *Psicoterapia*, *30*, 171–182.

Crowell, J. A., Keluskar, J., & Gorecki, A. (2019). Parenting behavior and the development of children with autism spectrum disorder. *Comprehensive Psychiatry*, *90*, 21–29. doi:10.1016/j.comppsych.2018.11.007 PMID:30658339

Dawson, G., Hill, D., Spencer, A., Galpert, L., & Watson, L. (1990). Affective exchanges between young autistic children and their mothers. *Journal of Abnormal Child Psychology, 18*(3), 335–345. doi:10.1007/BF00916569 PMID:2376657

Dawson, G., Jones, E. J., Merkle, K., Venema, K., Lowy, R., Faja, S., ... Smith, M. (2012). Early behavioral intervention is associated with normalized brain activity in young children with autism. *Journal of the American Academy of Child and Adolescent Psychiatry, 51*(11), 1150–1159. doi:10.1016/j.jaac.2012.08.018 PMID:23101741

Dawson, G., Rogers, S., Munson, J., Smith, M., Winter, J., Greenson, J., ... Varley, J. (2010). Randomized, controlled trial of an intervention for toddlers with autism: The Early Start Denver Model. *Pediatrics, 125*(1), 17–23. doi:10.1542/peds.2009-0958 PMID:19948568

De Wolff, M. S., & Van Ijzendoorn, M. H. (1997). Sensitivity and attachment: A meta-analysis on parental antecedents of infant attachment. *Child Development, 68*(4), 571–591. doi:10.1111/j.1467-8624.1997.tb04218.x PMID:9306636

Divan, G., Hamdani, S. U., Vajartkar, V., Minhas, A., Taylor, C., Aldred, C., ... Patel, V. (2015). Adapting an evidence-based intervention for autism spectrum disorder for scaling up in resource-constrained settings: The development of the PASS intervention in South Asia. *Global Health Action, 8*(1), 27278. doi:10.3402/gha.v8.27278 PMID:26243710

Dollberg, D., Feldman, R., & Keren, M. (2010). Maternal representations, infant psychiatric status, and mother–child relationship in clinic-referred and non-referred infants. *European Child & Adolescent Psychiatry, 19*(1), 25–36. doi:10.100700787-009-0036-5 PMID:19543936

Doussard-Roosevelt, J. A., Joe, C. M., Bazhenova, O., & Porges, S. W. (2003). Mother–child interaction in autistic and nonautistic children: Characteristics of maternal approach behaviors and child social responses. *Development and Psychopathology, 15*(2), 277–295. doi:10.1017/S0954579403000154 PMID:12931828

Dowrick, P. W. (1991). *Practical guide to using video in the behavioral sciences*. John Wiley & Sons.

Dunn, W. (2001). The sensations of everyday life: Empirical, theoretical, and pragmatic considerations. *The American Journal of Occupational Therapy, 55*(6), 608–620. doi:10.5014/ajot.55.6.608 PMID:12959225

Eisenhower, A. S., Baker, B. L., & Blacher, J. (2005). Preschool children with intellectual disability: Syndrome specificity, behavior problems, and maternal well-being. *Journal of Intellectual Disability Research*, *49*(9), 657–671. doi:10.1111/j.1365-2788.2005.00699.x PMID:16108983

Erba, H. W. (2000). Early intervention programs for children with autism: Conceptual frameworks for implementation. *The American Journal of Orthopsychiatry*, *70*(1), 82–94. doi:10.1037/h0087826 PMID:10702853

Factor, R. S., Ollendick, T. H., Cooper, L. D., Dunsmore, J. C., Rea, H. M., & Scarpa, A. (2019). All in the Family: A Systematic Review of the Effect of Caregiver-Administered Autism Spectrum Disorder Interventions on Family Functioning and Relationships. *Clinical Child and Family Psychology Review*, *22*(4), 433–457. doi:10.100710567-019-00297-x PMID:31363949

Fisch, G. S. (2012). Autism and epistemology III: Child development, behavioral stability, and reliability of measurement. *American Journal of Medical Genetics. Part A*, *158*(5), 969–979. doi:10.1002/ajmg.a.35269 PMID:22488915

Fisch, G. S. (2012, May). Nosology and epidemiology in autism: Classification counts. *American Journal of Medical Genetics. Part C, Seminars in Medical Genetics*, *160*(2), 91–103. doi:10.1002/ajmg.c.31325 PMID:22499526

Flippin, M., & Watson, L. R. (2015). Fathers' and mothers' verbal responsiveness and the language skills of young children with autism spectrum disorder. *American Journal of Speech-Language Pathology*, *24*(3), 400–410. doi:10.1044/2015_AJSLP-13-0138 PMID:25836377

Fombonne, E. (2009). Epidemiology of pervasive developmental disorders. *Pediatric Research*, *65*(6), 591–598. doi:10.1203/PDR.0b013e31819e7203 PMID:19218885

Fonagy, P., & Target, M. (1997). Attachment and reflective function: Their role in self-organization. *Development and Psychopathology*, *9*(4), 679–700. doi:10.1017/S0954579497001399 PMID:9449001

Fonagy, P., & Target, M. (1998). Mentalization and the changing aims of child psychoanalysis. *Psychoanalytic Dialogues*, *8*(1), 87–114. doi:10.1080/10481889809539235

Fountain, C., King, M. D., & Bearman, P. S. (2011). Age of diagnosis for autism: Individual and community factors across 10 birth cohorts. *Journal of Epidemiology and Community Health*, *65*(6), 503–510. doi:10.1136/jech.2009.104588 PMID:20974836

Fountain, C., King, M. D., & Bearman, P. S. (2011). Age of diagnosis for autism: Individual and community factors across 10 birth cohorts. *Journal of Epidemiology and Community Health, 65*(6), 503–510. doi:10.1136/jech.2009.104588 PMID:20974836

Frazier, T. W., Klingemier, E. W., Beukemann, M., Speer, L., Markowitz, L., Parikh, S., ... Ahuja, V. (2016). Development of an objective autism risk index using remote eye tracking. *Journal of the American Academy of Child and Adolescent Psychiatry, 55*(4), 301–309. doi:10.1016/j.jaac.2016.01.011 PMID:27015721

Gardener, H., Spiegelman, D., & Buka, S. L. (2011). Perinatal and neonatal risk factors for autism: A comprehensive meta-analysis. *Pediatrics, 128*(2), 344–355. doi:10.1542/peds.2010-1036 PMID:21746727

Gerdts, J., & Bernier, R. (2011). The broader autism phenotype and its implications on the etiology and treatment of autism spectrum disorders. *Autism Research and Treatment*. PMID:22937250

Gervais, H., Belin, P., Boddaert, N., Leboyer, M., Coez, A., Sfaello, I., ... Zilbovicius, M. (2004). Abnormal cortical voice processing in autism. *Nature Neuroscience, 7*(8), 801–802. doi:10.1038/nn1291 PMID:15258587

Giallo, R., Rose, N., & Vittorino, R. (2011). Fatigue, wellbeing and parenting in mothers of infants and toddlers with sleep problems. *Journal of Reproductive and Infant Psychology, 29*(3), 236–249. doi:10.1080/02646838.2011.593030 PMID:29517311

Green, J., Charman, T., McConachie, H., Aldred, C., Slonims, V., Howlin, P., ... Pickles, A. (2010). Parent-mediated communication-focused treatment in children with autism (PACT): A randomised controlled trial. *Lancet, 375*(9732), 2152–2160. doi:10.1016/S0140-6736(10)60587-9 PMID:20494434

Green, J., Pickles, A., Pasco, G., Bedford, R., Wan, M. W., Elsabbagh, M., ... Johnson, M. (2017). Randomised trial of a parent-mediated intervention for infants at high risk for autism: Longitudinal outcomes to age 3 years. *Journal of Child Psychology and Psychiatry, and Allied Disciplines, 58*(12), 1330–1340. doi:10.1111/jcpp.12728 PMID:28393350

Green, J., Rahman, A., Divan, G., Handani, S. U., Vajaratkar, M., Taylor, C., ... Patel, V. (2015). The effectiveness of the parent-mediated intervention for Autism Spectrum Disorders in South Asia (PASS) an RCT in India and Pakistan. *The Lancet. Psychiatry, 3*(2), 128–136. PMID:26704571

Green, V. A., Pituch, K. A., Itchon, J., Choi, A., O'Reilly, M., & Sigafoos, J. (2006). Internet survey of treatments used by parents of children with autism. *Research in Developmental Disabilities*, *27*(1), 70–84. doi:10.1016/j.ridd.2004.12.002 PMID:15919178

He, X., Sanders, S. J., Liu, L., De Rubeis, S., Lim, E. T., Sutcliffe, J. S., ... Devlin, B. (2013). Integrated model of de novo and inherited genetic variants yields greater power to identify risk genes. *PLOS Genetics*, *9*(8), e1003671. doi:10.1371/journal.pgen.1003671 PMID:23966865

Higgins, D. J., Bailey, S. R., & Pearce, J. C. (2005). Factors associated with functioning style and coping strategies of families with a child with an autism spectrum disorder. *Autism*, *9*(2), 125–137. doi:10.1177/1362361305051403 PMID:15857858

Holliday Willey, L. (1999). *Pretending to be normal: Living with Asperger's syndrome*. London: Jessica Kingsley.

Jordan, R. (2003). Social play and autistic spectrum disorders: A perspective on theory, implications and educational approaches. *Autism*, *7*(4), 347–360. doi:10.1177/1362361303007004002 PMID:14678675

Juffer, F., Bakermans-Kranenburg, M. J., & Van IJzendoorn, M. H. (2008). *Introduction and outline of the VIPP and VIPP-R program. Promoting positive parenting: An attachment-based intervention*. Mahwah, NJ: Erlbaum.

Juffer, F., Bakermans-Kranenburg, M. J., & van IJzendoorn, M. J. (2008). Promoting positive parenting: An introduction. In F. Juffer, M. J. Bakermans-Kranenburg, & M. J. van IJzendoorn (Eds.), Promoting positive parenting: An attachment based intervention. New York, NY: Taylor and Francis.

Kim, Y. S., Leventhal, B. L., Koh, Y. J., Fombonne, E., Laska, E., Lim, E. C., ... Song, D. H. (2011). Prevalence of autism spectrum disorders in a total population sample. *The American Journal of Psychiatry*, *168*(9), 904–912. doi:10.1176/appi.ajp.2011.10101532 PMID:21558103

Konstantareas, M. (2008). Temperament and internalizing disorders in children with Asperger's disorder: Implications for interventions. *International Journal of Psychology*, *43*(3-4), 544–564.

Krishnan, A., Zhang, R., Yao, V., Theesfeld, C. L., Wong, A. K., Tadych, A., ... Troyanskaya, O. G. (2016). Genome-wide prediction and functional characterization of the genetic basis of autism spectrum disorder. *Nature Neuroscience*, *19*(11), 1454–1462. doi:10.1038/nn.4353 PMID:27479844

Kuhn, J. C., & Carter, A. S. (2006). Maternal self-efficacy and associated parenting cognitions among mothers of children with autism. *The American Journal of Orthopsychiatry*, *76*(4), 564–575. doi:10.1037/0002-9432.76.4.564 PMID:17209724

Lord, C., Elsabbagh, M., Baird, G., & Veenstra-Vanderweele, J. (2018). Autism spectrum disorder. *Lancet*, *0*(0), 508–520. doi:10.1016/S0140-6736(18)31129-2 PMID:30078460

Losh, M., Martin, G. E., Lee, M., Klusek, J., Sideris, J., Barron, S., & Wassink, T. (2017). Developmental markers of genetic liability to autism in parents: A longitudinal, multigenerational study. *Journal of Autism and Developmental Disorders*, *47*(3), 834–845. doi:10.100710803-016-2996-x PMID:28070788

Lovaas, O. I., Koegel, R., Simmons, J. Q., & Long, J. S. (1970, June). Strengths and weaknesses of operant conditioning techniques for the treatment of autism. In *Proceedings of the conference and annual meeting of the National Society for Autistic Children* (pp. 30-41). Academic Press.

Magrelli, S., Jermann, P., Basilio, N., Ansermet, F., Hentsch, F., Nadel, J., & Billard, A. (2013). Social orienting of children with autism to facial expressions and speech: A study with a wearable eye-tracker in naturalistic settings. *Frontiers in Psychology*, *4*, 840. doi:10.3389/fpsyg.2013.00840 PMID:24312064

Makrygianni, M. K., & Reed, P. (2010). A meta-analytic review of the effectiveness of behavioral early intervention programs for children with autistic spectrum disorders. *Research in Autism Spectrum Disorders*, *4*(4), 577–593. doi:10.1016/j.rasd.2010.01.014

Malkova, N. V., Collin, Z. Y., Hsiao, E. Y., Moore, M. J., & Patterson, P. H. (2012). Maternal immune activation yields offspring displaying mouse versions of the three core symptoms of autism. *Brain, Behavior, and Immunity*, *26*(4), 607–616. doi:10.1016/j.bbi.2012.01.011 PMID:22310922

Masi, A., De Mayo, M. M., Glozier, N., & Guastella, A. J. (2017). An overview of autism spectrum disorder, heterogeneity and treatment options. *Neuroscience Bulletin*, *33*(2), 183–193. doi:10.100712264-017-0100-y PMID:28213805

Masi, A., Quintana, D. S., Glozier, N., Lloyd, A. R., Hickie, I. B., & Guastella, A. J. (2015). Cytokine aberrations in autism spectrum disorder: A systematic review and meta-analysis. *Molecular Psychiatry*, *20*(4), 440–446. doi:10.1038/mp.2014.59 PMID:24934179

McAuliffe, T., Thomas, Y., Vaz, S., Falkmer, T., & Cordier, R. (2019). The experiences of mothers of children with autism spectrum disorder: Managing family routines and mothers' health and wellbeing. *Australian Occupational Therapy Journal*, *66*(1), 68–76. doi:10.1111/1440-1630.12524 PMID:30264526

McConnell, S. R. (2002). Interventions to facilitate social interaction for young children with autism: Review of available research and recommendations for educational intervention and future research. *Journal of Autism and Developmental Disorders*, *32*(5), 351–372. doi:10.1023/A:1020537805154 PMID:12463515

McEvoy, R. E., Rogers, S. J., & Pennington, B. F. (1993). Executive function and social communication deficits in young autistic children. *Journal of Child Psychology and Psychiatry, and Allied Disciplines*, *34*(4), 563–578. doi:10.1111/j.1469-7610.1993.tb01036.x PMID:7685360

Mundy, P., Sigman, M., Ungerer, J., & Sherman, T. (1986). Defining the social deficits of autism: The contribution of non-verbal communication measures. *Journal of Child Psychology and Psychiatry, and Allied Disciplines*, *27*(5), 657–669. doi:10.1111/j.1469-7610.1986.tb00190.x PMID:3771682

Naber, F. B., Bakermans-Kranenburg, M. J., Van Ijzendoorn, M. H., Swinkels, S. H., Buitelaar, J. K., Dietz, C., ... Van Engeland, H. (2008). Play behavior and attachment in toddlers with autism. *Journal of Autism and Developmental Disorders*, *38*(5), 857–866. doi:10.100710803-007-0454-5 PMID:17896172

Naber, F. B. A., Bakermans-Kranenburg, M. J., van IJzendoorn, M. H., Dietz, C., van Daalen, E., Swinkels, S. H. M., ... van Engeland, H. (2008). Joint attention development in toddlers with autism. *European Journal of Child and Adolescent Psychiatry*, *17*(3), 143–152. doi:10.100700787-007-0648-6 PMID:17849078

Newschaffer, C. J., Croen, L. A., Daniels, J., Giarelli, E., Grether, J. K., Levy, S. E., ... Reynolds, A. M. (2007). The epidemiology of autism spectrum disorders. *Annual Review of Public Health*, *28*(1), 235–258. doi:10.1146/annurev.publhealth.28.021406.144007 PMID:17367287

Oono, I. P., Honey, E. J., & McConachie, H. (2013). Parent-mediated early intervention for young children with autism spectrum disorders (ASD). *Evidence-Based Child Health: A Cochrane Review Journal*, *8*(6), 2380–2479. doi:10.1002/ebch.1952 PMID:23633377

Oosterling, I. J., Wensing, M., Swinkels, S. H., Van Der Gaag, R. J., Visser, J. C., Woudenberg, T., ... Buitelaar, J. K. (2010). Advancing early detection of autism spectrum disorder by applying an integrated two-stage screening approach. *Journal of Child Psychology and Psychiatry, and Allied Disciplines*, *51*(3), 250–258. doi:10.1111/j.1469-7610.2009.02150.x PMID:19843319

Ospina, M. B., Seida, J. K., Clark, B., Karkhaneh, M., Hartling, L., Tjosvold, L., ... Smith, V. (2008). Behavioral and developmental interventions for autism spectrum disorder: A clinical systematic review. *PLoS One*, *3*(11), e3755. doi:10.1371/journal.pone.0003755 PMID:19015734

Ostfeld-Etzion, S., Golan, O., Hirschler-Guttenberg, Y., Zagoory-Sharon, O., & Feldman, R. (2015). Neuroendocrine and behavioral response to social rupture and repair in preschoolers with autism spectrum disorders interacting with mother and father. *Molecular Autism*, *6*(1), 11. doi:10.118613229-015-0007-2 PMID:25774280

Pajareya, K., & Nopmaneejumruslers, K. (2011). A pilot randomized controlled trial of DIR/Floortime™ parent training intervention for pre-school children with autistic spectrum disorders. *Autism*, *15*(5), 563–577. doi:10.1177/1362361310386502 PMID:21690083

Peters-Scheffer, N., Didden, R., Korzilius, H., & Sturmey, P. (2011). A meta-analytic study on the effectiveness of comprehensive ABA-based early intervention programs for children with autism spectrum disorders. *Research in Autism Spectrum Disorders*, *5*(1), 60–69. doi:10.1016/j.rasd.2010.03.011

Pickles, A., Le Couteur, A., Leadbitter, K., Salomone, E., Cole-Fletcher, R., Tobin, H., ... Aldred, C. (2016). Parent-mediated social communication therapy for young children with autism (PACT): Long-term follow-up of a randomised controlled trial. *Lancet*, *388*(10059), 2501–2509. doi:10.1016/S0140-6736(16)31229-6 PMID:27793431

Ploog, B. O. (2010). Stimulus overselectivity four decades later: A review of the literature and its implications for current research in autism spectrum disorder. *Journal of Autism and Developmental Disorders*, *40*(11), 1332–1349. doi:10.100710803-010-0990-2 PMID:20238154

Poslawsky, I. E., Naber, F. B., Bakermans-Kranenburg, M. J., De Jonge, M. V., Van Engeland, H., & Van IJzendoorn, M. H. (2014). Development of a Video-feedback Intervention to promote Positive Parenting for Children with Autism (VIPP-AUTI). *Attachment & Human Development*, *16*(4), 343–355. doi:10.1080/14616734.2014.912487 PMID:24972103

Poslawsky, I. E., Naber, F. B., Bakermans-Kranenburg, M. J., van Daalen, E., van Engeland, H., & van IJzendoorn, M. H. (2015). Video-feedback Intervention to promote Positive Parenting adapted to Autism (VIPP-AUTI): A randomized controlled trial. *Autism, 19*(5), 588–603. doi:10.1177/1362361314537124 PMID:24919961

Prior, V., & Glaser, D. (2006). *Understanding attachment and attachment disorders: Theory, evidence and practice*. Jessica Kingsley Publishers.

Rogers, S. J., & Vismara, L. A. (2008). Evidence-based comprehensive treatments for early autism. *Journal of Clinical Child and Adolescent Psychology, 37*(1), 8–38. doi:10.1080/15374410701817808 PMID:18444052

Rozga, A., Hesse, E., Main, M., Duschinsky, R., Beckwith, L., & Sigman, M. (2018). A short-term longitudinal study of correlates and sequelae of attachment security in autism. *Attachment & Human Development, 20*(2), 160–180. doi:10.1080/14616734.2017.1383489 PMID:28959921

Rutgers, A. H., Van Ijzendoorn, M. H., Bakermans-Kranenburg, M. J., Swinkels, S. H., Van Daalen, E., Dietz, C., ... Van Engeland, H. (2007). Autism, attachment and parenting: A comparison of children with autism spectrum disorder, mental retardation, language disorder, and non-clinical children. *Journal of Abnormal Child Psychology, 35*(5), 859–870. doi:10.100710802-007-9139-y PMID:17505877

Safe, A., Joosten, A., & Molineux, M. (2012). The experiences of mothers of children with autism: Managing multiple roles. *Journal of Intellectual & Developmental Disability, 37*(4), 294–302. doi:10.3109/13668250.2012.736614 PMID:23171310

Sasson, N. J., Lam, K. S., Parlier, M., Daniels, J. L., & Piven, J. (2013). Autism and the broad autism phenotype: Familial patterns and intergenerational transmission. *Journal of Neurodevelopmental Disorders, 5*(1), 11. doi:10.1186/1866-1955-5-11 PMID:23639131

Schaaf, C. P., & Zoghbi, H. Y. (2011). Solving the autism puzzle a few pieces at a time. *Neuron, 70*(5), 806–808. doi:10.1016/j.neuron.2011.05.025 PMID:21658575

Schopler, E. (1994). A statewide program for the treatment and education of autistic and related communication handicapped children (TEACCH). *Child and Adolescent Psychiatric Clinics, 3*(1), 91–103. doi:10.1016/S1056-4993(18)30517-0

Schwichtenberg, A., & Poehlmann, J. (2007). Applied behavior analysis: Does intervention intensity relate to family stressors and maternal well-being? *Journal of Intellectual Disability Research, 51*(8), 598–605. doi:10.1111/j.1365-2788.2006.00940.x PMID:17598873

Sigman, M., & Ungerer, J. A. (1984). Attachment behaviors in autistic children. *Journal of Autism and Developmental Disorders*, *14*(3), 231–244. doi:10.1007/BF02409576 PMID:6207163

Steele, M., Steele, H., Bate, J., Knafo, H., Kinsey, M., Bonuck, K., ... Murphy, A. (2014). Looking from the outside in: The use of video in attachment-based interventions. *Attachment & Human Development*, *16*(4), 402–415. doi:10.1080/14616734.2014.912491 PMID:24972107

Steiner, A. M., Koegel, L. K., Koegel, R. L., & Ence, W. A. (2012). Issues and theoretical constructs regarding parent education for autism spectrum disorders. *Journal of Autism and Developmental Disorders*, *42*(6), 1218–1227. doi:10.100710803-011-1194-0 PMID:21336525

Sucksmith, E., Roth, I., & Hoekstra, R. A. (2011). Autistic traits below the clinical threshold: Re-examining the broader autism phenotype in the 21st century. *Neuropsychology Review*, *21*(4), 360–389. doi:10.100711065-011-9183-9 PMID:21989834

Taylor, L. E., Swerdfeger, A. L., & Eslick, G. D. (2014). Vaccines are not associated with autism: An evidence-based meta-analysis of case-control and cohort studies. *Vaccine*, *32*(29), 3623–3629. doi:10.1016/j.vaccine.2014.04.085 PMID:24814559

Tronick, E. Z. (1989). Emotions and emotional communication in infants. *The American Psychologist*, *44*(2), 112–119. doi:10.1037/0003-066X.44.2.112 PMID:2653124

Vaillant, G. E. (1992). Ego mechanisms of defense: a guide for clinicans and researchers. American Psychiatric Pub.

Van IJzendoorn, M. H., Rutgers, A. H., Bakermans-Kranenburg, M. J., Swinkels, S. H., Van Daalen, E., Dietz, C., ... Van Engeland, H. (2007). Parental sensitivity and attachment in children with autism spectrum disorder: Comparison with children with mental retardation, with language delays, and with typical development. *Child Development*, *78*(2), 597–608. doi:10.1111/j.1467-8624.2007.01016.x PMID:17381792

Vernetti, A., Senju, A., Charman, T., Johnson, M. H., & Gliga, T. (2018). Simulating interaction: Using gaze-contingent eye-tracking to measure the reward value of social signals in toddlers with and without autism. *Developmental Cognitive Neuroscience*, *29*, 21–29. doi:10.1016/j.dcn.2017.08.004 PMID:28939027

Vik, K., & Rohde, R. (2014). Tiny moments of great importance: The Marte Meo method applied in the context of early mother–infant interaction and postnatal depression. Utilizing Daniel Stern's theory of 'schemas of being with' in understanding empirical findings and developing a stringent Marte Meo methodology. *Clinical Child Psychology and Psychiatry*, *19*(1), 77–89. doi:10.1177/1359104512468286 PMID:23242466

Wan, M. W., Green, J., Elsabbagh, M., Johnson, M., Charman, T., & Plummer, F. (2012). Parent–infant interaction in infant siblings at risk of autism. *Research in Developmental Disabilities*, *33*(3), 924–932. doi:10.1016/j.ridd.2011.12.011 PMID:22257674

Werling, D. M., & Geschwind, D. H. (2013). Sex differences in autism spectrum disorders. *Current Opinion in Neurology*, *26*(2), 146–153. doi:10.1097/WCO.0b013e32835ee548 PMID:23406909

Wetherby, A. M., Woods, J., Allen, L., Cleary, J., Dickinson, H., & Lord, C. (2004). Early indicators of autism spectrum disorders in the second year of life. *Journal of Autism and Developmental Disorders*, *34*(5), 473–493. doi:10.100710803-004-2544-y PMID:15628603

Wieder, S., & Greenspan, S. I. (2003). Climbing the symbolic ladder in the DIR model through floor time/interactive play. *Autism*, *7*(4), 425–435. doi:10.1177/1362361303007004008 PMID:14678681

Yaman, A., Mesman, J., van IJzendoorn, M. H., Bakermans-Kranenburg, M. J., & Linting, M. (2010). Parenting in an individualistic culture with a collectivistic cultural background: The case of Turkish immigrant families with toddlers in the Netherlands. *Journal of Child and Family Studies*, *19*(5), 617–628. doi:10.100710826-009-9346-y PMID:20835387

KEY TERMS AND DEFINITIONS

Attachment: Attachment is a system of behaviors and emotions connecting two individuals. According to Bowlby (1969), attachment can be described as the system of protection and socio-emotional needs of the child that are satisfied in proximity to the caregiver.

Broad Autism Phenotype: The Broad Autism Phenotype (BAP) is a concept that refers to the mild phenotypic expression of autism-related symptoms among relatives of individuals with ASD. These include cognitive, personality, social and language features.

Joint Attention: Joint attention is an individual's ability to share the focus of attention toward an object. It can be achieved by means of eye-gazing, pointing or through verbal indications. Joint attention was demonstrated to be a developmental precursor to many social and cognitive skills.

Parental Intrusiveness: Parental intrusiveness is enacted by caregivers who disrupt children's play patterns by excessively verbally and physically directing them, or even by replacing them when play-situations require specific tasks.

Parental Sensitivity: In 1978, Mary Ainsworth defined parental sensitivity as the parent's capacity to detect and interpret children's attachment signals and the ability to adequately provide answers on time.

Secure Base: Secure base refers to the parental role in the attachment system since the parent has to be a source of protection and a base to return to when the child interrupts exploration behaviors.

Still Face Paradigm: The Still Face, developed by Edward Tronick in 1978, is an experimental procedure consisting of a disruption to parent-baby face-to-face interactions; the parent abruptly stops communicating and reacting to the child's signals, by remaining still and emotionless in front of his/her son/daughter for a short time-interval.

Symbolic Play: Symbolic play represents a developmental milestone usually achieved at around two years of age. It is the ability to use objects or toys to represent other objects or actions during play sessions (i.e., to use a banana as if it were a mobile phone).

Chapter 10
The History and Evolution of Infant-Parental Attachment Security

Erika Nolan
Marymount Manhattan College, USA

ABSTRACT

From an ethological viewpoint, the term "attachment" refers to the affectional tie developed between two animals that creates a lasting bond. While the term generally refers to animals, for the purpose of this chapter, this term will be used to describe bonds among humans. Mainly, the word attachment will be used to analyze and describe the bond between an infant and his/her primary caregiver. One of the primary characteristics of attachment is the desire to maintain close proximity. This is accomplished through attachment behaviors, which are behaviors that support proximity to the attachment figure.

INTRODUCTION

The Origins of Attachment Theory

John Bowlby

Although there were many early contributors to attachment theory, John Bowlby is often considered to be the founder of the field and to be the most influential. He graduated from the University of Cambridge in 1928 and soon after, began working at a school for maladjusted children. There were two children at the school who

DOI: 10.4018/978-1-7998-2940-9.ch010

sparked his interest. The first lacked a consistent maternal figure and commonly displayed violent, delinquent behaviors. The second was a very shy and anxious young boy who tended to follow Bowlby while at work. These two children, while displaying very different personalities, inspired Bowlby to research how personality development is affected by family relationships. Soon after, Bowlby began work at the London Child Guidance Clinic. Here, he often met children who exhibited different types of behavioral problems linked with emotional disturbances. He slowly began to trace the origins of these emotional disturbances back to early familial experiences. This led to his first empirical study (Bretherton, 1992).

Bowlby gathered extensive notes on 44 children at the clinic. Similar to the children Bowlby met at his first job, the patients at the London Child Guidance Clinic often exhibited un-empathic behaviors such as lying and theft. After reviewing his notes, Bowlby began to theorize that the mischievous behavior displayed by his clients could possibly be related to maternal deprivation and separation. It was this research that introduced the idea that perhaps the answer to treating maladjusted children was to treat their parents. After World War II, Bowlby worked in the Children's Department of The Tavistock Clinic. This work provided Bowlby with the opportunity to gain expertise in statistical analysis that would later prove useful in conducting research and in developing his theories (Bretherton, 1992).

In 1948, Bowlby hired James Robertson to observe institutionalized and hospitalized children who had had experiences with parental separation. Previously, Robertson had worked under the direction of Anna Freud in a nursery for homeless children during World War II. Anna Freud required all of her employees to take notes on the children's behavior. In this way, Robertson was given the opportunity to gather experiences using naturalistic observation (Bretherton, 1992). This is a technique many researchers use that allows for a more accurate representation of behavior. It is accomplished by recording behavior made by an individual while in his/her natural habitat. Thus, the behavior of the subject may remain unmodified since they do not need to adapt to an unnatural environment or experience. The introduction of naturalistic observation to the field was a turning point in the development of attachment theory and will be further explained in the "Ainsworth Subsection" of this chapter (Bretherton, 1992).

Bowlby was then appointed to write about the effects of war on mental health in "the mental health of homeless children in postwar Europe" by the World Health Organization (WHO) in 1949. While preparing for the report, Bowlby was able to meet many people in his field who were also interested in attachment. Specifically, he met individuals who were interested in the mental health effects of maternal abandonment and neglect on children. The report was titled "Maternal Care and Mental Health," and published in 1951 (Bretherton, 1992).

In the report, Bowlby compares mental development to physical development. He emphasizes that there are critical periods in physical development that rely on exposure to correct stimuli. Similar to physical development, Bowlby argues that there are critical periods in mental development as well. He writes that the exposure needed during these critical periods is the presence of the mother, though Bowlby thought social networks, Economics, and health factors were also influential in the development of successful relationships between mothers and children (Bretherton, 1992).

Perhaps the principal point made in this report is the emphasis on the importance of mutual satisfaction between the mother and child. Bowlby theorized that the ability for a child to grow up mentally healthy relied heavily on experiencing a nurturing, tender, and consistent relationship with the mother. The concept of mutual satisfaction is applied to this idea by reiterating that the relationship must be equally rewarding to the child as it is to the mother (Bretherton, 1992). Bowlby's notion of mutual satisfaction would become one of the primary factors in establishing a secure attachment as a parent, as will be seen throughout this chapter.

The link between physical and mental development led Bowlby to begin to look at attachment from an ethological viewpoint. Prior to this, ethology, the study of animal behavior, had only mildly been linked to attachment. One of these links was made in an experiment conducted by Australian researcher Konrad Lorenz in 1935. Lorenz's work was a major influence in the development of Bowlby's ethological definition of attachment theory (Bretherton, 1992).

The purpose of Lorenz's experiment was to research the process of imprinting in a group of newborn ducklings. Imprinting is defined as the process in which certain avian species follow and form an attachment to the first moving object they perceive at birth. Naturally, this object of attachment is almost exclusively the bird's mother. (Vicedo, 2009).

Lorenz actively manipulated the ducklings' environments, so that he would be the first moving object the ducklings would see after hatching (Vicedo, 2009). This was critical for the evolution of Bowlby's theories for two reasons. The first was the indication that attachment did not rely on breastfeeding. This contradicted Freud's earlier theories that underlined the importance of oral gratification in forming attachments. The second way in which Lorenz's study shaped Bowlby's theories was due to the fact that Lorenz favored naturalistic observation from an ethological standpoint. Both of these qualities shaped the work that Bowlby would go on to pursue, thereby shaping the overall evolution of attachment theory (Bretherton, 1992).

Mary Salter Ainsworth

Mary Salter was introduced to security theory by a professor while pursuing a graduate degree at the University of Toronto. Security Theory is the idea that in order for children to have the ability to embark upon unfamiliar situations, they must have a secure dependence on parents. Salter highlights this theory in her dissertation entitled, "An Evaluation of Adjustment Based on the Concept of Security." She argues that this secure dependence forms the base upon which a child is able to develop interests and skills. If a child does not experience a secure base, his/her interest in exploration diminishes, which can result in the inability to develop in a normal way (Bretherton, 1992).

Mary Salter married and became Mary Ainsworth in 1950. She moved to London with her husband, where a job posting sparked her interest. The opportunity involved research on the effects that early childhood separation from the mother has on personality development. Ainsworth would work under the direction of John Bowlby. This collaboration, though not evident at the time, ultimately shaped the evolution of attachment theory (Bretherton, 1992).

Ainsworth was appointed to analyze the recorded observations made by James Robertson on the institutionalized and hospitalized children under Bowlby's direction. This was important in the development of attachment theory because it introduced Ainsworth to naturalistic observation techniques as a way of gathering data. She would later go on to use this method to conduct her own studies (Bretherton, 1992).

In 1953, Ainsworth conducted the first empirical study of infant attachment in Uganda. She used observational and longitudinal techniques to study the development of attachment between mothers and infants. Her participants included 26 families with children ages 1-24 months. She observed each dyad interact for two hours twice a week over a nine month period. Ainsworth was most interested in observing the quality of interactions between mothers and infants, specifically, the extent to which mothers effectively responded to their infants' signals. These signals are defined as behaviors displayed by an infant that indicate the desire for proximity to their mother. Ainsworth specifically noted when these proximity promoting behaviors were directed towards the mother (Bretherton, 1992).

Ainsworth's Uganda study lead to the classification of three diverse types of infant attachment. These attachment types were thought to describe the relationship of each dyad. Infants were defined as securely attached, insecurely attached, or not yet attached. The balance between the infant's crying and exploration of his/her environment was the basis of defining these attachment classifications. Infants with secure attachments did not cry often and contently explored their surroundings. Infants with insecure attachments were hesitant to explore their surroundings and cried regularly. Being held by their mothers often did not console these infants when they were upset. Unattached infants appeared to show complete indifference towards their mother (Bretherton, 1992).

The study's findings found a significant correlation between infant attachment and maternal sensitivity. Furthermore, children with secure attachments had mothers who tended to display higher levels of sensitivity. In short, mothers were described as having higher levels of sensitivity when they were more receptive to their child's behaviors that promoted proximity (Bretherton, 1992). A more in depth definition of maternal sensitivity can be found in the "Maternal Sensitivity Section" of this chapter.

In studies like these, it is important to note that the term correlation does not imply causation. It is possible that there are other reasons that children with more sensitive mothers tended to have more secure attachments. The study simply indicates that there is some significant relationship between the two. Ainsworth's Uganda Study also indicated a correlation between the maternal enjoyment of breastfeeding and infant security (Bretherton, 1992).

In 1956, Ainsworth and Bowlby worked on a paper along with Boston and Rosenbluth. Perhaps the greatest accomplishment in this work was the three classifications made by Ainsworth to categorize parent-child relationships. The classifications were "strong positive feelings toward their mothers," "uncertainty towards mothers," and "non-expressive, indifferent, or hostile relationships with the mother." These three classifications would evolve to become the basis of one of the most influential studies on attachment theory conducted by Mary Ainsworth (Bretherton, 1992).

In 1963, Ainsworth traveled to Baltimore to conduct her second empirical study. Similar to her study in Uganda, this study used naturalistic observational and longitudinal techniques to gather data. The sample was composed of 26 families. Ainsworth conducted 18 home visits once the infants reached one month of age. These visits extended throughout the infants' first year of life. To ensure that the utmost natural behavior was gathered, each visit was approximately four hours long. The purpose of incorporating a longer visit was to ensure the mothers' comfort with carrying out their usual daily routines, even while in the presence of an observer. Notes were written by hand every five minutes. (Bretherton, 1992).

Ainsworth expanded on her Uganda study to analyze more behaviors. She recorded "feeding situations, mother-infant face-to-face interaction, crying, infant greetings and following, attachment exploration balance, obedience, close bodily contact, approach behavior, and affectionate contact." Interestingly, the importance of maternal sensitivity was extremely evident during breastfeeding. When mothers were more aware of their infants' cues, the result was a harmonious experience for both parties. In contrast, there were mothers who had difficulties in adjusting and correctly interpreting the child's needs. This resulted in struggling, choking, or spitting up (Bretherton, 1992).

The effects of maternal sensitivity on attachment were also seen in this study as the relationship between mother and infant developed. Overall, higher levels of maternal sensitivity during the infant's first quarter of life, was linked to more harmonious infant-mother relationships in the last quarter. Furthermore, infants whose mothers were more attentive to their crying in the beginning of the year tended to cry less towards the end of the year. These findings discredit the fear that over-attending to an infant's cries could result in the child developing selfish or demanding personality traits. Similar results were found when analyzing bodily contact. Infants who received more affectionate holding during the beginning of the year tended to desire bodily contact less frequently. However, the contact made by these dyads were rated as more satisfying when they did occur (Bretherton, 1992).

Ainsworth's Strange Situation

Perhaps one of the most influential studies that shaped modern attachment theory was Ainsworth's "Strange Situation." Drawing from the Uganda and Baltimore Studies, the purpose of the study was to gather data that was unattainable through means of naturalistic observation. It was designed to examine infant attachment behaviors and exploratory tendencies when combined with an unfamiliar situation. The Strange Situation was comprised of eight episodes, and was meant to create a sense of novelty that would influence exploratory behavior. The sense of novelty, however, needed to be constructed without creating initial feelings of fear and alarm that could alter the study's findings (Ainsworth and Bell, 1970).

In the first episode, the mother and child are escorted by an observer to a semi-furnished room filled with toys. The mother places the child in a designated spot and sits in a chair, all the while not interacting unless the child actively seeks attention. This goes on for three minutes. A stranger enters and sits next to the mother in silence for one minute. The mother and stranger converse for one minute. The stranger then approaches the child with a toy for one minute as the mother leaves. The child and the stranger are left alone in the room for three minutes, during which the stranger's interaction with the child is determined by the child's response. This is the first separation episode and is the fourth episode of the overall situation (Ainsworth and Bell, 1970).

The first reunion episode begins when the mother reenters as the stranger leaves. The mother is instructed to allow the child to show some sort of response to her before consoling the child. Once the child is deemed relaxed and playing with toys, the mother leaves the room again. The child is left completely alone, which accounts for the second separation episode. This episode lasts up to three minutes, but the exact duration relies on the level of distress displayed by the child. The stranger reenters and attempts to engage in play with the child. The mother then returns as the stranger leaves, completing the situation (Ainsworth and Bell, 1970).

Data was collected by two unseen observers who recorded the child's behavior every 15 seconds, and coded two types of behaviors. Exploratory behavior including "locomotor, manipulatory, and visual exploration" were recorded along with "proximity and contact-seeking behaviors, contact-maintaining behaviors, proximity and interaction-avoiding behaviors, contact-and interaction resisting behaviors, and search behavior" (Ainsworth and Bell, 1970).

While the initial purpose of the study was to assess how the presence or absence of the mother influenced the child's exploratory behaviors, Ainsworth noticed that the study had other findings that perhaps would prove more beneficial to the study of attachment. This was the child's reaction to the return of his/her mother. Furthermore, she was able to link these specific behaviors to data drawn from her previous home observations (Ainsworth and Bell, 1970).

CLASSIFICATIONS OF ATTACHMENT

Ainsworth Strange Situation Findings

As stated previously, Ainsworth's Strange Situation resulted in three classifications of infant-mother attachment patterns. These classifications are secure, insecure avoidant, and insecure anxious/resistant. While there are many behaviors that contribute to the calculation of classifying a child, the classifications are largely distinguished by the behavior displayed during the separation episodes (Ainsworth, 1969).

Children with *secure attachments,* known by Ainsworth as Group B, displayed confidence that their mother would meet their needs. These children actively made attempts to gain proximity to her during the reunion episodes. Secure children tended to prefer interactions with the mother over the stranger. This is made clear in their child's behavior during the second separation. Their distraught feelings are due to the absence of the mother rather than due to being left alone, and while some may be comforted by the stranger during this episode, it is clear they want their mother (Ainsworth, 1969).

Generally, children with *insecure avoidant attachments* (Group A) do not show interest in gaining proximity or other forms of connection with their mothers. They appear ambivalent when held, and do not resist being put down or make any efforts to continue being held. Furthermore, they do not typically greet their mothers with warmth during the reunion episodes. Instead, they appear indifferent towards the mother's return (Ainsworth, 1969).

The primary distinction among infants with *insecure anxious resistant attachments,* referred to as Group C, is the lack of using their mother as a secure base from which to explore. This is especially notable during the first two episodes. While some children simply do not exhibit many exploratory behaviors, others do in fact seem to explore, but do not display behaviors of satisfaction while doing so (Ainsworth, 1969).

Modern Classifications of Attachment

Contemporary classifications of infant-child behavior are often still determined through a Strange Situation. Dr. Samantha Berkule, an expert in attachment theory and conductor of her own Strange Situations, highlights the importance of carrying out the episodes as Ainsworth initially intended. This is necessary in order for any findings to be considered valid. Similarly, the classifications of attachment are already fixed, as defined by Ainsworth in her original study. Current researchers, however, validate the disorganized attachment classification first established by Mary Main in 1990 (Berkule, 2019).

While it may seem that there are defining factors of each attachment type, Dr. Berkule underscores the notion that there is no specific behavior that creates or alters a classification. There are many behaviors that are coded throughout the Strange Situation, and these behaviors are combined to create an overall classification (Berkule, 2019). That being said, there have been patterns observed that can prove useful in defining the attachment types.

One of the primary characteristics of a secure attachment is often thought to be the confidence that the child has in his/her attachment figure. Since the attachment between the child and caregiver is a strong and positive one, the child possesses the ability to explore his/her surroundings. The child is able to do so with trust that the attachment figure will be available to help in instances of concern (McLeod, 2018). This confidence has as much to do with the caregiver as it does with the child. Many scholars agree that the key to a secure attachment is consistency. The child is able to trust their caregiver and use them as a secure base because their caregiver has consistently and successfully responded to their needs in the past (Johnson, 2019). This is seen in the reunion episodes of Ainsworth's Strange Situation. Secure children are easily consoled by their primary caregivers and are quickly able to return to play and exploration (Beebe and Lachmann, 2014). As previously stated in the "Bowlby Section" of this chapter, another important element of a secure attachment between a child and his/her primary caregiver is mutual satisfaction. The notion that the parent experiences feelings of fulfillment that are equal to those of the child is thought to be imperative (Bretherton, 1992).

In contrast, it is thought that children with insecure avoidant attachments have caregivers that are consistently unavailable. The child learns that they cannot rely on their caregiver and therefore, cannot use them as a secure base to explore (Hazan and Shaver, 1987). In the Strange Situation, these children typically experience high levels of stress during the reunion episodes. This includes increased heart rate and perspiration. It is also common for these children to not display any outward or visual signs of stress. Insecure avoidant children often appear relaxed, yet are extremely uneasy (Johnson, 2019).

Children with insecure anxious resistant attachments are thought to have caregivers that are not consistent. This leaves the child confused and unsure if they can use their caregiver as a secure base (Cassidy and Berlin, 1994). In the Strange Situation, insecure anxious resistant children often appear ambivalent towards the caregiver. This is most likely because they are unaware of what to expect from their caregiver (Johnson, 2019).

THE IMPORTANCE OF SECURE INFANT ATTACHMENT

Cognitive Implications of Early Attachment

As stated earlier, a primary characteristic of a secure attachment as classified by Ainsworth's Strange Situation is the idea of using the mother as a secure base in order to explore. A paper by Ainsworth and Bell (1970) emphasizes the importance of presence, but not necessarily the proximity of the mother in impacting the child's exploratory behaviors. Unfamiliar situations, people, or objects are thought to evoke feelings of either elusion and discomfort, or eagerness and curiosity. While the level of unfamiliarity is most relevant as opposed to the circumstances of the novelty itself, the presence of the attachment figure is also thought to impact how the child perceives and interacts with novelty (Ainsworth and Bell 1970).

Once there is a secure attachment established between an infant and his/her primary caregiver, the child begins to grow independently from his/her attachment figure through exploration of his/her environments. Over time, the child continues to grow farther apart from the caregiver. Throughout this gradual gain of independence, the child possesses the ability to learn from his or her environment. However, when situations of distress or danger arise, the child and attachment figures are reunited, making the bond even stronger (Ainsworth and Bell, 1970).

Stressful situations heighten the child's attachment behavior. His or her attention becomes fully directed towards the object of attachment. The child becomes less concerned with his/her surroundings and his/her sense of exploration diminishes. This idea suggests that since the child is no longer exploring his/her surroundings, his/her potential to learn and gather new information decreases. Researchers believe that prolonged periods of heightened attachment behavior are related to the disruption of the balance between attachment and exploration. It is possible that disruptions such as these can be the effect of extended periods of separation (Ainsworth and Bell, 1970).

There is evidence to suggest that face-to-face interactions between an infant and the primary caregiver influence attachment. These types of interactions at a young age are thought to influence a child's social and cognitive development. At this point in their lives, this is the most advanced form of communication an infant can experience. Years of research suggest that these interactions set the basis for the child's ability to relate to others (Beebe and Lachmann, 2014). Specific examples of how attachment is formed through this type of interaction will be further explained later in this chapter.

Social and Emotional Implications of Early Attachment

Previous research suggests links between infant attachment security on later social and emotional behaviors. Arguably, the basis of this revolves around the idea that once infants reach seven months of age, they establish certain expectations of the degree to which their primary caregivers will meet their emotional needs. These expectations are then thought to influence how infants regulate their own emotions. Infants who are more securely attached tend to be more well-behaved and attentive to paternal discipline. These individuals are also more likely to exhibit fewer behavioral issues, and have stronger, more frequent peer relationships. Secure toddlers are also thought to have higher levels of "coping competence" when presented with "novel stimuli." This includes behaviors such as "affective sharing, social referencing, and inquisitive vocalizing" (Braungart-Rieker, Garwood, Powers and Wang, 2001).

There is also research that indicates an association between mother-infant attachment behavior and emotion regulation. Furthermore, it is possible that emotion regulation is the basis of later socioemotional behaviors. Emotion regulation can be described as behaviors that adjust and control an individual's emotions. In infants, examples of such behaviors include the adjustment of gaze and self-soothing behaviors. Evidence suggests that these emotionally regulating behaviors reduce stress levels in infants. Typically, securely attached infants display suitable responses of emotional regulation of distress in situations that heighten attachment behaviors. Insecurely attached infants have been found to overregulate or under-regulate their emotions. The overregulation of emotions is associated with avoidant infants while the underregulation of emotions is linked to anxious-resistant infants (Braungart-Rieker et al., 2001).

Out of all three attachment types, infants with insecure anxious resistant attachments displayed the highest levels of distress during the Strange Situation overall. Secure infants displayed more appropriate levels of emotion regulation during reunion episodes than insecure anxious resistant infants. What is interesting about this finding is that infants of both classifications showed equal levels of distress during the separation episodes. Typically, insecure avoidant infants were less distressed during the separation episodes and displayed self-comforting behaviors. It is possible that these behaviors were used to regulate emotion. This finding strengthens the argument that infant attachment and emotion regulation are related (Braungart-Rieker et al., 2001).

Links to Adult Romantic Attachments

The attachment created between an infant and their primary caregiver is thought to influence all later attachments that the child will grow to have. This initial attachment gives children certain expectations of how attachment relationships typically work. This framework is referred to as an internal working model. If a child has been able to successfully rely on their primary caregiver, they will expect to be able to rely on future attachment figures. In contrast, if a child learns that their primary caregiver is inconsistent or unreliable, they will expect these qualities in future relationships (Bretherton, 1985).

When analyzing the relationship of child attachment to adult romantic attachment, it is important first to note the difference between generalized representations of attachment and romantic representations of attachment. Generalized representations of attachment are often used to describe the attachment between a child and his/her primary caregiver. This is usually the parent of the child, and most frequently the mother. The Adult Attachment Interview (AAI) is commonly used to evaluate and classify an individual's generalized representation of attachment. This is done by evaluating the effects of childhood experiences with caregivers. The two classifications of the test are secure-autonomous and non-autonomous. While analyzing the effect of childhood attachment on adult romantic relationships, secure-autonomous classifications have commonly been linked to more success in romantic functioning and relationship stability. In contrast, non-autonomous classifications are often related to poorer romantic functions and higher relationship instability and stress (Haydon, Collins, Salvatore, Simpson and Roisman, 2012).

Romantic representations of attachment are often analyzed by the Current Relationship Interview (CRI). The CRI possesses many similar qualities to the AAI. This is because it assesses "state of mind and coherence of discourse regarding romantic attachment experiences" and classifies an individual based on response. It differs, however, in that the CRI focuses on an individual's present romantic partner rather than on a previous caregiver. Similar to the AAI, the secure classification of the CRI has been associated with higher levels of romantic functioning and takes into account cognition and behavior (Haydon et al., 2012).

Early forms of attachment are thought to mold the base upon which all other relationships can be formed. This suggests an evident relationship in which the attachment created between an infant or child and their primary caregiver affects and predicts the romantic relationships that will be experienced throughout life. Furthermore, this theory can also suggest an interlocking dependence between romantic and generalized representations of attachment on account of their theorized shared basis in earlier experiences (Haydon et al., 2012).

In a recent study by Haydon et al. (2012), researchers examined the developmental basis of generalized and romantic attachment representations. The purpose of the study was to determine if the two representations have similar origins in development, or significant associations with romantic tendencies. The researchers hypothesized that both forms of attachment representations would have similar origins in parenting quality and infant attachment security. During the 1970s in Minneapolis, information was collected from 267 mothers who requested care from public health clinics. The children born to these mothers were extensively studied since birth. Once these children reached age 35, there were only 180 still actively participating in the study (Haydon et al., 2019).

The sample participated in Ainsworth's Strange Situation at 12 months of age, and were classified as secure, insecure avoidant, or insecure anxious resistant. Parenting quality was then assessed when the sample was 24 months of age. In order to code, the participants were presented with a series of problems dictated through an interactive video, and were given tools in order to complete the increasingly challenging tasks in a laboratory setting. The tasks dictated by the video were designed to gradually become more difficult and require the help of the mother in order to complete the set task. The behaviors of the mothers were coded to assess parenting quality and to highlight how sensitive she was to her child's emotional and developmental needs (Haydon et al., 2012).

Ego resiliency was assessed at age 54 months through a series of tests taken in a laboratory setting that measured how effectively the sample could adaptively regulate their attention and behavior in response to their changing environments. Once the participants reached age 16, the quality of their adolescent friendships was evaluated. This was conducted via an interview format wherein participants were asked to describe their closest friendships. Individual scores were provided to assess the dictated relationship's security, disclosure, and closeness. These scores were then combined to calculate a single score to categorize adolescent friendship quality (Haydon et al., 2012).

Four measures were assessed when participants were between ages 20 and 21, and again between the ages of 26 to 28. The first were couples assessment procedures and were completed with the participant's current romantic partner of at least 4 months. At both ages, the couples separately completed the CRI and described their perception of the relationship. The couples then completed the Markman-Cox Procedure in which they identify an obstacle in their relationship and seek to come to a mutual agreement within ten minutes. They also completed the Ideal Couple Q-sort in which couples were asked to identify characteristics of an ideal relationship by sorting 45 cards (Haydon et al., 2012).

The second measure taken during this age range was observed romantic behavior. Observers collected behavioral data while each couple completed the assessment procedures previously defined. These observers looked for conflict resolution, secure base processes, and negative reciprocity. Secure base process is referred to as the degree to which the couples exhibited caregiving or care-seeking roles. Negative reciprocity describes negative demands made by one partner directed towards the other (Haydon et al., 2012).

Positive relationship feelings were also measured at this age, and were gathered using the Relationship Assessment Scale, The Emotional Tone Index, and The Subjective Closeness Index. The first gathered information to assess the satisfaction or lack thereof felt by the participant in the current relationship. The Emotional Tone index identified ten positive emotions typically felt in the relationship and measured their frequency. The Subject Closeness Index evaluated the participant's impressions of relationship closeness. The AAI and CRI were used to evaluate participants' general and romantic representations of attachment (Haydon et al., 2019).

The study by Haydon et al. (2012) did indeed find that security-autonomy for both generalized and romantic representations of attachment were positively correlated with early parenting quality. However, only romantic attachment security was associated with ego resiliency at the preschool age. Interestingly, the study found that neither generalized nor romantic security, were associated with infant attachment security. (Haydon, 2012).

The findings of the study also indicated that secure generalized and romantic representations of attachment were positively correlated with efficient conflict resolution. Secure representations of generalized attachments were also positively correlated with secure base behavior, while secure romantic representations were only mildly associated. Neither secure forms of attachment were linked with infant attachment security. This indicates that although early forms of secure attachment are indeed critical for an individual to have successful relationships throughout his/her life, it is possible that it is the attachments formed during the toddler years and beyond that have the most influence on these later relationships (Haydon, 2012).

The findings of the study indicate that both secure representations are indeed linked to early parenting quality. Higher levels of parenting quality were related to forming early secure representations with caregivers. Higher parenting quality was also related to secure representations with participants' later romantic partners. These findings emphasize the importance of forging secure relationships with caregivers at a young age, and how these relationships influence attachments formed with others throughout development (Haydon, 2012).

ESTABLISHING A SECURE ATTACHMENT AS A PARENT

Bodily Contact and Warmth

Some of the earliest data about the formation of infant attachments can be seen in Ainsworth's work. Early evidence has found that mothers of infants with secure attachments picked up their children more affectionately and more frequently than mothers of insecurely attached infants. In this case, the word "affectionately" refers to specific behaviors such as hugging and kissing in addition to general holding (Tracey and Ainsworth, 1981).

Mothers of infants with insecure avoidant attachments were found to be generally more rejecting towards their infants. This idea of rejection is defined as the degree to which a mother's feelings of positivity towards her child are overshadowed by negative feelings of irascibility or resentment. These feelings are caused by the extent to which the child imposes him/herself in the mother's daily routine, interfering with her other interests and activities. Mothers of insecure avoidant infants also display more opposition to or less interest in close bodily contact with their children than mothers of secure and anxious resistant infants (Tracey and Ainsworth, 1981).

The purpose of a study by Tracey and Ainsworth (1981) was to examine maternal affectionate behavior and differentiate the behaviors made by mothers of infants within each form of attachment. Specifically, the researchers were interested in discriminating the behaviors of mothers with infants that had insecure avoidant attachments. The sample included 23 mother-infant dyads in white, middle class families. The sample was observed during the first 12 months of the infant's life. These observations were comprised of four hour visits that occurred every three weeks. The sample participated in a Strange Situation once they turned one year of age (Tracey and Ainsworth, 1981).

Maternal affectionate behavior was divided into four categories. These were "kissing, hugging/cuddling, patting/stroking, and other." The frequency of general affectionate acts made by the mother, were recorded separately from the frequency of acts made within each individual category. The final measure taken was the percentage of each category present in the mother's overall number of affectionate acts. The infant's first year was separated into quarters due to the hypothesis that maternal affectionate behavior would evolve as the child grew (Tracey and Ainsworth, 1981).

The study found that mothers of secure infants showed more total affectionate behaviors than mothers of insecure infants. Mothers of infants with insecure avoidant attachments displayed more affectionate acts than mothers with insecure anxious resistant infants. The data also showed that mothers of insecure avoidant infants kissed their children more frequently than mothers of secure children. However, mothers of secure infants kissed their children more frequently than mothers of insecure anxious resistant infants. Interestingly, kissing comprised a larger percentage of the total affectionate acts displayed by mothers of insecure avoidant infants. This was especially noticeable during the second half of the infant's first year (Tracey and Ainsworth, 1981).

Hugging and cuddling was not a common act of affection among mothers of insecure avoidant infants. In fact, this specific type of affection behavior continued to decrease in the second half of the infant's first year. This decrease created a large gap which distinguished mothers of infants with this type of attachment versus the other two groups. Although the total number of affectionate acts displayed by mothers of insecure anxious resistant infants was relatively low, hugging and cuddling made up for the majority of their affectionate acts overall. This distinguished them from mothers of insecure avoidant infants, but not from mothers of secure infants (Tracey and Ainsworth, 1981).

The fact that mothers of avoidant infants were more likely to kiss their children as a sign of affection whereas mothers of anxious resistant infants were more likely to initiate close bodily contact is important to note. In the Strange Situation, it is the children with insecure avoidant attachments that feel very distressed yet seem unfazed by the separation from their mothers. It is possible that this is because when these infants sought this type of contact in the past, their needs were not met. This possibly resulted in the child not openly searching for these interactions in the future due to the fact that unpleasant feelings were experienced when their needs were not previously met (Tracey and Ainsworth, 1981).

It is important to point out, as well, that hugging and cuddling are often considered a more affectionate act than kissing. During the separation episodes of the Strange Situation, the children's attachment behaviors are heightened. It is bodily contact that the children crave when the mother reenters. All of this emphasizes the importance of bodily contact between an infant and primary caregiver in developing a secure attachment. This evidence also suggests that a lack thereof can lead to an insecure avoidant attachment (Tracey and Ainsworth, 1981).

The importance of bodily contact and warmth and its impact on attachment is a topic that has been heavily discussed. There have been many studies over the past decade that link intimacy to temperature. Specifically, there is evidence to suggest that warmer temperatures are associated with perceptions of social proximity. A study conducted by Vess (2012) analyzed the relationship between intimacy and temperature. The participants were comprised of 56 individuals with an average age of 33 years. Their levels of attachment avoidance and attachment anxiety were measured. The participants were then randomly assigned to two different conditions. In the first, participants were instructed to recall a romantic breakup. Participants in the second condition were asked to remember some sort of random event. They were then asked to rate the degree to which they desired different refreshments. These included warm and room-temperature items such as hot chocolate, pie, crakers, and pretzels (Vess, 2012).

Vess (2012) found that attachment anxiety and the desire for warm temperature refreshments were positively correlated among individuals that described a previous romantic breakup. In contrast, the two measures were unrelated among individuals who described ordinary events. Additionally, participants with higher levels of attachment anxiety were far more likely to desire warm temperature refreshments while reflecting on a romantic breakup than those with lower levels of anxiety. These findings suggest that people with more prominent attachment anxiety are more likely to associate warmer temperatures with physical intimacy (Vess, 2012).

Face to Face Interactions

In addition to warmth and close bodily contact, there is evidence to suggest that face-to-face interactions made between an infant and his/her primary caregiver influence attachment. There has been a lot of research that assesses mother and infant face-to-face interactions at four months of age. This is used to predict the attachment classification most likely displayed by the child during Ainsworth's Strange Situation at one year. In these studies, mothers and infants are seated facing each other in a laboratory setting. Typically, there are cameras aimed at the mother and the infant. This is to gather simultaneous data. The interaction typically lasts 5-10 minutes (Beebe and Lachmann, 2014).

Face-to-face interaction is a continuous process that requires mutual effort by each party. The overall interaction is entirely based around the degree and nature in which the infant and caregiver respond to each other's behaviors in order to create a singular coherent experience. These behaviors created by either party can be engaging or disengaging, yet either type yields some sort of response from the other (Beebe and Lachmann, 2014).

These behaviors are also reflected and influenced by self and interactive regulation separately experienced by both caregiver and infant. These internal thoughts are also combined with personal expectations as to how the chosen behaviors will be interpreted by the other, and how the behaviors of the other will be interpreted by the experiencer. The overall experience of the interaction revolves around the mutual satisfaction it creates among the dyad (Beebe and Lachmann, 2014).

This finding was evident in Ainsworth's Baltimore study. Face-to-face interactions had more mutual satisfaction when mothers combined their playful behavior with that of their infants. In contrast, non-playful face-to-face interactions initiated by the mother were met with a similar response by the infant. If the mother was silent or did not smile, the infant typically mirrored her expressions (Bretherton, 1992).

These studies of face-to-face interaction at age four months are then paired with Ainsworth's Strange Situation. Once again, the classification of attachment type displayed by the child largely relies on the extent to which children are able to explore the unfamiliar environment while simultaneously using their mother as a safe haven to do so (Beebe and Lachmann, 2014).

Maternal Sensitivity

The term maternal sensitivity has been used throughout this chapter, but will now be fully defined and elaborated since it is a highly relevant factor in a child's attachment development. Maternal sensitivity refers to a few things. The overlapping quality is how attentive or inattentive the mother is to her infant's needs. This includes responding to a child's needs promptly and effectively. Meeting a child's needs in this regard also includes the ability to resolve a conflict in a mutually satisfying way. Children with secure attachments often have mothers who exhibit higher levels of emotional sensitivity. While research suggests that parental sensitivity plays a critical role in the type of attachment a child develops, it is not the sole cause (Beebee and Lachmann, 2014).

There have been research studies with similar findings in attachment pertaining to paternal sensitivity. In these specific studies however, the link between paternal sensitivity and infant-father attachment were not as significant as that of maternal sensitivity and infant-mother attachment (Braungart-Rieker et al., 2001). It is important to reiterate once again, that although much of the information in this chapter is based around mother and infant interactions in predicting, describing, and maintaining attachment, attachment is not influenced by gender. The majority of studies examining infant attachment include the infant's mother solely because the primary caregiver is more frequently female rather than male. There are many possible reasons for this, such as the act of breastfeeding or the societal acceptance of maternal leave rather than paternal leave. Nevertheless, attachment is attachment, and there is no evidence to suggest that a child's attachment classification would be altered if his/her primary caregiver identified with a gender other than female. The purpose of presenting the information disclosed in this way is to describe the evidence in the most accurate way possible.

CONCLUSION

As stated earlier, John Bowlby and Mary Ainsworth are considered the pioneers of the development of attachment theory. Bowlby's observational work with children, as well as his papers for WHO, were revolutionary to the field. Ainsworth's work also shaped attachment theory through her empirical studies. Specifically, her Strange Situation and corresponding attachment classifications are still used today to study infant attachment. These three classifications are based on behavioral patterns displayed by infants. The primary characteristic of a secure attachment is confidence in a primary caregiver. In contrast, insecure attachments are categorized by a lack of confidence in a primary caregiver. There has been evidence to suggest that attachments formed between an infant and a primary caregiver can have lasting impacts on the child's social and emotional wellbeing.

There is a crucial emphasis on the importance of face-to-face interactions, bodily contact, parental sensitivity, and mutual satisfaction in the development of secure attachments. Evidence suggests that not only the frequency, but the quality of these interactions, are both important. Face-to-face interactions between parents and children are most successful when both playful personalities are combined to create a fun interaction that is mutually satisfying. Bodily contact is most beneficial when it provides a sense of warmth. While warm contact between a parent and child is positive, research suggests that acts of hugging and holding are superior to kissing. It is important that parents are able to recognize and appropriately respond to their children's signals. Lastly, the love that is exchanged between a parent and child must be equal in order for the child to be securely attached.

REFERENCES

Ainsworth, M. S. (1969). *Individual Differences in Strange-Situational Behaviour of One-Year-Olds*. Academic Press.

Ainsworth, M. S., & Bell, S. M. (1970). Attachment, Exploration, and Separation: Illustrated by the Behavior of One-Year-Olds in a Strange Situation. *Child Development*, *41*(1), 49–67. doi:10.2307/1127388 PMID:5490680

Beebe, B., & Lachmann, F. M. (2014). The origins of relatedness: Film illus trations. In The Origins of Attachment: Infant Research and Adult Treatment (pp. 3-22). Routledge.

Braungart-Rieker, J. M., Garwood, M. M., Powers, B. P., & Wang, X. (2001). Parental Sensitivity, Infant Affect, and Affect Regulation: Predictors of Later Attachment. *Child Development*, *72*(1), 252–270. doi:10.1111/1467-8624.00277 PMID:11280483

Bretherton, I. (1985). Attachment theory: Retrospect and prospect. *Monographs of the Society for Research in Child Development*, *50*(1/2), 3–35. doi:10.2307/3333824

Bretherton, I. (1992). The origins of attachment theory: John Bowlby and Mary Ainsworth. *Developmental Psychology*, *28*, 759–775. Retrieved from http://www.psychology.sunysb.edu/attachment/online/inge_origins.pdf

Haydon, K. C., Collins, W. A., Salvatore, J., Simpson, J. E., & Roisman, G. I. (2012). Shared and distinctive origins and correlates of adult attachment representations: The developmental organization of romantic functioning. *Child Development*, *83*(5), 1689–1702. doi:10.1111/j.1467-8624.2012.01801.x PMID:22694197

Hazan, C., & Shaver, P. (1987). Romantic love conceptualized as an attachment process. *Journal of Personality and Social Psychology*, *52*(3), 511.

McLeod, S. (2018). *Mary Ainsworth*. Retrieved from https://www.simplypsychology.org/mary ainsworth.html

Tracy, R. L., & Ainsworth, M. D. S. (1981). Maternal Affectionate Behavior and Infant-Mother Attachment Patterns. *Child Development*, *52*(4), 1341–1343. doi:10.2307/1129529 PMID:7318528

Vess, M. (2012). Warm thoughts: attachment anxiety and sensitivity to temperature cues. *Psychological Science, 23*(5), 472-474. Retrieved from http://www.jstor.org/stable/414899727

Vicedo, M. (2009). The Father of Ethology and the Foster Mother of Ducks: Konrad Lorenz as Expert on Motherhood. *Isis*, *100*(2), 263–291. doi:10.1086/599553 PMID:19653490

KEY TERMS AND DEFINITIONS

Attachment Behaviors: Behaviors that support proximity to an attachment figure.

Correlation: A relationship between two variables.

Ego Resiliency: How effectively children can adaptively regulate their attention and behavior in response to their changing environments.

Emotion Regulation: Behaviors that adjust and control an individual's emotion.

Ethology: The study of animal behavior.

Generalized Representations of Attachment: The attachment forged between a child and his/her primary caregiver.

Imprinting: The process in which certain avian species follow and form an attachment to the first moving object they perceive at birth.

Insecure Anxious Resistant Attachment: A form of attachment between a child and his/her primary caregiver in which the child does not use the attachment figure as a secure base to explore. The caregiver has inconsistently met the child's needs. The child appears ambivalent towards the caregiver.

Insecure Avoidant Attachment: A form of attachment between a child and his/her primary caregiver in which the child does not use the attachment figure as a secure base to explore. The caregiver has consistently not met the child's needs.

Maternal Sensitivity: How attentive or inattentive a mother is to her infant's needs.

Mutual Satisfaction: A relationship is equally rewarding to a child as it is to his/her primary caregiver.

Naturalistic Observation: A research technique in which a researcher records behavior made by an individual while in the subject's natural habitat.

Romantic Representations of Attachment: The attachment between adults and their romantic partners.

Secure Attachment: A form of attachment between a child and his/her primary caregiver that emphasizes the ability for children to use their attachment figure as a secure base to explore their environment. The caregiver has consistently met the child's needs.

Security Theory: A theory that suggests that in order for children to have the ability to embark upon unfamiliar situations, they must have a secure dependence on parents.

Strange Situation: A study conducted by Mary Ainsworth that was comprised of eight episodes and was meant to create a sense of novelty that would influence exploratory behavior in a child.

Chapter 11
Parenting Practices in Botswana:
A Nexus of Legal and Sociocultural Discourses

Poloko Nuggert Ntshwarang
University of Botswana, Botswana

Odireleng Mildred Shehu
University of Botswana, Botswana

ABSTRACT

As in other Sub-Saharan countries, the legal reforms that occur in Botswana have significant effects on family functioning and how parenting occurs. Parenting practices such as strategies for supporting, monitoring, and disciplining children have significant effects on children's physical, social, psychological, emotional, and behavioral wellbeing. An important section of the structural system that affects parenting practices is the law. Botswana's Children's Act is an overriding law that informs any children's policy and program as well as parenting behaviors. Children's laws in the country are influenced by both socio-cultural discourses as well as the international bodies that Botswana is signatory to such as the Convention for the Rights of the Child (CRC). The authors adopt a critical discourse analysis (CDA) to examine how Botswana's Children's Act of 2009 contributes to parenting practices in the country and the impact of socio-cultural discourses in understanding and implementing the act. Implications for social work practice, research, and policy are highlighted.

DOI: 10.4018/978-1-7998-2940-9.ch011

INTRODUCTION

Parenting is a concept that is understood globally, but it is difficult to attach an exact meaning to it because nowadays a parent no longer necessarily means an individual with a biological tie to the child. For example, parenting can refer to a fostering situation including individual(s) or the state. The definition of parenting varies depending on the context in which it is used. Parenting commonly refers to child rearing behavior and parental beliefs, and attitudes such as perceptions, expectations, knowledge, ideas, goals, and values (Smith, 2011). That is, parenting denotes activities endorsed by parents when they interact with their child or children to enable physical, social, psychological, emotional, and behavioral wellbeing throughout the child's lifespan (Liang, Fuller, & Singer, 2000; Danford, Schultz & Marvicsin, 2015). Parenting practices are noticeable behaviors, activities, decisions, and methods that are part and parcel of the parenting process implemented by parents to socialize and care for children (Liang, Fuller, & Singer, 2000; Bornstein, Hahn, & Haynes, 2011). Examples of parenting practices include parental involvement, support, monitoring, and disciplining of children.

Children's exposure to various parenting practices speaks to their developmental processes (Williamson, Dutch & Clawson, 2010: Myers, Shoffner & Briggs, 2002). Positive parenting practices have affirmative behavioral outcomes such as delayed sexual debut (Wamoyi, Fenwick, Urassa, Zaba & Stones, 2011). Sexual debut is the age at which people have sexual intercourse for the first time in their life time (National AIDS Coordinating Agency-NACA, 2004). Negative parenting practices are associated with several behavioral challenges such as delinquency (Demuth & Brown, 2004) and depression (Garbarino, Vorrasi & Kostelny, 2002; Gershoff, 2010). For example, on the one hand, socio-cultural parenting practices such as physical discipline tend to be in conflict with legal parenting expectations since they often result in poor mental health development, and on the other hand those that encourage communal child care affirm legal expectations since they promote children's security and protection that enhance children's developmental needs.

Therefore the effects of structural factors on family structure and functioning as well as parenting practices cannot be over-emphasized. As in other sub-Saharan countries, the structural changes that occur in Botswana have significant effects on family structures and on how parenting occurs. Given the changes that occur at a family level as a result of economic and social development, one would expect that parenting issues would be given priority in research and social practice. However, limited literature on parenting implies that the issues pertaining to parenting practices are not given adequate attention in Botswana, especially in the research agenda. Culture and poverty play a significant role in the functioning of the family as well as in parenting practices (McDaniel & Zulu 1996; Ruiz-Casares 2009; Gaisie

2000; Dintwa 2010) even though they are often discussed in general terms. Another important section of the political and social context that affects family functioning and parenting but often receives minimal attention is public law.

The law, policy and programs, play a pivotal role in parenting and the lives of families (Ntshwarang, 2017). According to Paglioca, Meltou, Lyongs & Weisz (2002) the law interferes with family functioning daily by controlling parent-child relationships. Even though parents are said to be the legal and social primary authority figures in children's upbringing (Paglioca, Meltou, Lyongs & Weisz, 2002), their parenting practices are regulated by social policy and the law. Public policy also monitors, regulates family life, sets parameters for parental responsibility and prioritizes the rights and needs of family members (Garbarino, Vorrasi & Kostelny, 2002). The effects of social policy on parenting ultimately positively or negatively influences children's development (Garbarino, Vorrasi & Kostelny, 2002). Thus the law cannot be dismissed to have the same effects as it plays a major role in the formulation of social policies. Hence it is the intention of the paper to critically analyze the Children's Act of 2009 (an overarching children's law) to determine and discuss how it contributes to parenting behavior (parenting practices) in the country. Implications for social work practice, research and policy are highlighted in the paper.

PARENTING PRACTICES, CHILDREN'S PROGRAMS AND LAWS IN THE CONTEXT OF BOTSWANA

Botswana is currently rated as an upper middle income country because of improved and rapid development characterized by infrastructure and society's enhanced access to social services (UNICEF, 2011). It is a landlocked country located in southern Africa with an estimated population of 2 million (Statistics Botswana, 2011), sharing borders with South Africa, Namibia, Zimbabwe, and Zambia. As in other African countries and elsewhere, parenting practices in Botswana are influenced by cultural and traditional norms to a larger extent. Such parenting practices include corporal punishment (CP), gendered roles as well as limited participation of children in decision making (Ntshwarang, 2017). Corporal punishment is the deliberate infliction of physical pain on others as a way to discipline them (Lansford, 2010). As Ntshwarang and Sewpaul (forthcoming) noted, CP is practiced in both western and non-western countries. Parents often use CP to get rid of perceived unacceptable behaviors. Ntshwarang and Sewpaul (forthcoming) highlight that family religious beliefs and appreciation of physical punishment at a legal level play a major role in the application of corporal discipline as a relevant parenting practice in Botswana. In addition, parenting practices are mostly gendered. Gendered parenting practices mostly manifest in two ways: (a) fathers being excluded from actively participating in child care especially when children are young. (b) The gendered division of household roles where children are allocated chores based on whether they are boys or girls. In most situations, the girls are given caring and indoor activities such as cooking and cleaning, whereas the boys will be given outdoor activities such as gardening or fixing broken items. Such practice is also responsible for the tendency of families to render men a provider status, and women caring roles (Maharaj & Sewpaul, 2016). Furthermore, the level of children's participation and decision making at different levels of society in the country is insignificant (UNICEF, 2011), a situation that is highly influenced by cultural and religious beliefs by a majority of the population.

Botswana does not have any family-focused social policies but, rather compartmentalized social security programs and policies that target different vulnerable and needy individuals. This mainly aims at the eradication of poverty, examples being the Destitute Persons Program, The World War II Veterans Program, the Old Age Pension Scheme, and The Community Home Based Care and Remote Area Development Program (RADP) (Ntseane & Solo, 2007). Poverty is more prevalent in households with children under four years of age (UNICEF, 2011), a situation that government attempts to address by providing an infant feeding Program where supplementary food is given to children aged one to five years on a monthly basis as well as to school children (Ntseane & Solo, 2007). In addition, the National Plan of Action for Orphans and Vulnerable Children (2010-2016) also aims at meeting the needs of such children in the country. Orphans and vulnerable children are given the necessary items they need for survival such as food, clothing and shelter, depending on their specific needs.

Whereas the above social security programs provide different basic needs for needy children, different laws also exist that serve various purposes for parents, families and children. Botswana has laws that somehow impact the welfare of children and parenting practices such as the (a) Adoption of Children's Act (b) Children's Act (c) Married Persons Property Act (d) Employment Act and (e) Marriage Act. However the overarching law that specifically focuses on the status of children and seems to have had a significant impact on parenting practices in Botswana is the Children's Act of 2009 because it raises issues that relate to parent-child relationships, parental responsibilities, and issues pertaining to child survival, development, participation, and protection as well as the roles of different institutions in improving the general wellbeing of children.

METHODOLOGY

The article adopts a critical discourse analysis (CDA) to examine how The Children's Act of 2009 affects parenting practices in Botswana. Discourse analysis has its roots in critical linguistics analysis (CLA) and the two concepts are often used interchangeably (Wodak, 2001). According to Sheyholislami (2001), critical linguistics adopts the stance that language has the following purposes: (1) speech is influenced by the speaker's experiences, personal attitudes, and evaluation of the phenomena they present; (2) speech yields a relationship between speakers and listeners; and (3) speakers are able to produce information understandable to listeners. It is more interested in the relationship between language and power. CDA was developed in the early 1990s and its proponents are Teun Vann Dijk, Norman Fairclough, Gunther Kress, Theo Vann Leeuwen, and Ruth Wodak (Wodak, 2001). CDA is a multidisciplinary approach that seeks to analyze the relationship between social structures and discourse (Wodak, 1999; Van Dijk, 2001). CDA takes a multidisciplinary approach because the formulation of theory, problem, and applications are closely intertwined and mutually inspiring (Van Dijk, 2001: 96).

Embedded within CDA are philosophical ideas of critique, ideology, and power (Wodak, 2001). Critique implies that the researcher takes a socio-political stance when analyzing data; ideology focuses on the ways in which meaning is constructed and conveyed, facilitating how power is developed and maintained by discourse; and power is at the core of CDA because it recognizes that power is embedded in discourse and that inequalities are linked to social structures (Wodak, 2001; Leitch & Palmer 2010). Critical discourse analysis is a method of discourse analysis that acknowledges that social problems are rooted within power dynamics and inequalities which can be understood through the analysis of text (Leitch & Palmer 2010).

CDA connects to a structural social work approach because it is concerned about how social practices, institutions, and individuals shape behavior by making it easy to understand a situation in a particular way as well as comprehending how institutional practices shape behavior (Hodges, Kuper, & Reeves, 2008). It aims to analyze social interactions that are easily noticeable and those that are hard to notice with the view that discourse is socially produced and conditioned (Blommaert & Bulcaen, 2000). According to the authors, discourse can be text or social practice. Discourse as text is written while as practice it is produced, circulated, distributed, and consumed in society. As social practice, it is composed of sociopolitical effects that occur within dominant processes in which discourse occurs (Blommaert & Bulcaen, 2000). Sociopolitical effects include effects of dominant structural systems such as social injustice that are embedded within the approved social, economic and political context. Discourse as text determines the behavior of people who are subjected to it; hence it is the goal of CDA to analyze the relations between discourse and social meaning (Blommaert & Bulcaen, 2000).

From a socio-political stance, CDA attempts to understand social issues by studying and analyzing written and spoken texts to identify causes or sources of power, injustice, and inequalities (Van Dijk, 1993; Van Dijk 2001; Sheyholislami,

2001; Wodak, 2001). Inequality can be in the form of unequal access to discourse and communication (Van Dijk, 1993). It is against that background that CDA recognizes that people sometimes take for granted power and dominance that is endorsed and reproduced by subtle text and talk that often appear natural and acceptable to society. Hence it is the goal of CDA to examine such issues (Wodak, 2001). Some of the critiques of CDA are that different readers have different understanding and interpretations of the same texts and, because they are influenced by their background and knowledge about the phenomena discussed, readers are unlikely to critique texts (Sheyholislami, 2001) and simply take them as they appear to them without critically analyzing them.

The goals and principles of CDA uphold structural social work theory's view that society, through its different systems, affects people's behavior and their quality of life (Blau 1960; Mullaly 1997). Both CDA and structural social work theory acknowledge that society is embedded with interrelated forms of oppression, discrimination, and exploitation (Carniol 1992; Mullaly 1997) which are often unrecognized unless they are brought to the surface through critical analysis of social structures. CDA is achieved through analyzing written and spoken texts to reveal the interrelationships between discourse practices, social practices, and social structures, the ultimate goal being to identify sources of power, dominance, and inequality at different levels of society (Van Dijk, 1993; Van Dijk, 2001; Sheyholislami, 2001; Wodak, 2001). The paper acknowledges Leitch and Palmer's (2010) argument that scholars frequently overlook the main issues and challenges in connecting specific texts to specific contexts and the authors' call for objectivity in CDA methodology. The current paper adopts a flexible and less systematic approach to analyze the Botswana Children's Act, 2009 as text to highlight the power dynamics and inequalities that come to play in developing family and children's policies, which ultimately may have an impact on parenting practices. According to Chouliaraki and Fairclough (2010) flexible and pervious CDA methodologies are necessary to create opportunities for interdisciplinary research and to help cultivate a stronger understanding of the link between social problems and power dynamics, especially in organizational research.

BOTSWANA CHILDREN'S ACT OF 2009 AND PARENTING PRACTICES

Botswana Children's Act of 2009 is an Act of Parliament whose goal is to uphold and protect the rights of children, and to enhance children's developmental needs through the establishment of structures to support the goal (Republic of Botswana, 2009). Section 4 outlines the objectives of the Act as promoting the well-being of children, families, and communities in Botswana; provide for the protection and care of children where their parents fail; protect children from harm; acknowledge parents and families as primary caregivers; acknowledge communities as allies in child welfare, support them in their roles and protect children from illegal and harmful labor practices. In analyzing the Act, the authors attempt to consider the following critical aspects in CDA as noted by Van Dijk (1993): discourse and access, power enactment and discourse production, and power and dominance and how they are represented in the Children's Act of 2009, with a focus on selected sections within the Act as well as their interrelationship with some of the socio-cultural discourses.

Discourse and Access

It is important to note that only parents who have access to the Children's Act of 2009 will be able to modify their parenting practices and re-set their parental goals to ensure that they adopt those that fulfill the expectations of the Act. Parents who do not know how to read and write and those who do not have readily available community resources such as libraries or information centers are at a disadvantage. From a CDA perspective, the Act offers only privileged access to discourse and communication (Van Dijk, 1993) because it does not state how parents are going to be educated about their duties, responsibilities, and rights. Rather, it states that the functions of the village children's committees should educate people about child abuse and monitor the welfare of children in those communities (Section 33, sub section 1).What is also paramount is that the village children's committees may not be available in most villages in Botswana, making it difficult to educate parents about child abuse and monitoring the welfare of children in such villages.

Given that the parent may have his or her own religious beliefs that may guide his/her parenting practices; these may be in conflict with those of the child. Section 7, article (g) reads that "decisions about a child shall be consistent with cultural, ethnic, and religious values and traditions relevant to the child." From a parental lens, the cultural, ethnic, and religious values and traditions that children adopt are those of the parent and family because parental practices are influenced by the parent's background which is his or her culture, ethnicity, religion, and value system. Ntshwarang & Sewpaul (forthcoming) caution that legal reform should not be interpreted as an assurance to protect and uphold human rights but should be viewed as an enabling mechanism because cultural and religious beliefs of families are often a source of negative parenting practices that perpetuate child abuse. However, sections 21 and 22 of the Act emphasize that the child has the right to freedom of religion and to choose her/his preferred association, while section 23 emphasizes the child's right to privacy (Republic of Botswana, 2009). Section 23: 1-2 of the Children's Act of 2009 states:

"(1) Every child has a right to have his or her privacy protected. (2) The right to privacy shall be exercised subject to the child's best interests taking into account (a) the child's age, maturity and level of understanding; (b) the need for guidance and to protect the child from pornography and other influences which may cause emotional, physical. psychological or moral harm to the child; (c) the public interest, national security, public morality, public health and the rights and freedoms of other people."

One would be naïve to think that children and parents are unlikely to interpret such statements differently given that they might have differing world views of situations, especially at the adolescent stage of development. It is so at the adolescent stage because this is a state of development when adolescents discover the world through their own lens, which may also be in conflict with those of their parents. For example, Maundeni and Jacques (2012) highlighted that during meetings they conducted to educate communities in Botswana about the Children's Act of 2019, some community members raised concerns that some children intentionally engage in delinquent behaviors because the Act has a provision that children have no capacity for criminal responsibility. While on one hand there was concern over children's deviant behavior, on the other hand, adults were also noted as taking advantage of the aforementioned provision by using children to commit crimes. One community member was quoted as having lamented:

"When these children are questioned by the police, they say that some adults requested them to sell such drugs in exchange for money. Because the law is lenient with children, those children are usually not imprisoned. Yet the sale of illegal drugs is a serious offence…So something should be done about these scenarios, otherwise we going to see more and more children being used by adults to commit crime." (Maundeni & Jacques, 2012:p.78)

Furthermore, both parents and children are likely to understand the concept of "the best interest of the child" differently. The Act constructively outlines factors to consider in determining the best interests of the child in sections 5 and 6. However, those factors are also likely to be interpreted differently by parents, children and child welfare workers such as social workers. There is available literature (Jacobs 1996; Kelly, 1997; Tirri, & Husu, 2002; Peskind, 2004) demonstrating that professionals also have difficulty in making decisions about what is in the best interest of the child, and thus the concept is likely to be extremely difficult for lay persons to grasp. The question therefore arises as to whose interpretation of the "the child's best interest" parents should adopt in their pursuit of parenting practices suitable for children.

As a result, parents may find themselves having to adopt parenting practices that suit both their religious beliefs as well as those of their children. It is possible that, in some families, especially in the context of Botswana, parents will impose practices that are in line with their religious and/or cultural beliefs and this may create conflict between them and their children. Some young people who have access to information on the Children's Act are likely to misunderstand or misinterpret the discourse and reject the guidance and control of parents. Such a response would be a sign that they have limited accessibility to, and understanding of, the goals of the Act.

Power Enactment and Discourse Production

Even though the Children's Act of 2009 acknowledges the importance of relatives, guardians, foster parents, and adoptive parents in the care of children, it tends to overlook the fact that the family is the primary unit of socialization for children. There is no section in the Act that concentrates on the duties of the family as a unit. Instead there is more emphasis on persons, parents, relatives, and guardians. Therefore it tends to overlook that structures such as the family play a critical role in determining parenting practices. A family can take different forms and definitions but is usually perceived as a social unit that is organized based on societal norms, affinity, reproduction and socialization of children (Amoateng & Richter, 2007). This is an indication that Botswana's Children's Act of 2009 presents a biased approach towards parenting and child rearing in Botswana. The significance of the family in parenting practices is very important because the family harbors cultural practices and norms that represent the institutionalization of male supremacy over women and children (Kidd, 1997). Such dominant cultural norms and practices preserve social injustice and internalization of discrimination in families (Sewpaul, 2013). Therefore the need to focus on families as the basic unit of a child's up-bringing is critical since law reform that aims at improving family lifestyles has the potential to improve the children's social environment as well as to enhance the fulfilment of the developmental needs of children as well as the promotion of their general wellbeing (Garbarino, Vorrasi & Kostelny, 2002).

A positive aspect of the Act is that it recognizes the importance of community in the upbringing of children. The Act expects community leaders to discuss issues of concern regarding the wellbeing of children in the community. Part V, Section 30 highlights:

"A community leader shall have a duty to receive and have discussed in Kgotla or similar gatherings matters that may be affecting or may affect the common well-being of children in his or her community."

The term Kgotla refers to an assembly court yard and a traditional law court headed by the village chief used for peaceful dialogues about issues of concern in the village or community (Maundeni & Jacques, 2012). It is perceived as an inclusive place because every member of the community is allowed to air his or her view without intimidation. However it is important to note that children seldom take part in Kgotla meetings and they are hardly allowed to speak in such public gatherings.

Section 33 calls for the establishment of village child protection committees whose functions should be to educate community members about child abuse and to monitor the welfare of the concerned children. The approach is in line with a common belief among African people that every child belongs to his or her community and thus every community member should take responsibility for these children in their care (Ntarangwi, 2012). The Children's Act, therefore, is considerate of the collectivist nature of Botswana communities as opposed to the individualist approach that is adopted in many western countries.

Moreover, the 2009 Act attempted to avoid discrimination with regard to the composition of the village child committees by gender and age, since children, women and men are represented (Republic of Botswana, 2009). That is, most of the proposed community committees that are supposed to spearhead the promotion of children's rights are expected to include children, women and men. However, the Act omitted the teacher in the composition of village child committees despite the fact that, currently children start school at a young age and often spend more time at school than in their homes. The fact that children in Botswana spend almost eight hours a day in school (Mmonadibe, 2009) is an indication that teachers are likely to have more interaction with children than some of the children's parents and thus their participation is critical for the functioning of the village child committees. Teachers have insight about children's behavior that can assist parents and other people responsible for the upbringing of children to critically examine their choice of parenting practices. The school system is therefore more likely to have a significant influence on parenting practices.

As a result of such omissions, one may question whether adequate consultation with people at local and community levels was carried out prior to passing the Bill in parliament. This begs the question as to whether local people had the power to make contributions to the design of the Children's Act on whether major decisions were made by authority figures and endorsed by members of parliament. The issues discussed above validate the meaningful argument that policy and law makers are mostly authority figures whose frame of reference is based on western and urbanized principles (Ntarangwi, 2012) and that power and dominance should be institutionalized and supported by legislation (Van Dijk, 1993).

Power and Dominance

Sections 27 to 29 of the Children's Act of 2009 define the duties and rights of parents. The Act enforces these parental duties since it clearly states that the "Act takes precedence" over any other legislation unless its decisions may cause harm to the child (section 3). Although the act provides a protective dimension for the parents by stipulating their rights the Act imposes duties on parents because it overrides their cultural and religious backgrounds as well as their wisdom as primary caregivers in the upbringing of children. Section 28 (1) of the Children's Act:

" Subject to the best interests of the child... every parent shall have the right in relation to that child, to (a) have the child live with him or her; (b) control and guide the child's upbringing; (c) maintain personal relations with, and have access to, the child if the child does not live with him or her; (d) represent the child in all contractual and other legal matters regarding the child's property and other interests; participate, in the prescribed manner, in court and other proceedings related to his or her child; (f) appoint a guardian or revoke the appointment of a guardian where one has been appointed, subject to the court's approval; and (g) have access to parenting skills programmes put in place in terms of this Act or any other law."

The initial Children's Act of 1989 had flaws that were not in line with international standards regarding the survival, protection, and rights of children. Therefore the Children's Act of 2009 was designed to meet the standards of International treaties such as the United Nations Convention on the Rights of the Child (CRC) of 1989, and the African Charter on the Rights and Welfare of the Child (ACRWC). Such an approach could undermine the participation of parents and people at grassroots levels in the establishment of public law and social policy.

While to some extent the Children's Act of 2009 facilitates positive parenting by providing guidelines on what a parent should do in the best interest of the child, it also constrains parenting practices and freedoms in allowing parents to raise their children independently. The duties of parents outlined in the Act reflect Garbarino, Vorrasi & Kostelny (2002)'s notion that policy restricts parental performance because most of the time the law shapes the outcome of policies. For example, if parents were to engage in parental practices that do not align with what is stipulated by the Act or do something that is not in the 'best interest of the child' they are likely to lose their parental rights. Given that the Act takes precedence over other existing legislation and programs (Republic of Botswana, 2009), it is relevant to highlight that to some extent, law influences parenting practices because it is the ultimate tool that monitors and guides how parents are supposed to discipline and care for their children. But the final decision has to be proven in a court of law so that there are checks and balances.

IMPLICATIONS FOR SOCIAL WORK PRACTICE, RESEARCH, AND POLICY

Family-Focused Policies

There is a need for social and economic policies that target families. Such policies are important in enhancing positive parenting practices. The availability of economic resources such as prioritization of employment provisions to families with children has the potential to enhance parental self-efficacy that will assist parents in establishing parental goals that improve the wellbeing of their children (Garbarino, Vorrasi & Kostelny, 2002). This is relevant because UNICEF (2011) has indicated that families with children under the age of five are more impoverished than other families. One of the objectives of the Children's Act of 2009 is to help parents and families care for and protect children but the act does not outline specific activities and ways to achieve that role.

The establishment of family-focused policy will also help social workers and other professionals working with families and children to provide services that are designed to meet the needs of both children and other family members. Further, family policies will provide opportunities to ensure that the family as a primary and critical unit of children's socialization constitutes a platform for the development of positive parenting practices. The family focused approach is important because it discourages a situation where matters of concern to the family are indirectly attended to through policies that have been enacted for individuals such as the destitute policy. For example, the Children's Act of 2009, Part 1, Section 2, defines a fit person as 'an individual of good repute and right standing in the society who is emotionally, physically, mentally and financially capable of caring for, maintaining, guiding and controlling a child.' However it is common in practice that when an unemployed parent is financially incapacitated and struggles to provide the basic needs of the family, the social worker registers that particular parent for destitution. Therefore, the argument is that the government should develop programs that are specifically designed to assist families with children in all areas of life such as financially, spiritually, psychologically and socially to support positive child development. Thus registering the needy parent as a destitute only partially addresses the needs of the child.

Research for Evidence Based Practice and Social Policy

There is also a need for further research to examine how structural factors such as public law and policy influence parenting practices within African countries such as Botswana. Empirical evidence is likely to contribute to the development of family-focused programs and social policies that are based on the experiences of parents and families to enhance parenting skills, practices, and ultimately the developmental needs of children as well as their general wellbeing.

Given that critical discourse analysis of the Children's Act of 2009 points to likely possibilities that there was inadequate consultation with local people and communities prior to its enactment, research should be actively used as a tool or mechanism to involve local people in decision making and in the development of public law and policy. Research to examine whether the Children's Act of 2009 is acknowledged and understood by both children and parents is greatly needed. Further examination of how structural forces affect parenting could help formulate policies and programs that are not in conflict with the culture of communities. This would help policy-makers to harmoniously and clearly specify how culture, policy and the law support each other in advancing the rights of children, attending to the needs of parents, and promoting positive parenting skills and practices.

Consultative and Educational Forums

The experience of engaging in critical discourse analysis (CDA) of the Children's Act of 2009 raises an awareness that sometimes laws and policies are enacted with the assumption that they will be easily understood by implementers, as well as beneficiaries. Therefore rigorous outreach work is necessary to educate both parents and children about the Children's Act, and other policies relevant to their wellbeing. Such outreach work will provide opportunities for dialogue, critical analysis of issues, and identification of gaps in the implementation and operationalization of the Act. UNICEF (2011) also highlights the fact that there is a need to operationalize the Children's Act of 2009 in a holistic manner and to provide public education if the welfare of children is to be effectively promoted.

CONCLUSION

The paper attempted to illustrate how Botswana's Children's Act of 2009 affects parenting practices by using critical discourse analysis (CDA) to examine the interrelationship of the Act and socio-cultural discourses on parenting and parenting practices. It is important to note that more research and dialogue with the community in regard to the Act is necessary. Gaps in accessibility to relevant information, lack of adequate community consultation prior to establishment of the Act and issues pertaining to power, discrimination, and dominance were identified. There are notable positive aspects of Botswana's Children's Act of 2009 such as its attempt to protect both the rights of parents and children as well as to ensure equal participation of people of different ages and genders in the village children's committee. The paper proposes family-oriented laws and policies as opposed to individualistic ones to enhance positive parenting practices and to meet the developmental needs of children as well as to ensure the wellbeing of all family members.

REFERENCES

Amoateng, A. Y., & Richter, L. M. (2007). *Social and economic context of families and households in South Africa*. Pretoria: HSRC.

Blau, P. M. (1960). Structural Effects. *American Sociological Review*, *25*(2), 178–193. doi:10.2307/2092624

Blommaert, J., & Bulcaen, C. (2000). Critical Discourse Analysis. *Annual Review of Anthropology*, *29*(1), 447–466. doi:10.1146/annurev.anthro.29.1.447

Bornstein, M. H., Hahn, C. S., & Haynes, O. M. (2011). Maternal personality, parenting cognitions, and parenting practices. *Developmental Psychology*, *47*(3), 658–675. doi:10.1037/a0023181 PMID:21443335

Carniol, B. (1992). Structural social work: Maurice Moreau's challenge to social work practice. *Journal of Progressive Human Services*, *3*(1), 1–20. doi:10.1300/J059v03n01_01

Chouliaraki, L., & Fairclough, N. (2010). Critical discourse analysis in organizational studies: Towards an integrationist methodology. *Journal of Management Studies*, *47*(6), 1213–1218. doi:10.1111/j.1467-6486.2009.00883.x

Danford, C. A., Schultz, C. M., & Marvicsin, D. (2015). Parental roles in the development of obesity in children: Challenges and opportunities. *Research and Reports in Biology*, 6.

Dintwa, K. F. (2010). Changing Family Structure in Botswana. *Journal of Comparative Family Studies*, *41*(3), 281–297. doi:10.3138/jcfs.41.3.281

Gaisie, S. K. (2000). Family structure, gender and fertility in Botswana, *Pula: Botswana. Journal of African Studies*, *14*(2).

Garbarino, J., Vorrasi, J. A., & Kostelny, K. (2002). Parenting and Public Policy. In Handbook of Parenting: Vol. 5. Practical Issues in Parenting (2nd ed.; pp. 487-507). London: Lawrence Erlbaum Associates.

Hodges, B. D., Kuper, A., & Reeves, S. (2008). Qualitative Research: Discourse Analysis. *British Medical Journal*, *337*(7669), 570–572.

Jacobs, S. B. (1996). Hidden Gender Bias behind the Best Interest of the Child Standard in Custody Decisions. *The Ga. St. UL Rev.*, *13*, 845.

Kelly, J. B. (1997). The best interests of the child. *Family Court Review*, *35*(4), 377–387. doi:10.1111/j.174-1617.1997.tb00480.x

Kidd, P. E. (1997). *Botswana families and women's rights in a changing environment*. Gaborone: Women and Law in Southern Africa.

Lansford, J. E. (2010). The special problem of cultural differences in effects of corporal punishment. *Law and Contemporary Problems*, *73*(2), 89–106.

Leitch, S., & Palmer, I. (2010). Analysing texts in context: Current practices and new protocols for critical discourse analysis in organization studies. *Journal of Management Studies*, *47*(6), 1194–1212. doi:10.1111/j.1467-6486.2009.00884.x

Liang, X., Fuller, B., & Singer, J. D. (2000). Ethnic differences in child care selection: The Influence of family structure, parenting practices, and home language. *Early Childhood Research Quarterly*, *15*(3), 357–384. doi:10.1016/S0885-2006(00)00071-5

Maharaj, S., & Sewpaul, V. (2016). Accidental burns in children under five years of age: The gendered burden of care and socio-economic deprivation. *Children and Youth Services Review*, *68*, 51–58. doi:10.1016/j.childyouth.2016.06.014

Maundeni, T., & Jacques, G. (2012). "… and a little child shall lead them": Utilising Kgotla meetings to empower children and the communities that nurture them. *Thari ya Bana: Reflections on Children in Botswana*, 74-80.

McDaniel, A., & Zulu, E. (1996). Women, Fathers, and Children: Regional Patterns in Child-Parent Residence in Sub-Saharan Africa. *African Population Studies*, 11.

Mmonadibe, P. N. (2009). Orphaned HIV-positive children in Botswana: Challenges and prospects. In C. M. Fombad, R. Mupedziswa, T. Maundeni, & G. Mookodi (Eds.), *HIV and AIDS, Vulnerable groups, Human Rights and Development in Botswana* (pp. 155–167). OSSREA.

Mullaly, R. P. (1997). *Structural social work: Ideology, theory, and practice* (2nd ed.). New York: Oxford University Press.

National AIDS Coordinating Agency-NACA. (2004). *Botswana AIDS Impact Survey II: Statistical report*. Gaborone: Central Statistics Office.

Ntarangwi, M. (2012). Introduction: Parents' Involvement in Children's Lives in Africa. *Africa Development. Afrique et Developpement*, *37*(3), 1–18.

Ntseane, D., & Solo, K. (2007). *Social security & social protection in Botswana*. Gaborone: Bay Publishers.

Ntshwarang, P. N. (2017). Parenting and parenting practices among contemporary families in Botswana: Does government policy matter? In R. Mupedzisa, G. Jacques, & L-K, Mwansa (Eds.), Social Work and Social Development in Botswana: Issues, Challenges & Prospects. IFSW.

Ntshwarang, P. N., & Sewpaul, V. (forthcoming). When national law and culture coalesce: Challenges for children's rights in Botswana with specific reference to corporal punishment. In V. Sewpaul, L. Kreitzer, & T. Raniga (Eds.), Culture, Human Rights and Social Work: African Perspectives. Calgary: Calgary University Press.

Paglioca, P. M., Meltou, B. G., Lyons, P. M. Jr, & Weisz, V. (2002). Parenting and the Law. In M. H. Bornstein (Ed.), Handbook of Parenting: Vol. 5. *Practical Issues in Parenting* (2nd ed.; pp. 463–486). London: Lawrence Erlbaun Associates.

Peskind, S. N. (2004). Determining the Undeterminable: The Best Interest of the Child Standard as an Imperfect but Necessary Guidepost to Determine Child Custody. *N. Ill. UL Rev.*, *25*, 449.

Renzaho, A., Green, J., Mellor, D., & Swinburn, B. (2011). Parenting, family functioning and lifestyle in a new culture: The case of African migrants in Melbourne, Victoria, Australia. *Child & Family Social Work*, *16*(2), 228–240. doi:10.1111/j.1365-2206.2010.00736.x

Republic of Botswana. (2008). *National Situation Analysis on Orphans and Vulnerable Children in Botswana, Ministry of Local Government Department of Social Services*. Gaborone: Government Printers.

Republic of Botswana. (2009). *Children's Act*. Gaborone: Government Printers.

Republic of Botswana. (2010). *Improving the quality of life in Botswana: National Plan for Orphans and Vulnerable Children 2010-2016*. Gaborone: Ministry of Local Government.

Ruiz-Casares, M., & Heymann, J. (2009). Children home alone unsupervised: Modeling parental decisions and associated factors in Botswana, Mexico, and Vietnam. *Child Abuse & Neglect*, *33*(5), 312–323. doi:10.1016/j.chiabu.2008.09.010 PMID:19477517

Sewpaul, V. (2013). Inscribed in our blood: Challenging the ideology of sexism and racism. *Affilia*, *28*(2), 116–125. doi:10.1177/0886109913485680

Sheyholislami, J. (2001). *Critical Discourse Analysis*. Retrieved from http://www.carleton.ca/~jsheyhol/cda.htm

Smith, M. (2011). Measures for assessing parenting in research and practice. *Child and Adolescent Mental Health, 16*(3), 158–166. doi:10.1111/j.1475-3588.2010.00585.x

Statistics Botswana. (2011). *Population and housing census 2011, analytical report.* Gaborone: Department of Printing & Publishing Services.

Tirri, K., & Husu, J. (2002). Care and Responsibility in 'The Best Interest of the Child': Relational voices of ethical dilemmas in teaching. *Teachers and Teaching, 8*(1), 65–80. doi:10.1080/13540600120110574

UNICEF. (2011). *The situation analysis of children and their families in Botswana. Summary Report: Findings and recommendations to policy makers 2010/2011.* Gaborone: UNICEF Botswana Country Office.

Van Dijk, T. A. (1993). Principles of critical discourse analysis. *Discourse & Society, 4*(2), 249–283. doi:10.1177/0957926593004002006

Van Dijk, T. A. (2001). Multidisciplinary CDA: a plea for diversity. In Methods of critical discourse analysis. London: Sage Publications.

Wodak, R. (1999). Critical discourse analysis at the end of the 20th century. *Research on Language and Social Interaction, 32*(1-2), 185–193. doi:10.1080/08351813.1999.9683622

Wodak, R. (2001). What CDA is about-a summary of its history, important concepts and its development. In Methods of critical discourse analysis. London: Sage Publications.

KEY TERMS AND DEFINITIONS

Act: A legally binding order passed by the state's parliamentary body.

Child: Any person under the age of 18 years old (Botswana Children's Act of 2009).

Critical Discourse Analysis (CDA): Is a multidisciplinary approach that seeks to analyze the relationship between social structures and discourse (Wodak, 1999; Van Dijk, 2001). Critical discourse analysis is a method of discourse analysis that acknowledges that social problems are rooted within power dynamics and inequalities which can be understood through the analysis of text (Leitch & Palmer 2010).

Family: An organized social institution that takes different forms but is usually perceived as a social unit that is based on societal norms, affinity and reproduction, whose main aim is to socialize children (Amoateng & Richter, 2007).

Kgotla: A traditional and cultural place found in villages and small communities where community members gather to discuss different issues of interest to the community.

Negative Parenting Practices: Parenting practices associated with several behavioral challenges such as delinquency (Demuth & Brown, 2004).

Parenting: Parental behaviors influenced by beliefs, norms and attitudes such as perceptions, expectations, knowledge, ideas, goals, and values to facilitate child rearing (Smith, 2011).

Parenting Practices: Noticeable behaviors, activities, decisions, and techniques that are part and parcel of the parenting process implemented by parents to socialize and care for children (Liang, Fuller, & Singer, 2000; Bornstein, Hahn, & Haynes, 2011).

Positive Parenting Practices: Favorable behavioral outcomes that affect positive child behavior (Wamoyi, Fenwick, Urassa, Zaba, & Stones, 2011).

Sexual Debut: The age at which people have sexual intercourse for the first time in their lifetime (National AIDS Coordinating Agency, 2004).

Compilation of References

Adamson, L. B., Bakeman, R., Deckner, D. F., & Nelson, P. B. (2012). Rating parent–child interactions: Joint engagement, communication dynamics, and shared topics in autism, Down syndrome, and typical development. *Journal of Autism and Developmental Disorders*, *42*(12), 2622–2635. doi:10.100710803-012-1520-1 PMID:22466689

Ainsworth, M. D. S., Blehar, M., Waters, E., & Wall, S. (1978). Patterns of attachment: Observations in the Strange Situation and at home. Hillsdale, NJ: Erlbaum.

Ainsworth, M. S. (1969). *Individual Differences in Strange-Situational Behaviour of One-Year-Olds*. Academic Press.

Ainsworth, M. S., & Bell, S. M. (1970). Attachment, Exploration, and Separation: Illustrated by the Behavior of One-Year-Olds in a Strange Situation. *Child Development*, *41*(1), 49–67. doi:10.2307/1127388 PMID:5490680

Ainsworth, M. S., & Bowlby, J. (1991). An ethological approach to personality development. *The American Psychologist*, *46*(4), 333–341. doi:10.1037/0003-066X.46.4.333

Akbag, M., & Ümmet, D. (2017). Predictive Role of Grit and Basic Psychological Needs Satisfaction on Subjective Well-Being for Young Adults. *Online Submission*, *8*(26), 127–135.

Akinin, L. B., Hamlin, J. K., & Dunn, E. W. (2012). Giving Leads to Happiness in Young Children. *PLoS One*, *7*(6), e39211. doi:10.1371/journal.pone.0039211 PMID:22720078

Akos, P., & Kretchmar, J. (2017). Investigating grit at a non-cognitive predictor of college success. *The Review of Higher Education*, *40*(2), 163–186. doi:10.1353/rhe.2017.0000

Alan, C. (2012). Psychiatric Rehabilitation Journal. *Trustees of Boston University.*, *35*(4), 335–358. doi:10.2975/35.42012.355.358

Aldred, C., Taylor, C., Wan, M. W., & Green, J. (2018). Using video feedback strategies in parent-mediated early autism intervention. In *Handbook of Parent-Implemented Interventions for Very Young Children with Autism* (pp. 221–239). Cham: Springer. doi:10.1007/978-3-319-90994-3_14

Alegre, A. (2011). Parenting styles and children's emotional intelligence: What do we know? *The Family Journal*, *19*(1), 56–62. doi:10.1177/1066480710387486

American Psychiatric Association. (2013). *Diagnostic and statistical manual of mental disorders* (5th ed.). Washington, DC: Author.

Amoateng, A. Y., & Richter, L. M. (2007). *Social and economic context of families and households in South Africa*. Pretoria: HSRC.

Anderson, C., Turner, A. C., Heath, R. D., & Payne, C. M. (2016). On the meaning of grit… and hope… and fate control… and alienation… and locus of control… and… self-efficacy… and… effort optimism… and…. *The Urban Review*, *48*(2), 198–219. doi:10.100711256-016-0351-3

Anschutz, D. J., Van Strien, T., & Engels, R. C. (2011). *Exposure to slim images in mass media: Television commercials as reminders of restriction in restrained eaters*. Academic Press.

Argyros, G., & Johnson, C. (2018). *Psychological Resilience in Higher Education Students: A Systematic Investigation of Predictive Factors*. Academic Press.

Arseniev-Koehler, A., Lee, H., McCormick, T., & Moreno, M. A. (2016). # Proana: Pro-eating disorder socialization on Twitter. *The Journal of Adolescent Health*, *58*(6), 659–664. doi:10.1016/j.jadohealth.2016.02.012 PMID:27080731

Arya, B., & Lal, D. S. (2018). Grit and sense of coherence as predictors of well- being. *Indian Journal of Positive Psychology*, *9*(1), 169–172. doi:10.15614/ijpp.v9i01.11766

Asher, S. R., & Coie, J. D. (1990). *Peer Rejection in Childhood*. Cambridge University Press.

Bai, S., Repetti, R. L., & Sperling, J. B. (2016). Children's expressions of positive emotion are sustained by smiling, touching, and playing with parents and siblings: A naturalistic observational study of family life. *Developmental Psychology*, *52*(1), 88–101. doi:10.1037/a0039854 PMID:26524382

Baker, V.A. (1991). *Changing attitudes of children in grades three to six towards persons with disabilities via the 'Kids on the Block' program*. Academic Press.

Banaschewski, T., Brandeis, D., Heinrich, H., Albrecht, B., Brunner, E., & Rothenberger, A. (2003). Association of ADHD and conduct disorder–brain electrical evidence for the existence of a distinct subtype. *Journal of Child Psychology and Psychiatry, and Allied Disciplines*, *44*(3), 356–376. doi:10.1111/1469-7610.00127 PMID:12635966

Bandura, A. (1982). Self-efficacy mechanism in human agency. *The American Psychologist*, *37*(2), 122–147. doi:10.1037/0003-066X.37.2.122

Baptiste, D. R., Tolou-Shams, M., Miller, S. R., Mcbride, C. K., & Paikoff, R. L. (2007). Determinants of parental monitoring and preadolescent sexual risk situations among African American families living in urban public housing. *Journal of Child and Family Studies*, *16*(2), 261–274. doi:10.100710826-006-9083-4

Bariso, J. (2018, Feb. 28). 13 Signs of High Emotional Intelligence: Wonder what emotional intelligence looks like in everyday life? *Inc.,* 1-5.

Barkin, S., Ip, E., Richardson, I., Klinepeter, S., Finch, S., & Krcmar, M. (2006). Parental media mediation styles for children aged 2 to 11 years. *Archives of Pediatrics & Adolescent Medicine, 160*(4), 395–401. doi:10.1001/archpedi.160.4.395 PMID:16585485

BarOn, R. (1997). *The BarOn Emotional Quotient inventory* (BarOn EQ-i). Author.

Baron-Cohen, S., & Hammer, J. (1997). Parents of children with Asperger syndrome: What is the cognitive phenotype? *Journal of Cognitive Neuroscience, 9*(4), 548–554. doi:10.1162/jocn.1997.9.4.548 PMID:23968217

Baron-Cohen, S., Lombardo, M. V., Auyeung, B., Ashwin, E., Chakrabarti, B., & Knickmeyer, R. (2011). Why are autism spectrum conditions more prevalent in males? *PLoS Biology, 9*(6), e1001081. doi:10.1371/journal.pbio.1001081 PMID:21695109

Beebe, B., & Lachmann, F. M. (2014). The origins of relatedness: Film illus trations. In The Origins of Attachment: Infant Research and Adult Treatment (pp. 3-22). Routledge.

Beebe, B. (2010). Mother–infant research informs mother–infant treatment. *Clinical Social Work Journal, 38*(1), 17–36. doi:10.100710615-009-0256-7

Bekhet, A. K., Johnson, N. L., & Zauszniewski, J. A. (2012). Resilience in family members of persons with autism spectrum disorder: A review of the literature. *Issues in Mental Health Nursing, 33*(10), 650–656. doi:10.3109/01612840.2012.671441 PMID:23017040

Bell, S. K., & Morgan, S. B. (2000). Children's attitudes and behavioral intentions toward a peer pre- sented as obese: Does a medical explanation for the obesity make a difference? *Journal of Pediatric Psychology, 25*(3), 137–145. doi:10.1093/jpepsy/25.3.137 PMID:10780140

Benjak, T., Vuletić Mavrinac, G., & Pavić Šimetin, I. (2009). Comparative study on selfperceived health of parents of children with autism spectrum disorders and parents of nondisabled children in croatia. *Croatian Medical Journal, 50*(4), 403–409. doi:10.3325/cmj.2009.50.403 PMID:19673041

Benson, P. R., & Karlof, K. L. (2009). Anger, stress proliferation, and depressed mood among parents of children with ASD: A longitudinal replication. *Journal of Autism and Developmental Disorders, 39*(2), 350–362. doi:10.100710803-008-0632-0 PMID:18709548

Benzies, K. M., Magill-Evans, J. E., Hayden, K. A., & Ballantyne, M. (2013). Key components of early intervention programs for preterm infants and their parents: A systematic review and meta-analysis. *BMC Pregnancy and Childbirth, 13*(1Suppl 1), S10. doi:10.1186/1471-2393-13-S1-S10 PMID:23445560

Bernier, M., & O'Hare, J. (Eds.). (2005). *Puppetry in Education and Therapy: Unlocking the Doors to the Mind and Heart.* Bloomington, IN: AuthorHouse.

Bettelheim, B. (1967). *The empty fortress.* New York: Free Press.

Biederman, J., Faraone, S. V., Milberger, S., Jetton, J. G., Chen, L., Mick, E., ... Russell, R. L. (1996). Is childhood oppositional defiant disorder a precursor to adolescent conduct disorder? Findings from a four-year follow-up study of children with ADHD. *Journal of the American Academy of Child and Adolescent Psychiatry*, *35*(9), 1193–1204. doi:10.1097/00004583-199609000-00017 PMID:8824063

Binfet, J.T. & Schonert-Reichl, K. A. (2015). Measuring kindness at school: Psychometric properties of a school kindness scale for children and adolescents. *Psychology in the Schools, 0*, 1–16.

Binfet, J.-T., & Passmore, H.-A. (2017). Teachers' Perceptions of Kindness at School. *The International Journal of Emotional Education*, *9*(1), 37–53. https://files.eric.ed.gov/fulltext/EJ1137976.pdf

Biringen, Z. (2000). Emotional availability: Conceptualization and research findings. *The American Journal of Orthopsychiatry*, *70*(1), 104–114. doi:10.1037/h0087711 PMID:10702855

Biringen, Z., Robinson, J. L., & Emde, R. N. (2000). Appendix B: The emotional availability scales; an abridged infancy/early childhood version). *Attachment & Human Development*, *2*(2), 256–270. doi:10.1080/14616730050085626

Blanchard, V. (2018). *Doctoral Program Completion: Grit, Goal setting, Social Support*. Seton Hall University Dissertations and Theses (ETDs). 2552.

Blau, P. M. (1960). Structural Effects. *American Sociological Review*, *25*(2), 178–193. doi:10.2307/2092624

Block, H. (1984). *School Learning Activities More Playlike: Flow and Mastery Learning*. The University of Chicago Press.

Blommaert, J., & Bulcaen, C. (2000). Critical Discourse Analysis. *Annual Review of Anthropology*, *29*(1), 447–466. doi:10.1146/annurev.anthro.29.1.447

Bloom, C., & Bloom, L. (2014). *Got Grit?* Retrieved from https://www.psychologytoday.com/us/blog/stronger-the-broken-places/201410/got-grit

Blumberg, F. C., Blades, M., & Oates, C. (2015). Youth and new media. *Zeitschrift fur Psychologie mit Zeitschrift fur Angewandte Psychologie*.

Boduszek, D., Belsher, R., Dhingra, K., & Ioannou, M. (2014). Psychosocial correlates of recidivism in a sample of ex-prisoners: The role of oppositional defiant disorder and conduct disorder. *Journal of Forensic Psychiatry & Psychology*, *25*(1), 61–76. doi:10.1080/14789949.2013.862293

Bögels, S., Hoogstad, B., van Dun, L., de Schutter, S., & Restifo, K. (2008). Mindfulness training for adolescents with externalizing disorders and their parents. *Behavioural and Cognitive Psychotherapy*, *36*(2), 193–209. doi:10.1017/S1352465808004190

Boggess, A. J., Rahman, G. M., Pamukcu, M., Faber, S., & Kingston, H. S. (2014). An accurate and transferable protocol for reproducible quantification of organic pollutants in human serum using direct isotope dilution mass spectrometry. *Analyst (London)*, *139*(23), 6223–6231. doi:10.1039/C4AN00851K PMID:25302342

Boniel-Nissim, M., Tabak, I., Mazur, J., Borraccino, A., Brooks, F., Gommans, R., ... Finne, E. (2015). Supportive communication with parents moderates the negative effects of electronic media use on life satisfaction during adolescence. *International Journal of Public Health*, *60*(2), 189–198. doi:10.100700038-014-0636-9 PMID:25549611

Booker, J. A., Ollendick, T. H., Dunsmore, J. C., & Greene, R. W. (2016). Perceived parent–child relations, conduct problems, and clinical improvement following the treatment of Oppositional Defiant Disorder. *Journal of Child and Family Studies*, *25*(5), 1623–1633. doi:10.100710826-015-0323-3 PMID:27284234

Bornstein, M. H., Hahn, C. S., & Haynes, O. M. (2011). Maternal personality, parenting cognitions, and parenting practices. *Developmental Psychology*, *47*(3), 658–675. doi:10.1037/a0023181 PMID:21443335

Borresen, K. (2019). *How to prevent a home renovation from wrecking your relationship*. Retrieved from https://www.huffpost.com/entry/home-renovation-relationship-marriage_1_5cae1371e4b03ab9f24f4604

Borzekowski, D. L., Schenk, S., Wilson, J. L., & Peebles, R. (2010). e-Ana and e-Mia: A content analysis of pro–eating disorder websites. *American Journal of Public Health*, *100*(8), 1526–1534. doi:10.2105/AJPH.2009.172700 PMID:20558807

Bossaert, G., Colpin, H., Pijl, S. P., & Petry, K. (2011). Loneliness among students with special educational needs in mainstream seventh grade. *Research in Developmental Disabilities*, *33*(6), 1888–1897. doi:10.1016/j.ridd.2012.05.010 PMID:22705912

Bowlby, J. (1969). Attachment and loss: Vol. 1. *Attachment*. London: Hogarth.

Bowman, N. A., Hill, P. L., Denson, N., & Bronkema, R. (2015). Keep on truckin'or stay the course? Exploring grit dimensions as differential predictors of educational achievement, satisfaction, and intentions. *Social Psychological & Personality Science*, *6*(6), 639–645. doi:10.1177/1948550615574300

Bradberry, T. (2014). Emotional Intelligence. *Forbes*.

Braungart-Rieker, J. M., Garwood, M. M., Powers, B. P., & Wang, X. (2001). Parental Sensitivity, Infant Affect, and Affect Regulation: Predictors of Later Attachment. *Child Development*, *72*(1), 252–270. doi:10.1111/1467-8624.00277 PMID:11280483

Breath, J. (2016). *The Importance of Meditation Breaks for Kids*. Retrieved from https://www.healthychildren.org/English/healthy-living/emotional-wellness/Pages/Just-Breathe-The-Importance-of-Meditation-Breaks-for-Kids.aspx

Bretherton, I. (1985). Attachment theory: Retrospect and prospect. *Monographs of the Society for Research in Child Development, 50*(1/2), 3–35. doi:10.2307/3333824

Bretherton, I. (1992). The origins of attachment theory: John Bowlby and Mary Ainsworth. *Developmental Psychology, 28*, 759–775. Retrieved from http://www.psychology.sunysb.edu/attachment/online/inge_origins.pdf

Buck, R. (1984). *The Communication of Emotion*. New York: The Guilford Press.

Buggey, T., & Ogle, L. (2012). Video self-modeling. *Psychology in the Schools, 49*(1), 52–70. doi:10.1002/pits.20618

Bulimia nervosa. (2018, May 10). Retrieved from https://www.mayoclinic.org/diseases-conditions/bulimia/symptoms-causes/syc-20353615

Burke, J. D., Loeber, R., & Birmaher, B. (2004). Oppositional defiant disorder and conduct disorder: A review of the past 10 years, part II. *Focus (San Francisco, Calif.), 41*(4), 1275–1576. PMID:12410070

Butner, D. (2017, November). The World's Happiest Places. *National Geographic: The Search For Happiness, 232*(5), 30–59.

Cameron, L., & Rutland, A. (2006). Extended contact through story reading in school: Reducing children's prejudice toward the disabled. *The Journal of Social Issues, 62*(3), 469–488. doi:10.1111/j.1540-4560.2006.00469.x

Campbell, J., Gilmore, L., & Cuskelly, M. (2003). Changing student teachers' attitudes towards disability and inclusion. *Journal of Intellectual & Developmental Disability, 28*(4), 369–379. doi:825031000161 6407 doi:10.1080/1366

Campbell, J. M., Ferguson, J. E., Herzinger, C. V., Jackson, J. N., & Marino, C. A. (2004). Combined descriptive and explanatory information improves peers' perceptions of autism. *Research in Developmental Disabilities, 25*(4), 321–339. doi:10.1016/j.ridd.2004.01.005 PMID:15193668

Campbell, K., & Peebles, R. (2014). Eating disorders in children and adolescents: State of the art review. *Pediatrics, 134*(3), 582–592. doi:10.1542/peds.2014-0194 PMID:25157017

Carey, B. (2014). *How we learn*. Random House.

Carniol, B. (1992). Structural social work: Maurice Moreau's challenge to social work practice. *Journal of Progressive Human Services, 3*(1), 1–20. doi:10.1300/J059v03n01_01

Cavazos, J. Jr, Johnson, M. B., Fielding, C., Cavazos, A. G., Castro, V., & Vela, L. (2010). A qualitative study of resilient Latina/o college students. *Journal of Latinos and Education, 9*(3), 172–188. doi:10.1080/15348431003761166

Çelik, İ., & Sariçam, H. (2018). The Relationships between Positive Thinking Skills, Academic Locus of Control and Grit in Adolescents. *Universal Journal of Educational Research, 6*(3), 392–398. doi:10.13189/ujer.2018.060305

Chang, W. (2014). *Grit and Academic Performance: Is Being Grittier Better?* Retrieved from https://scholarlyrepository.miami.edu/oa_dissertations/1306

Charney, D. (2004). *Psychobiological mechanism of resilience and vulnerability: Implications for successful adaptation to extreme stress.* Retrieved from doi:10.1176/appi.ajp.161.2.195

Chaste, P., & Leboyer, M. (2012). Autism risk factors: Genes, environment, and gene-environment interactions. *Dialogues in Clinical Neuroscience*, *14*(3), 281. PMID:23226953

Cherry, K. (2019). *How Social Support Contributes to Psychological Health.* Retrieved from https://www.verywellmind.com/social-support-for-psychological-health-4119970

Chilcott, L., Birtel, M., & Guggenheim, D. (2010). *Waiting for "Superman"*. Paramount Studios.

Chouliaraki, L., & Fairclough, N. (2010). Critical discourse analysis in organizational studies: Towards an integrationist methodology. *Journal of Management Studies*, *47*(6), 1213–1218. doi:10.1111/j.1467-6486.2009.00883.x

Clement, S., Schauman, O., Graham, T., Maggioni, F., Evans-Lacko, S., Bezborodovs, N., & Thornicroft, G. (2015). What is the impact of mental health-related stigma on help-seeking? A systematic review of quantitative and qualitative studies. *Psychological Medicine*, *45*(1), 11–27. doi:10.1017/S0033291714000129 PMID:24569086

Coffey, J. K. (2019). *Cascades of infant happiness: Infant positive affect predicts childhood IQ and adult educational attainment. Emotion.* Retrieved from https://slb.mmm.edu:2208/10.1037/emo0000640

Collingwood, J. (2018). *Building resilience.* Retrieved from https://psychcentral.com/lib/building-resilience/

Collins, K., & Barber, H. (2005). Female athletes' perceptions of parental influences. *Journal of Sport Behavior*, *28*(4), 295.

Collins, N. L., & Read, S. J. (1990). Adult attachment, working models, and relationship quality in dating couples. *Journal of Personality and Social Psychology*, *58*(4), 64. doi:10.1037/0022-3514.58.4.644 PMID:14570079

Constantin, T., Holman, A., & Hojbotă, M. A. (2011). Development and validation of a motivational persistence scale. *Psihologija (Beograd)*, *45*(2), 99–120. doi:10.2298/PSI1202099C

Corrigan, P. (2004). How stigma interferes with mental health care. *The American Psychologist*, *59*(7), 614–625. doi:10.1037/0003-066X.59.7.614 PMID:15491256

Corrigan, P. W., Lurie, B. D., Goldman, H. H., Slopen, N., Medasani, K., & Phelan, S. (2005). How adolescents perceive the stigma of mental illness and alcohol abuse. *Psychiatric Services*, *56*(5), 544–550. doi:10.1176/appi.ps.56.5.544 PMID:15872162

Cory, D. (2019). *EQ-i Certification Course.* The Emotional Intelligence Training Company Inc.

Covey, F. (2015). *Using Stephen R. Covey's The 7 Habits of Highly Effective People in Education.* Retrieved from https://www.theleaderinme.org/uploads/Documents/results/7_Habits_Lit_Review_for_Ed ucation.pdf

Covey, S. R. (1989). *The seven habits of highly effective people.* New York: Free Press.

Cozolino, L. (2014). *The neuroscience of human relationships: Attachment and the developing social brain.* WW Norton & Company.

Credé, M., Tynan, M. C., & Harms, P. D. (2017). Much ado about grit: A meta-analytic synthesis of the grit literature. *Journal of Personality and Social Psychology, 113*(3), 492–511. doi:10.1037/pspp0000102 PMID:27845531

Crittenden, P. M. (2005). Attachment theory, psychopathology and psychotherapy: The dynamic-maturational approach. *Psicoterapia, 30,* 171–182.

Crowell, J. A., Keluskar, J., & Gorecki, A. (2019). Parenting behavior and the development of children with autism spectrum disorder. *Comprehensive Psychiatry, 90,* 21–29. doi:10.1016/j.comppsych.2018.11.007 PMID:30658339

Csikszentmihalyi, M., & Wong, M. M.-H. (1991). The situational and personal correlates of happiness: A cross-national comparison. In F. Strack, M. Argyle, & N. Schwarz (Eds.), International series in experimental social psychology, Vol. 21. Subjective well-being: An interdisciplinary perspective (pp. 193-212). Elmsford, NY, US: Pergamon Press.

Csikszentmihalyi, M. (1990). *Flow: The psychology of optimal experience.* New York: Harper & Row.

Csikszentmihalyi, M. (2014). *Flow and the foundations of positive psychology* (1st ed.). doi:10.1007/978-94-017-9088-8

Csikszentmihalyi, M., & Csikszentmihalyi, I. (1988). *Optimal Experience: Psychological Studies of Flow in Consciousness.* Cambridge University Press. doi:10.1017/CBO9780511621956

Csikszentmihalyi, M., & Graef, R. (2014). The Experience of Freedom in Daily Life. In *Flow and the Foundations of Positive Psychology.* Dordrecht: Springer. doi:10.1007/978-94-017-9088-8_4

Csikszentmihalyi, M., Montijo, M. N., & Mouton, A. R. (2018). Flow theory: Optimizing elite performance in the creative realm. In S. I. Pfeiffer, E. Shaunessy-Dedrick, M. Foley-Nicpon, & S. I. Pfeiffer (Eds.), *APA Handbook of Giftedness and Talent* (pp. 215–229). Washington, DC: American Psychological Association. doi:10.1037/0000038-014

Csikszentmihalyi, M., & Rathunde, K. (1993). The measurement of flow in everyday life. *Nebraska Symposium on Motivation, 40,* 57–97. PMID:1340523

Csikszentmihaly, M. (1996). *Creativity Flow and The Psychology of Discovery and Invention.* New York, NY: Harper Collins.

Damasio, A. R. (1994). *Descartes' error: emotion, reason, and the human brain.* New York: GP Putnam's Sons.

Danford, C. A., Schultz, C. M., & Marvicsin, D. (2015). Parental roles in the development of obesity in children: Challenges and opportunities. *Research and Reports in Biology*, 6.

Datu, J. A. D. (2017). Sense of relatedness is linked to higher grit in a collectivist setting. *Personality and Individual Differences, 105*, 135–138. Retrieved from org.proxy.wexler.hunter.cuny.edu/10.1016/j.paid.2016.09.039

Dawson, G., Hill, D., Spencer, A., Galpert, L., & Watson, L. (1990). Affective exchanges between young autistic children and their mothers. *Journal of Abnormal Child Psychology, 18*(3), 335–345. doi:10.1007/BF00916569 PMID:2376657

Dawson, G., Jones, E. J., Merkle, K., Venema, K., Lowy, R., Faja, S., ... Smith, M. (2012). Early behavioral intervention is associated with normalized brain activity in young children with autism. *Journal of the American Academy of Child and Adolescent Psychiatry, 51*(11), 1150–1159. doi:10.1016/j.jaac.2012.08.018 PMID:23101741

Dawson, G., Rogers, S., Munson, J., Smith, M., Winter, J., Greenson, J., ... Varley, J. (2010). Randomized, controlled trial of an intervention for toddlers with autism: The Early Start Denver Model. *Pediatrics, 125*(1), 17–23. doi:10.1542/peds.2009-0958 PMID:19948568

De Clercq, B., Van Leeuwen, K., De Fruyt, F., Van Hiel, A., & Mervielde, I. (2008). Maladaptive personality traits and psychopathology in childhood and adolescence: The moderating effect of parenting. *Journal of Personality, 76*(2), 357–383. doi:10.1111/j.1467-6494.2007.00489.x PMID:18331276

De Lepeleere, S., DeSmet, A., Verloigne, M., Cardon, G., & De Bourdeaudhuij, I. (2013). What practices do parents perceive as effective or ineffective in promoting a healthy diet, physical activity, and less sitting in children: Parent focus groups. *BMC Public Health, 13*(1), 1067. doi:10.1186/1471-2458-13-1067 PMID:24219513

De Wolff, M. S., & Van Ijzendoorn, M. H. (1997). Sensitivity and attachment: A meta-analysis on parental antecedents of infant attachment. *Child Development, 68*(4), 571–591. doi:10.1111/j.1467-8624.1997.tb04218.x PMID:9306636

Deci, E., & Ryan, R. (2000). Self-determination theory and the facilitation of intrinsic motivation, social development, and well-being. *American Psychological Association. Inc., 55*(1), 68–67.

Delle Fave, A. (2009). Optimal Experience and Meaning: Which Relationship? *Psihologijske Teme*, 18.

Diamond, K. E. (1994). Evaluating preschool children's sensitivity to developmental differences. *Topics in Early Childhood Special Education, 14*(1), 49–63. doi:10.1177/027112149401400107

Diamond, K. E., & Stacey, S. (2000). The other children at preschool: Experiences of typically developing children in inclusive programs. In S. Sandall & M. Ostrosky (Eds.), *Natural Environments and Inclusion* (pp. 59–68). Frederick, CO: Sopris West.

Diener, E., & Oishi, S. (2005). *The nonobvious social psychology of happiness.* Taylor Francis.

Diener, E., Lucas, R. E., & Scollon, C. N. (2006). Beyond the hedonic treadmill: Revising the adaptation theory of well-being. *The American Psychologist, 61*(4), 305–314. doi:10.1037/0003-066X.61.4.305 PMID:16719675

Dintwa, K. F. (2010). Changing Family Structure in Botswana. *Journal of Comparative Family Studies, 41*(3), 281–297. doi:10.3138/jcfs.41.3.281

Disabato, D. J., Goodman, F. R., & Kashdan, T. B. (2019). Is grit relevant to well-being and strengths? Evidence across the globe for separating perseverance of effort and consistency of interests. *Journal of Personality, 87*(2), 194–211. doi:10.1111/jopy.12382 PMID:29573415

Divan, G., Hamdani, S. U., Vajartkar, V., Minhas, A., Taylor, C., Aldred, C., ... Patel, V. (2015). Adapting an evidence-based intervention for autism spectrum disorder for scaling up in resource-constrained settings: The development of the PASS intervention in South Asia. *Global Health Action, 8*(1), 27278. doi:10.3402/gha.v8.27278 PMID:26243710

Dollberg, D., Feldman, R., & Keren, M. (2010). Maternal representations, infant psychiatric status, and mother–child relationship in clinic-referred and non-referred infants. *European Child & Adolescent Psychiatry, 19*(1), 25–36. doi:10.100700787-009-0036-5 PMID:19543936

Doussard-Roosevelt, J. A., Joe, C. M., Bazhenova, O., & Porges, S. W. (2003). Mother–child interaction in autistic and nonautistic children: Characteristics of maternal approach behaviors and child social responses. *Development and Psychopathology, 15*(2), 277–295. doi:10.1017/S0954579403000154 PMID:12931828

Dowrick, P. W. (1991). *Practical guide to using video in the behavioral sciences.* John Wiley & Sons.

Duckworth, A. (2016). *Grit: The power of passion and perseverance.* New York: Scribner.

Duckworth, A. L., & Eskreis-Winkler, L. (2013). True grit. *APS Observer, 26*(4).

Duckworth, A. L., Peterson, C., Matthews, M. D., & Kelly, D. R. (2007). Grit: Perseverance and passion for long-term goals. *Journal of Personality and Social Psychology, 92*(6), 1087–1101. doi:10.1037/0022-3514.92.6.1087 PMID:17547490

Duckworth, A. L., & Quinn, P. D. (2009). Development and validation of the Short Grit Scale (GRIT–S). *Journal of Personality Assessment, 91*(2), 166–174. doi:10.1080/00223890802634290 PMID:19205937

Duckworth, A., Gendler, T., & Gross, J. (2014). Self-control in school-age children. *Educational Psychologist, 49*(3), 199–217. doi:10.1080/00461520.2014.926225

Duckworth, A., Quinn, P., & Seligman, M. (2009). Positive predictors of teacher effectiveness. *The Journal of Positive Psychology, 4*(6), 540–547. doi:10.1080/17439760903157232

Dunn, W. (2001). The sensations of everyday life: Empirical, theoretical, and pragmatic considerations. *The American Journal of Occupational Therapy*, *55*(6), 608–620. doi:10.5014/ajot.55.6.608 PMID:12959225

Dunst, C. J. (2014). Meta-analysis of the effects of puppet shows on attitudes toward and knowledge of individuals with disabilities. *Exceptional Children*, *80*(2), 136–148. doi:10.1177/001440291408000201

Dweck, C. S. (2009). Developing Talent Through a Growth Mindset. *Olympic Coach, 21*(1).

Dymond, R. F. (1949). A scale for the measurement of empathic ability. *Journal of Consulting Psychology*, *13*(2), 127–133. doi:10.1037/h0061728 PMID:18118267

Dziobek, I., Rogers, K., Fleck, S., Bahnemann, M., Heekeren, H. R., Wolf, O. T., & Convit, A. (2008). Dissociation of cognitive and emotional empathy in adults with Asperger syndrome using the Multifaceted Empathy Test (MET). *Journal of Autism and Developmental Disorders, 38*(3), 464–473. doi:10.100710803-007-0486

Eisenberg, N., Eggum, N. D., & Di Giunta, L. (2010). Empathy-related responding: Associations with prosocial behavior, aggression, and intergroup relations. *Social Issues and Policy Review*, *4*(1), 143–180. doi:10.1111/j.1751-2409.2010.01020.x PMID:21221410

Eisenhower, A. S., Baker, B. L., & Blacher, J. (2005). Preschool children with intellectual disability: Syndrome specificity, behavior problems, and maternal well-being. *Journal of Intellectual Disability Research*, *49*(9), 657–671. doi:10.1111/j.1365-2788.2005.00699.x PMID:16108983

Erba, H. W. (2000). Early intervention programs for children with autism: Conceptual frameworks for implementation. *The American Journal of Orthopsychiatry*, *70*(1), 82–94. doi:10.1037/h0087826 PMID:10702853

Eskreis-Winkler, L., Duckworth, A. L., Shulman, E. P., & Beal, S. (2014). The grit effect: Predicting retention in the military, the workplace, school and marriage. *Frontiers in Psychology*, *5*, 36. doi:10.3389/fpsyg.2014.00036 PMID:24550863

Evans, S., Ling, M., Hill, B., Rinehart, N., Austin, D., & Sciberras, E. (2007). Systematic review of meditation-based intervention for children with ADHD. *European Child Adolescent Psychiatry, 27*, 9-27.

Factor, R. S., Ollendick, T. H., Cooper, L. D., Dunsmore, J. C., Rea, H. M., & Scarpa, A. (2019). All in the Family: A Systematic Review of the Effect of Caregiver-Administered Autism Spectrum Disorder Interventions on Family Functioning and Relationships. *Clinical Child and Family Psychology Review*, *22*(4), 433–457. doi:10.100710567-019-00297-x PMID:31363949

Fairbrother, N. (2011). *Social support*. Retrieved from http://www.heretohelp.bc.ca/sites/default/files/images/visions-ss.pdf

Fatum, B. (2013). Healthy Classrooms, Emotional Intelligence, and Brain Research. *Six seconds: The emotional intelligence network.* Retrieved from http://www.6seconds. org/2013/05/29/healthy-classrooms-emotionalintelligence-and-brain-research

Favazaa, P. C., & Odom, S. L. (1997). Promoting Positive Attitudes of Kindergarten-Age Children toward People with Disabilities. *Exceptional Children*, *63*(3), 405–418. doi:10.1177/001440299706300308

Feinman, J., & Feldman, R. (1982). Decoding Children's Expressions of Affect. *Child Development*, *53*(3), 710–716. doi:10.2307/1129384

Feldman, S., & Nash, S. (1984). The transition from expectancy to parenthood: Impact of the firstborn children on men and women. *Sex Roles*, *11*(1–2), 61–78. doi:10.1007/BF00287441

Fisch, G. S. (2012). Autism and epistemology III: Child development, behavioral stability, and reliability of measurement. *American Journal of Medical Genetics. Part A*, *158*(5), 969–979. doi:10.1002/ajmg.a.35269 PMID:22488915

Fisch, G. S. (2012, May). Nosology and epidemiology in autism: Classification counts. *American Journal of Medical Genetics. Part C, Seminars in Medical Genetics*, *160*(2), 91–103. doi:10.1002/ajmg.c.31325 PMID:22499526

Flippin, M., & Watson, L. R. (2015). Fathers' and mothers' verbal responsiveness and the language skills of young children with autism spectrum disorder. *American Journal of Speech-Language Pathology*, *24*(3), 400–410. doi:10.1044/2015_AJSLP-13-0138 PMID:25836377

Fombonne, E. (2009). Epidemiology of pervasive developmental disorders. *Pediatric Research*, *65*(6), 591–598. doi:10.1203/PDR.0b013e31819e7203 PMID:19218885

Fonagy, P., & Target, M. (1997). Attachment and reflective function: Their role in self-organization. *Development and Psychopathology*, *9*(4), 679–700. doi:10.1017/S0954579497001399 PMID:9449001

Fonagy, P., & Target, M. (1998). Mentalization and the changing aims of child psychoanalysis. *Psychoanalytic Dialogues*, *8*(1), 87–114. doi:10.1080/10481889809539235

Forgas, J. P. (1992). Affect in social judgments and decisions: A multiprocess model. *Advances in Experimental Social Psychology*, *25*, 227–275. doi:10.1016/S0065-2601(08)60285-3

Forgas, J. P., Bower, G. H., & Moylan, S. J. (1990). Praise or blame? Affective influences on attributions for achievement. *Journal of Personality and Social Psychology*, *59*(4), 809–819. doi:10.1037/0022-3514.59.4.809 PMID:2254856

Fountain, C., King, M. D., & Bearman, P. S. (2011). Age of diagnosis for autism: Individual and community factors across 10 birth cohorts. *Journal of Epidemiology and Community Health*, *65*(6), 503–510. doi:10.1136/jech.2009.104588 PMID:20974836

France, S. (2016). *The Fixed Mindset vs. The Growth Mindset*. Retrieved from http://executivesecretary.com/the-fixed-mindset-vs-the-growth-mindset/

Franklin, P., & Volk, A. A. (2018). A review of infants' and children's facial cues' influence on adults' perceptions and behaviors. *Evolutionary Behavioral Sciences*, *12*(4), 296–321. doi:10.1037/ebs0000108

Frazier, T. W., Klingemier, E. W., Beukemann, M., Speer, L., Markowitz, L., Parikh, S., ... Ahuja, V. (2016). Development of an objective autism risk index using remote eye tracking. *Journal of the American Academy of Child and Adolescent Psychiatry*, *55*(4), 301–309. doi:10.1016/j.jaac.2016.01.011 PMID:27015721

Frigda, N. H. (1988). The laws of emotion. *The American Psychologist*, *43*(5), 349–358. doi:10.1037/0003-066X.43.5.349 PMID:3389582

Funderburk, B. W., Eyberg, S. M., Newcomb, K., McNeil, C. B., Hembree-Kigin, T., & Capage, L. (1998). Parent-child interaction therapy with behavior problem children: Maintenance of treatment effects in the school setting. *Child & Family Behavior Therapy*, *20*(2), 17–38. doi:10.1300/J019v20n02_02

Gaisie, S. K. (2000). Family structure, gender and fertility in Botswana, *Pula: Botswana. Journal of African Studies*, *14*(2).

Galantino, M. L., & Quinn, L. (2008). Therapeutic effects of yoga for children: A systematic review of the literature. *Pediatric Physical Therapy*, *20*(1), 66–80. doi:10.1097/PEP.0b013e31815f1208 PMID:18300936

Galla, B., & Duckworth, A. (2013). More than resisting temptation: Habits mediate the association between self-control and positive life outcomes. *Journal of Personality and Social Psychology*, *109*(3), 508–525. doi:10.1037/pspp0000026 PMID:25643222

Garbarino, J., Vorrasi, J. A., & Kostelny, K. (2002). Parenting and Public Policy. In Handbook of Parenting: Vol. 5. Practical Issues in Parenting (2nd ed.; pp. 487-507). London: Lawrence Erlbaum Associates.

Gardener, H., Spiegelman, D., & Buka, S. L. (2011). Perinatal and neonatal risk factors for autism: A comprehensive meta-analysis. *Pediatrics*, *128*(2), 344–355. doi:10.1542/peds.2010-1036 PMID:21746727

Gerdts, J., & Bernier, R. (2011). The broader autism phenotype and its implications on the etiology and treatment of autism spectrum disorders. *Autism Research and Treatment*. PMID:22937250

Gervais, H., Belin, P., Boddaert, N., Leboyer, M., Coez, A., Sfaello, I., ... Zilbovicius, M. (2004). Abnormal cortical voice processing in autism. *Nature Neuroscience*, *7*(8), 801–802. doi:10.1038/nn1291 PMID:15258587

Giallo, R., Rose, N., & Vittorino, R. (2011). Fatigue, wellbeing and parenting in mothers of infants and toddlers with sleep problems. *Journal of Reproductive and Infant Psychology*, *29*(3), 236–249. doi:10.1080/02646838.2011.593030 PMID:29517311

Gibbs, N. (2001, June 24). The EQ Factor. *TIME*. Retrieved from http://content.time.com/time/magazine/article/0,9171,133181,00.html

Goffman, E. (1963). *Stigma: Notes on the management of spoiled identity*. New York: Simon and Schuster.

Goleman, D. (1995). *Emotional intelligence*. New York: Academic Press.

Graham, P. (2003). *Mark Parker Follett: Prohpet of Management*. Washington, DC: Beard Books.

Grayson, R. (2012). *Social, developmental, & organizational psychology applied to camp*. Retrieved from www.visionrealization.com

Green, J., Charman, T., McConachie, H., Aldred, C., Slonims, V., Howlin, P., ... Pickles, A. (2010). Parent-mediated communication-focused treatment in children with autism (PACT): A randomised controlled trial. *Lancet*, *375*(9732), 2152–2160. doi:10.1016/S0140-6736(10)60587-9 PMID:20494434

Green, J., Pickles, A., Pasco, G., Bedford, R., Wan, M. W., Elsabbagh, M., ... Johnson, M. (2017). Randomised trial of a parent-mediated intervention for infants at high risk for autism: Longitudinal outcomes to age 3 years. *Journal of Child Psychology and Psychiatry, and Allied Disciplines*, *58*(12), 1330–1340. doi:10.1111/jcpp.12728 PMID:28393350

Green, J., Rahman, A., Divan, G., Handani, S. U., Vajaratkar, M., Taylor, C., ... Patel, V. (2015). The effectiveness of the parent-mediated intervention for Autism Spectrum Disorders in South Asia (PASS) an RCT in India and Pakistan. *The Lancet. Psychiatry*, *3*(2), 128–136. PMID:26704571

Green, V. A., Pituch, K. A., Itchon, J., Choi, A., O'Reilly, M., & Sigafoos, J. (2006). Internet survey of treatments used by parents of children with autism. *Research in Developmental Disabilities*, *27*(1), 70–84. doi:10.1016/j.ridd.2004.12.002 PMID:15919178

Grieger, R. (2014). *Happiness with Others: Practice Win–Win*. Retrieved from https://www.psychologytoday.com/us/blog/happiness-purpose/201407/happiness-others-practice-win-win

Gruber, J., Mauss, I., & Tamir, M. (2011). A dark side of happiness? How, when and why happi ness is not always good. *Sage (Atlanta, Ga.)*, *6*(3), 222–233. doi:10.1177/1745691611406927 PMID:26168514

Guerrero, L. R., Dudovitz, R., Chung, P. J., Dosanjh, K. K., & Wong, M. D. (2016). Grit: A potential protective factor against substance use and other risk behaviors among Latino adolescents. *Academic Pediatrics*, *16*(3), 275–281. doi:10.1016/j.acap.2015.12.016 PMID:26796576

Guralnick, M. J. (1999). Family and child influences on the peer-related social competence of young children with developmental delays. *Mental Retardation and Developmental Disabilities Research Reviews*, *5*(1), 21–29. doi:<2 doi:10.1002/(SICI)1098-2779(1999)5:1

Haimovitz, K., & Dweck, C. S. (2016). What predicts children's fixed and growth intelligence mind-sets? Not their parents' views of intelligence but their parents' views of failure. *Psychological Science*, *27*(6), 859–869. doi:10.1177/0956797616639727 PMID:27113733

Happiness, C. (n.d.). *More Than Just Child's Play*. Retrieved from https://www.psychologytoday.com/us/blog/longing-nostalgia/201201/childhood-happiness-more-just-childs-play

Harrison, K., & Cantor, J. (1997). The relationship between media consumption and eating disorders. *Journal of Communication*, *47*(1), 40–67. doi:10.1111/j.1460-2466.1997.tb02692.x

Harvey, J., & Pauwels, B. (2003). The Ironies of Positive Psychology. *Psychological Inquiry*, *14*(2), 125–128. Retrieved from http://www.jstor.org/stable/1449818

Haydon, K. C., Collins, W. A., Salvatore, J., Simpson, J. E., & Roisman, G. I. (2012). Shared and distinctive origins and correlates of adult attachment representations: The developmental organization of romantic functioning. *Child Development*, *83*(5), 1689–1702. doi:10.1111/j.1467-8624.2012.01801.x PMID:22694197

Hazan, C., & Shaver, P. (1987). Romantic love conceptualized as an attachment process. *Journal of Personality and Social Psychology*, *52*(3), 511.

Heim, J. (2016). *Finland's schools were once the envy of the world. Now, they're slipping*. Retrieved from https://www.washingtonpost.com/local/education/finlands-schools-were-once-the-envy-of-the-world-now-theyre-slipping/2016/12/08/dcfd0f56-bd60-11e6-91ee-1adddfe36cbe_story.html

Henggeler, S. W., & Sheidow, A. J. (2012). Empirically supported family-based treatments for conduct disorder and delinquency in adolescents. *Journal of Marital and Family Therapy*, *38*(1), 30–58. doi:10.1111/j.1752-0606.2011.00244.x PMID:22283380

He, X., Sanders, S. J., Liu, L., De Rubeis, S., Lim, E. T., Sutcliffe, J. S., ... Devlin, B. (2013). Integrated model of de novo and inherited genetic variants yields greater power to identify risk genes. *PLOS Genetics*, *9*(8), e1003671. doi:10.1371/journal.pgen.1003671 PMID:23966865

Higgins, D. J., Bailey, S. R., & Pearce, J. C. (2005). Factors associated with functioning style and coping strategies of families with a child with an autism spectrum disorder. *Autism*, *9*(2), 125–137. doi:10.1177/1362361305051403 PMID:15857858

Hochanadel, A., & Finamore, D. (2015). Fixed and growth mindset in education and how grit helps students persist in the face of adversity. *Journal of International Education Research*, *11*(1), 47–50.

Hodges, B. D., Kuper, A., & Reeves, S. (2008). Qualitative Research: Discourse Analysis. *British Medical Journal*, *337*(7669), 570–572.

Hogan, M. J., & Strasburger, V. C. (2008). *Media and prosocial behavior in children and adolescents. In Handbook of Moral and Character Education* (pp. 537–553). Mahwah, NJ: Lawrence Erlbaum.

Holliday Willey, L. (1999). *Pretending to be normal: Living with Asperger's syndrome*. London: Jessica Kingsley.

Honig, Miller, & Church. (2019). *Ages & Stages: Helping Happiness Along*. Retrieved from https://www.scholastic.com/teachers/articles/teaching-content/ages-stages-helping-happiness-along/

Howard, J. M., Nicholson, B. C., & Chesnut, S. R. (2019). Relationships Between Positive Parenting, Overparenting, Grit, and Academic Success. *Journal of College Student Development*, *60*(2), 189–202. doi:10.1353/csd.2019.0018

Isen, A. M., Daubman, K. A., & Nowicki, G. P. (1987). Positive affect facilitates creative problem solving. *Journal of Personality and Social Psychology, 52*(6), 1122–1131. doi:10.1037/0022-3514.52.6.1122 PMID:3598858

Jachimowicza, J., Wihlerb, A., Baileya, E., & Galinskya, A. (2018). Why grit requires perseverance and passion to positively predict performance. *Proceedings of the National Academy of Sciences of the United States of America Journal*, 115(40). 10.1073/pnas.1803561115

Jackson, S., Steptoe, A., & Wardle, J. (2015). The Influence of Partner's Behavior on Health Behavior Change The English Longitudinal Study of Ageing. *JAMA Internal Medicine, 175*(3), 385–392. doi:10.1001/jamainternmed.2014.7554 PMID:25599511

Jacobs, S. B. (1996). Hidden Gender Bias behind the Best Interest of the Child Standard in Custody Decisions. *The Ga. St. UL Rev., 13*, 845.

Jaggernath, J. (2019). *How to Talk to Your Spouse About Setting Financial Goals- Money & Relationships.* Retrieved from https://www.mymoneycoach.ca/blog/communicate-about-money-with-spouse-set-financial-goals.html

Jairam, D., & Kahl, D. (2012). Navigating the doctoral experience: The role of social support in the successful degree completion. *International Journal of Doctoral Studies, 7*. doi:10.28945/1700

Jiang, W., Xiao, Z., Liu, Y., Guo, K., Jiang, J., & Du, X. (2019). Reciprocal relations between grit and academic achievement: A longitudinal study. *Learning and Individual Differences, 71*, 13–22. doi:10.1016/j.lindif.2019.02.004

Jordan, R. (2003). Social play and autistic spectrum disorders: A perspective on theory, implications and educational approaches. *Autism, 7*(4), 347–360. doi:10.1177/1362361303007004002 PMID:14678675

Jorm, A. F. (2012). Mental health literacy: Empowering the community to take action for better mental health. *The American Psychologist, 67*(3), 231–243. doi:10.1037/a0025957 PMID:22040221

Jorm, A. F., Korten, A. E., Jacomb, P. A., Christensen, H., Rodgers, B., & Pollitt, P. (1997). "Mental health literacy": A survey of the public's ability to recognize mental disorders and their beliefs about the effectiveness of treatment. *The Medical Journal of Australia, 166*(4), 182–186. doi:10.5694/j.1326-5377.1997.tb140071.x PMID:9066546

Joyce, A. (2019, April 21). *Are you raising nice kids? A Harvard psychologist gives 5 ways to raise them to be kind.* Retrieved from: https://www.washingtonpost.com/news/parenting/wp/2014/07/18/are-you-raising-nice-kids-a-harvard-psychologist-gives-5-ways-to-raise-them-to-be-kind/

Juffer, F., Bakermans-Kranenburg, M. J., & van IJzendoorn, M. J. (2008). Promoting positive parenting: An introduction. In F. Juffer, M. J. Bakermans-Kranenburg, & M. J. van IJzendoorn (Eds.), Promoting positive parenting: An attachment based intervention. New York, NY: Taylor and Francis.

Juffer, F., Bakermans-Kranenburg, M. J., & Van IJzendoorn, M. H. (2008). *Introduction and outline of the VIPP and VIPP-R program. Promoting positive parenting: An attachment-based intervention.* Mahwah, NJ: Erlbaum.

Kahn, D. (2003). Montessori and optimal experience research: Toward building a comprehensive education reform. *The NAMTA Journal, 28*, 1–9.

Kannangara, C. S., Allen, R. E., Waugh, G., Nahar, N., Khan, S. Z. N., Rogerson, S., & Carson, J. (2018). All that glitters is not grit: Three studies of grit in university students. *Frontiers in Psychology*, 9. PMID:30210389

Kaplan, D. M., DeBlois, M., Dominguez, V., & Walsh, M. E. (2016). Studying the teaching of kindness: A conceptual model for evaluating kindness education programs in schools. *Evaluation and Program Planning, 58*, 160–170.

Kelly, J. B. (1997). The best interests of the child. *Family Court Review, 35*(4), 377–387. doi:10.1111/j.174-1617.1997.tb00480.x

Kelly, M. (2005). Psychological adaptation to graduate school: How to smell the roses while burning the midnight oil. *Behavior Therapist, 28*, 57–59.

Kesebir, P., & Diener, E. (2008). *In pursuit of happiness: Empirical answers to philosophical questions.* Sage Publications, Inc.

Kessler, R. C., Price, R. H., & Wortman, C. B. (1985). Social factors in psychopathology: Stress, social support, and coping processes. *Annual Review of Psychology, 36*(1), 531–572. doi:10.1146/annurev.ps.36.020185.002531 PMID:3883893

Kidd, P. E. (1997). *Botswana families and women's rights in a changing environment.* Gaborone: Women and Law in Southern Africa.

Kids & Tech: Tips for Parents in the Digital Age. (2018). Retrieved from https://www.healthychildren.org/English/family-life/Media/Pages/Tips-for-Parents-Digital-Age.aspx

Kim, Y. S., Leventhal, B. L., Koh, Y. J., Fombonne, E., Laska, E., Lim, E. C., ... Song, D. H. (2011). Prevalence of autism spectrum disorders in a total population sample. *The American Journal of Psychiatry, 168*(9), 904–912. doi:10.1176/appi.ajp.2011.10101532 PMID:21558103

Konstantareas, M. (2008). Temperament and internalizing disorders in children with Asperger's disorder: Implications for interventions. *International Journal of Psychology, 43*(3-4), 544–564.

Kotler, J. A., Schiffman, J. M., & Hanson, K. G. (2012). The influence of media characters on children's food choices. *Journal of Health Communication, 17*(8), 886–898. doi:10.1080/10810730.2011.650822 PMID:22475307

Kral, T. V., & Rauh, E. M. (2010). Eating behaviors of children in the context of their family environment. *Physiology & Behavior, 100*(5), 567–573. doi:10.1016/j.physbeh.2010.04.031 PMID:20457172

Krebs, D. (1975). Empathy and altruism. *Journal of Personality and Social Psychology*, *32*(6), 1134–1146. doi:10.1037/0022-3514.32.6.1134 PMID:1214217

Krishnan, A., Zhang, R., Yao, V., Theesfeld, C. L., Wong, A. K., Tadych, A., ... Troyanskaya, O. G. (2016). Genome-wide prediction and functional characterization of the genetic basis of autism spectrum disorder. *Nature Neuroscience*, *19*(11), 1454–1462. doi:10.1038/nn.4353 PMID:27479844

Krueger, R. F., Hicks, B. M., Patrick, C. J., Carlson, S. R., Iacono, W. G., & McGue, M. (2002). Etiologic connections among substance dependence, antisocial behavior and personality: Modeling the externalizing spectrum. *Journal of Abnormal Psychology*, *111*(3), 411–424. doi:10.1037/0021-843X.111.3.411 PMID:12150417

Kuhn, J. C., & Carter, A. S. (2006). Maternal self-efficacy and associated parenting cognitions among mothers of children with autism. *The American Journal of Orthopsychiatry*, *76*(4), 564–575. doi:10.1037/0002-9432.76.4.564 PMID:17209724

Lahey, B. B., Applegate, B., Barkley, R. A., Garfinkel, B., McBurnett, K., Kerdyk, L., ... Biederman, J. (1994). DSM-IV field trials for oppositional defiant disorder and conduct disorder in children and adolescents. *The American Journal of Psychiatry*, *151*(8), 1163–1171. doi:10.1176/ajp.151.8.1163 PMID:8037251

Langer, E. J. (2000). *Mindful learning*. Sage Publications, Inc.

Lansford, J. E. (2010). The special problem of cultural differences in effects of corporal punishment. *Law and Contemporary Problems*, *73*(2), 89–106.

Larsen, J. T., & McKibban, A. R. (2008). *Is happiness having what you want, wanting what you have, or both?* Association for Psychological Science.

Latham, G. P. (2003). Goal setting: A five-step approach to behavior change. *Organizational Dynamics*, *32*(3), 309–318. doi:10.1016/S0090-2616(03)00028-7

Laurent, V., Nidich, S., Wendt, S., Jamie, G., & Nidich, R. (2019). Effect of Meditation on Social- emotional Learning in Middle School Students. *Project Innovation, 139*(3), 111-119.

Lavigne, J. V., Dahl, K. P., Gouze, K. R., LeBailly, S. A., & Hopkins, J. (2015). Multi-domain predictors of oppositional defiant disorder symptoms in preschool children: Cross-informant differences. *Child Psychiatry and Human Development*, *46*(2), 308–319. doi:10.100710578-014-0472-4 PMID:24997089

Lazarus, R. (2003). Does the Positive Psychology Movement Have Legs? *Psychological Inquiry*, *14*(2), 93–109. doi:10.1207/S15327965PLI1402_02

Leech, R. M., McNaughton, S. A., & Timperio, A. (2014). The clustering of diet, physical activity and sedentary behavior in children and adolescents: A review. *The International Journal of Behavioral Nutrition and Physical Activity*, *11*(1), 4. doi:10.1186/1479-5868-11-4 PMID:24450617

Leitch, S., & Palmer, I. (2010). Analysing texts in context: Current practices and new protocols for critical discourse analysis in organization studies. *Journal of Management Studies, 47*(6), 1194–1212. doi:10.1111/j.1467-6486.2009.00884.x

Lenoir, F. (2015). *Happiness: A Philosopher's Guide*. Brooklyn, NY: Melville House.

Levy, J. M., & Steele, H. (2011). Attachment and grit: Exploring possible contributions of attachment styles (from past and present life) to the adult personality construct of grit. *Journal of Social and Psychological Sciences, 4*(2), 16–49.

Liang, X., Fuller, B., & Singer, J. D. (2000). Ethnic differences in child care selection: The Influence of family structure, parenting practices, and home language. *Early Childhood Research Quarterly, 15*(3), 357–384. doi:10.1016/S0885-2006(00)00071-5

Lin, C. L. S., & Chang, C. Y. (2017). Personality and Family Context in Explaining Grit of Taiwanese High School Students. *Eurasia Journal of Mathematics. Science and Technology Education, 13*(6), 2197–2213.

LiveScience. (2015). *Couples who set health goals together have more success, study suggests.* Retrieved from https://www.foxnews.com/health/couples-who-set-health-goals-together-have-more-success-study-suggests

Locke, E. A., & Latham, G. P. (1990). *A theory of goal setting and task performance*. Academic Press.

Locke, E. A., & Latham, G. P. (2002). Building a practically useful theory of goal setting and task motivation. *The American Psychologist, 57*(9), 705–717. doi:10.1037/0003-066X.57.9.705 PMID:12237980

Loeber, R., Burke, J. D., Lahey, B. B., Winters, A., & Zera, M. (2000). Oppositional defiant and conduct disorder: A review of the past 10 years, part I. *Journal of the American Academy of Child and Adolescent Psychiatry, 39*(12), 1468–1484. doi:10.1097/00004583-200012000-00007 PMID:11128323

Lopez, S., & Snyder, C. (2009). *The oxford handbook of positive psychology* (2nd ed.). Oxford, UK: Oxford University Press.

Lord, C., Elsabbagh, M., Baird, G., & Veenstra-Vanderweele, J. (2018). Autism spectrum disorder. *Lancet, 0*(0), 508–520. doi:10.1016/S0140-6736(18)31129-2 PMID:30078460

Losh, M., Martin, G. E., Lee, M., Klusek, J., Sideris, J., Barron, S., & Wassink, T. (2017). Developmental markers of genetic liability to autism in parents: A longitudinal, multigenerational study. *Journal of Autism and Developmental Disorders, 47*(3), 834–845. doi:10.100710803-016-2996-x PMID:28070788

Lovaas, O. I., Koegel, R., Simmons, J. Q., & Long, J. S. (1970, June). Strengths and weaknesses of operant conditioning techniques for the treatment of autism. In *Proceedings of the conference and annual meeting of the National Society for Autistic Children* (pp. 30-41). Academic Press.

Loveless, T. (2017). *The 2017 Brown Center Report on American Education: How Well Are American Students Learning?* Brown Center on Education Policy at Brookings. Retrieved from https://www.brookings.edu/wp-content/uploads/2017/03/2017-brown-center-report-on-american-education.pdf

Lunenburg, F. (2011). Goal-setting theory of motivation. *International Journal of Management, Business, and Administration, 15*(1), 5.

Luthar, S. S. (2015). Resilience in development: A synthesis of research across five decades. Developmental Psychopathology: Volume Three: Risk, Disorder, and Adaptation, 739-795

Lyubomirsky, S. (2008). *The how of happiness: A scientific approach to getting the life you want.* New York: Penguin Press.

Lyubomirsky, S., King, L. A., & Diener, E. (2005). The benefits of frequent positive affect: Does happiness lead to success? *Psychological Bulletin, 131*(6), 803–855. doi:10.1037/0033-2909.131.6.803 PMID:16351326

Lyubomirsky, S., Sheldon, K. M., & Schkade, D. (2005). Pursuing happiness: The architecture of sustainable change. *Review of General Psychology, 9*(2), 111–113. doi:10.1037/1089-2680.9.2.111

Magrelli, S., Jermann, P., Basilio, N., Ansermet, F., Hentsch, F., Nadel, J., & Billard, A. (2013). Social orienting of children with autism to facial expressions and speech: A study with a wearable eye-tracker in naturalistic settings. *Frontiers in Psychology, 4*, 840. doi:10.3389/fpsyg.2013.00840 PMID:24312064

Maharaj, S., & Sewpaul, V. (2016). Accidental burns in children under five years of age: The gendered burden of care and socio-economic deprivation. *Children and Youth Services Review, 68*, 51–58. doi:10.1016/j.childyouth.2016.06.014

Makrygianni, M. K., & Reed, P. (2010). A meta-analytic review of the effectiveness of behavioral early intervention programs for children with autistic spectrum disorders. *Research in Autism Spectrum Disorders, 4*(4), 577–593. doi:10.1016/j.rasd.2010.01.014

Malkova, N. V., Collin, Z. Y., Hsiao, E. Y., Moore, M. J., & Patterson, P. H. (2012). Maternal immune activation yields offspring displaying mouse versions of the three core symptoms of autism. *Brain, Behavior, and Immunity, 26*(4), 607–616. doi:10.1016/j.bbi.2012.01.011 PMID:22310922

Masi, A., De Mayo, M. M., Glozier, N., & Guastella, A. J. (2017). An overview of autism spectrum disorder, heterogeneity and treatment options. *Neuroscience Bulletin, 33*(2), 183–193. doi:10.100712264-017-0100-y PMID:28213805

Masi, A., Quintana, D. S., Glozier, N., Lloyd, A. R., Hickie, I. B., & Guastella, A. J. (2015). Cytokine aberrations in autism spectrum disorder: A systematic review and meta-analysis. *Molecular Psychiatry, 20*(4), 440–446. doi:10.1038/mp.2014.59 PMID:24934179

Maundeni, T., & Jacques, G. (2012). "… and a little child shall lead them": Utilising Kgotla meetings to empower children and the communities that nurture them. *Thari ya Bana: Reflections on Children in Botswana*, 74-80.

McAuliffe, T., Thomas, Y., Vaz, S., Falkmer, T., & Cordier, R. (2019). The experiences of mothers of children with autism spectrum disorder: Managing family routines and mothers' health and wellbeing. *Australian Occupational Therapy Journal*, *66*(1), 68–76. doi:10.1111/1440-1630.12524 PMID:30264526

McConnell, S. R. (2002). Interventions to facilitate social interaction for young children with autism: Review of available research and recommendations for educational intervention and future research. *Journal of Autism and Developmental Disorders*, *32*(5), 351–372. doi:10.1023/A:1020537805154 PMID:12463515

McDaniel, A., & Zulu, E. (1996). Women, Fathers, and Children: Regional Patterns in Child-Parent Residence in Sub-Saharan Africa. *African Population Studies*, 11.

McEvoy, R. E., Rogers, S. J., & Pennington, B. F. (1993). Executive function and social communication deficits in young autistic children. *Journal of Child Psychology and Psychiatry, and Allied Disciplines*, *34*(4), 563–578. doi:10.1111/j.1469-7610.1993.tb01036.x PMID:7685360

McLeod, S. (2018). *Mary Ainsworth*. Retrieved from https://www.simplypsychology.org/mary ainsworth.html

McLeod, M. (2018). *The ultimate happiness: An exclusive interview with the Dalai Lama* (2nd ed.). Lions Roar Foundation.

Meadows, H. D. (2008). *Thinking in Systems: A Primer*. White River Junction, VT: Chelsea Green Publishing Company.

Medina, J. (2008). *Brain rules*. Seattle, WA: Pear Press.

Mehrabian, A., & Epstein, N. (1972). A measure of emotional empathy 1. *Journal of Personality*, *40*(4), 525–543. doi:10.1111/j.1467-6494.1972.tb00078.x PMID:4642390

Miller-Johnson, S., Coie, J. D., Maumary-Gremaud, A., & Bierman, K. (2002). Peer rejection and aggression and early starter models of conduct disorder. *Journal of Abnormal Child Psychology*, *30*(3), 217–230. doi:10.1023/A:1015198612049 PMID:12041708

Mindset Works. (2015). *Dr. Dweck's discovery of fixed and growth mindsets have shaped our understanding of learning*. Retrieved from https://www.mindsetworks.com/science/

Mmonadibe, P. N. (2009). Orphaned HIV-positive children in Botswana: Challenges and prospects. In C. M. Fombad, R. Mupedziswa, T. Maundeni, & G. Mookodi (Eds.), *HIV and AIDS, Vulnerable groups, Human Rights and Development in Botswana* (pp. 155–167). OSSREA.

Mogilner, C., Aaker, J., & Kamvar, S. (2012). How Happiness Affects Choice. *The Journal of Consumer Research*, *39*(2), 429–443. doi:10.1086/663774

Mogro-Wilson, C. (2008). The influence of parental warmth and control on Latino adolescent alcohol use. *Hispanic Journal of Behavioral Sciences*, *30*(1), 89–105. doi:10.1177/0739986307310881

Mooradian, T., Matzler, K., Uzelac, B., & Bauer, F. (2016). Perspiration and inspiration: Grit and innovativeness as antecedents of entrepreneurial success. *Journal of Economic Psychology*, *56*, 232–243. doi:10.1016/j.joep.2016.08.001

Morgan, S. B., & Wisely, D. W. (1996). Children's attitudes and behavioral intentions toward a peer presented as physically handicapped: A more positive view. *Journal of Developmental and Physical Disabilities*, *8*(1), 29–42. doi:10.1007/BF02578438

Morris, W. N. (1989). *Mood: The frame of mind*. New York: Springer-Verlag. doi:10.1007/978-1-4612-3648-1

Muenks, K., Wigfield, A., Yang, J. S., & O'Neal, C. R. (2017). How true is grit? Assessing its relations to high school and college students' personality characteristics, self-regulation, engagement, and achievement. *Journal of Educational Psychology*, *109*(5), 599–620. doi:10.1037/edu0000153

Mullaly, R. P. (1997). *Structural social work: Ideology, theory, and practice* (2nd ed.). New York: Oxford University Press.

Mundy, P., Sigman, M., Ungerer, J., & Sherman, T. (1986). Defining the social deficits of autism: The contribution of non-verbal communication measures. *Journal of Child Psychology and Psychiatry, and Allied Disciplines*, *27*(5), 657–669. doi:10.1111/j.1469-7610.1986.tb00190.x PMID:3771682

Murray, J., & Farrington, D. P. (2010). Risk factors for conduct disorder and delinquency: Key findings from longitudinal studies. *Canadian Journal of Psychiatry*, *55*(10), 633–642. doi:10.1177/070674371005501003 PMID:20964942

Myers, C. A., Wang, C., Black, J. M., Bugescu, N., & Hoeft, F. (2016). The matter of motivation: Striatal resting-state connectivity is dissociable between grit and growth mindset. *Social Cognitive and Affective Neuroscience*, *11*(10), 1521–1527. doi:10.1093can/nsw065 PMID:27217105

Naber, F. B. A., Bakermans-Kranenburg, M. J., van IJzendoorn, M. H., Dietz, C., van Daalen, E., Swinkels, S. H. M., ... van Engeland, H. (2008). Joint attention development in toddlers with autism. *European Journal of Child and Adolescent Psychiatry*, *17*(3), 143–152. doi:10.100700787-007-0648-6 PMID:17849078

Naber, F. B., Bakermans-Kranenburg, M. J., Van Ijzendoorn, M. H., Swinkels, S. H., Buitelaar, J. K., Dietz, C., ... Van Engeland, H. (2008). Play behavior and attachment in toddlers with autism. *Journal of Autism and Developmental Disorders*, *38*(5), 857–866. doi:10.100710803-007-0454-5 PMID:17896172

Nakumara, J., & Csikszentmihaly, M. (2009). The concept of flow. In C. R. Snyder & S. J. Lopez (Eds.), *Oxford handbook of positive psychology* (pp. 89–105). Oxford University Press.

Narvaez, D. (2013). *New Moms Need Social Support*. Retrieved from https://www.psychologytoday.com/us/blog/moral-landscapes/201301/new-moms-need-social-support

Narvaez, D., Panksepp, J., Schore, A., & Gleason, T. (Eds.). (2013). *Evolution, Early Experience and Human Development: From Research to Practice and Policy*. New York: Oxford University Press.

National AIDS Coordinating Agency-NACA. (2004). *Botswana AIDS Impact Survey II: Statistical report*. Gaborone: Central Statistics Office.

National Center for Education Statistics. (2016). *Children and youth with disabilities*. Author.

National Childbirth Trust (NCT). (2019). *Changes in your relationships after having a baby*. Retrieved from https://www.nct.org.uk/life-parent/your-relationship-couple/relationship-changes/changes-your-relationships-after-having-baby

National Research Council. (2001). *Eager to Learn: Educating Our Preschoolers*. Washington, DC: National Academy Press.

Nelson, S., Kushlev, K., & Lyubomirsky, S. (2014). The pains and pleasures of parenting: When, why, and how is parenthood associated with more or less well-being? *Psychological Bulletin*, *140*(3), 846–895. doi:10.1037/a0035444 PMID:24491021

Newschaffer, C. J., Croen, L. A., Daniels, J., Giarelli, E., Grether, J. K., Levy, S. E., ... Reynolds, A. M. (2007). The epidemiology of autism spectrum disorders. *Annual Review of Public Health*, *28*(1), 235–258. doi:10.1146/annurev.publhealth.28.021406.144007 PMID:17367287

Nowicki, E. A., & Sandieson, R. (2002). A meta-analysis of school-age children's attitudes towards persons with physical or intellectual disabilities. *International Journal of Disability Development and Education*, *49*(3), 243–265. doi:10.1080/1034912022000007270

Ntarangwi, M. (2012). Introduction: Parents' Involvement in Children's Lives in Africa. *Africa Development. Afrique et Developpement*, *37*(3), 1–18.

Ntseane, D., & Solo, K. (2007). *Social security & social protection in Botswana*. Gaborone: Bay Publishers.

Ntshwarang, P. N. (2017). Parenting and parenting practices among contemporary families in Botswana: Does government policy matter? In R. Mupedzisa, G. Jacques, & L-K, Mwansa (Eds.), Social Work and Social Development in Botswana: Issues, Challenges & Prospects. IFSW.

Ntshwarang, P. N., & Sewpaul, V. (forthcoming). When national law and culture coalesce: Challenges for children's rights in Botswana with specific reference to corporal punishment. In V. Sewpaul, L. Kreitzer, & T. Raniga (Eds.), Culture, Human Rights and Social Work: African Perspectives. Calgary: Calgary University Press.

O'Brien, C. (2008). Sustainable happiness: How happiness studies can contribute to a more sustainable future. *Canadian Psychology*, *49*(4), 289–295. doi:10.1037/a0013235

O'Gara, J. L., Calzada, E. J., & Kim, S. Y. (2019). The father's role in risk and resilience among Mexican-American adolescents. *The American Journal of Orthopsychiatry*. PMID:30628806

O'Neal, C. R., Espino, M. M., Goldthrite, A., Morin, M. F., Weston, L., Hernandez, P., & Fuhrmann, A. (2016). Grit under duress: Stress, strengths, and academic success among non-citizen and citizen Latina/o first-generation college students. *Hispanic Journal of Behavioral Sciences, 38*(4), 446–466. Retrieved from org.proxy.wexler.hunter.cuny.edu/10.1177/0739986316660775

Odenweller, K. G., Booth-Butterfield, M., & Weber, K. (2014). Investigating helicopter parenting, family environments, and relational outcomes for millennials. *Communication Studies, 65*(4), 407–425. doi:10.1080/10510974.2013.811434

Odom, S., Zercher, C., Li, S., Marquart, J., Sandall, S., & Brown, W. (2006). Social acceptance and rejection of preschool children with disabilities: A mixed-method analysis. *Journal of Educational Psychology, 98*(4), 807–823. doi:10.1037/0022-0663.98.4.807

Okoro, C. A., Hollis, N. D., Cyrus, A. C., & Griffin-Blake, S. (2018). Prevalence of disabilities and health care access by disability status and type among adults—United States, 2016. *Morbidity and Mortality Weekly Report, 67*(32), 882–887. doi:10.15585/mmwr.mm6732a3 PMID:30114005

Oono, I. P., Honey, E. J., & McConachie, H. (2013). Parent-mediated early intervention for young children with autism spectrum disorders (ASD). *Evidence-Based Child Health: A Cochrane Review Journal, 8*(6), 2380–2479. doi:10.1002/ebch.1952 PMID:23633377

Oosterling, I. J., Wensing, M., Swinkels, S. H., Van Der Gaag, R. J., Visser, J. C., Woudenberg, T., ... Buitelaar, J. K. (2010). Advancing early detection of autism spectrum disorder by applying an integrated two-stage screening approach. *Journal of Child Psychology and Psychiatry, and Allied Disciplines, 51*(3), 250–258. doi:10.1111/j.1469-7610.2009.02150.x PMID:19843319

Ortiz, J., & Raine, A. (2004). Heart rate level and antisocial behavior in children and adolescents: A meta-analysis. *Journal of the American Academy of Child and Adolescent Psychiatry, 43*(2), 154–162. doi:10.1097/00004583-200402000-00010 PMID:14726721

Ospina, M. B., Seida, J. K., Clark, B., Karkhaneh, M., Hartling, L., Tjosvold, L., ... Smith, V. (2008). Behavioral and developmental interventions for autism spectrum disorder: A clinical systematic review. *PLoS One, 3*(11), e3755. doi:10.1371/journal.pone.0003755 PMID:19015734

Ostfeld-Etzion, S., Golan, O., Hirschler-Guttenberg, Y., Zagoory-Sharon, O., & Feldman, R. (2015). Neuroendocrine and behavioral response to social rupture and repair in preschoolers with autism spectrum disorders interacting with mother and father. *Molecular Autism, 6*(1), 11. doi:10.118613229-015-0007-2 PMID:25774280

Padilla-Walker, L. M., Day, R. D., Dyer, W. J., & Black, B. C. (2013). "Keep on Keeping On, Even When It's Hard!" Predictors and Outcomes of Adolescent Persistence. *The Journal of Early Adolescence, 33*(4), 433–457. doi:10.1177/0272431612449387

Paglioca, P. M., Meltou, B. G., Lyons, P. M. Jr, & Weisz, V. (2002). Parenting and the Law. In M. H. Bornstein (Ed.), Handbook of Parenting: Vol. 5. *Practical Issues in Parenting* (2nd ed.; pp. 463–486). London: Lawrence Erlbaun Associates.

Pajareya, K., & Nopmaneejumruslers, K. (2011). A pilot randomized controlled trial of DIR/ Floortime™ parent training intervention for pre-school children with autistic spectrum disorders. *Autism, 15*(5), 563–577. doi:10.1177/1362361310386502 PMID:21690083

Palmitotto, J. (2018). *Patience and Your Relationships*. Retrieved from https://familyguidanceandtherapy.com/patience-and-your-relationships/

Paolini, S., Hewstone, M., Cairns, E., & Voci, A. (2004). Effects of direct and indirect cross-group friendships on judgments of Catholics and Protestants in Northern Ireland: The mediating role of an anxiety-reduction mechanism. *Personality and Social Psychology Bulletin, 30*(6), 770–786. doi:10.1177/0146167203262848 PMID:15155040

Park, D., Yu, A., Baelen, R. N., Tsukayama, E., & Duckworth, A. L. (2018). Fostering grit: Perceived school goal-structure predicts growth in grit and grades. *Contemporary Educational Psychology, 55*, 120–128. doi:10.1016/j.cedpsych.2018.09.007

Parker, K., & Wang, W. (2013). *Modern parenthood: Roles of moms and dads converge as they balance work and family*. Retrieved from http://www.pewsocialtrends.org/2013/03/14/ modern-parenthood-roles-of-moms-and-dads-converge-as-they-balance-workand-family/

Park, S., Kwak, K., & Kim, Y. (2018). Psychological variables related to grit among adolescents in South Korea: A longitudinal study from age 4 to 14. *Current Psychology,* 1–6.

Parks, A., Della Porta, M. D., Pierce, R. S., Zilca, R., & Lyubomirsky, S. (2012). Pursuing happiness in everyday life: The characteristics and behaviors of online happiness seekers. *Emotion (Washington, D.C.), 12*(6), 1222–1234. doi:10.1037/a0028587 PMID:22642345

Pascale, R., & Primavera, L. (2017). *Time Together and Time Apart*. Retrieved from https://www.psychologytoday.com/us/blog/so-happy-together/201702/time-together-and-time-apart

Peck, S. C., Roeser, R. W., Zarrett, N., & Eccles, J. S. (2008). Exploring the roles of extracurricular activity quantity and quality in the educational resilience of vulnerable adolescents: Variable-and pattern-centered approaches. *The Journal of Social Issues, 64*(1), 135–156. doi:10.1111/j.1540-4560.2008.00552.x PMID:19543445

Pérez-Álvarez, M. (2016). The science of happiness: As felicitous as it is fallacious. *Journal of Theoretical and Philosophical Psychology, 36*(1), 1–19. doi:10.1037/teo0000030

Perkins-Gough, D. (2013). The Significance of Grit: A Conversation with Angela Lee Duckworth. *Resilience and Learning, 71*, 14-20.

Perkins-Gough, D. (2013). The significance of grit: A conversation with Angela Lee Duckworth. *Educational Leadership, 71*(1), 14–20.

Peskind, S. N. (2004). Determining the Undeterminable: The Best Interest of the Child Standard as an Imperfect but Necessary Guidepost to Determine Child Custody. *N. Ill. UL Rev., 25*, 449.

Peters-Scheffer, N., Didden, R., Korzilius, H., & Sturmey, P. (2011). A meta-analytic study on the effectiveness of comprehensive ABA-based early intervention programs for children with autism spectrum disorders. *Research in Autism Spectrum Disorders*, *5*(1), 60–69. doi:10.1016/j.rasd.2010.03.011

Petrides, K. V. (2011). Ability and trait emotional intelligence. In The Wiley- Blackwell handbook of individual differences, (pp. 656–678). Chichester, UK: Wiley-Blackwell.

Petrides, K. V., & Furnham, A. (2003). Trait emotional intelligence: Behavioural validation in two studies of emotion recognition and reactivity to mood induction. *European Journal of Personality*, *17*(1), 39–57. doi:10.1002/per.466

Pettigrew, T. F., & Tropp, L. R. (2000). Does inter-group contact reduce prejudice: Recent meta-analytic findings. In S. Oskamp (Ed.), *Reducing prejudice and discrimination. The Claremont Symposium on Applied Social Psychology* (pp. 93–114). Mahwah, NJ: Lawrence Erlbaum Associates, Publishers.

Pickles, A., Le Couteur, A., Leadbitter, K., Salomone, E., Cole-Fletcher, R., Tobin, H., ... Aldred, C. (2016). Parent-mediated social communication therapy for young children with autism (PACT): Long-term follow-up of a randomised controlled trial. *Lancet*, *388*(10059), 2501–2509. doi:10.1016/S0140-6736(16)31229-6 PMID:27793431

Piña-Watson, B., López, B., Ojeda, L., & Rodriguez, K. M. (2015). Cultural and cognitive predictors of academic motivation among Mexican American adolescents: Caution against discounting the impact of cultural processes. *Journal of Multicultural Counseling and Development*, *43*(2), 109–121. doi:10.1002/j.2161-1912.2015.00068.x

Ploog, B. O. (2010). Stimulus overselectivity four decades later: A review of the literature and its implications for current research in autism spectrum disorder. *Journal of Autism and Developmental Disorders*, *40*(11), 1332–1349. doi:10.100710803-010-0990-2 PMID:20238154

Pocock, M., Trivedi, D., Wills, W., Bunn, F., & Magnusson, J. (2010). Parental perceptions regarding healthy behaviours for preventing overweight and obesity in young children: A systematic review of qualitative studies. *Obesity Reviews*, *11*(5), 338–353. doi:10.1111/j.1467-789X.2009.00648.x PMID:19780989

Polanczyk, G. V., Willcutt, E. G., Salum, G. A., Kieling, C., & Rohde, L. A. (2014). ADHD prevalence estimates across three decades: An updated systematic review and meta-regression analysis. *International Journal of Epidemiology*, *43*(2), 434–442. doi:10.1093/ije/dyt261 PMID:24464188

Poslawsky, I. E., Naber, F. B., Bakermans-Kranenburg, M. J., De Jonge, M. V., Van Engeland, H., & Van IJzendoorn, M. H. (2014). Development of a Video-feedback Intervention to promote Positive Parenting for Children with Autism (VIPP-AUTI). *Attachment & Human Development*, *16*(4), 343–355. doi:10.1080/14616734.2014.912487 PMID:24972103

Poslawsky, I. E., Naber, F. B., Bakermans-Kranenburg, M. J., van Daalen, E., van Engeland, H., & van IJzendoorn, M. H. (2015). Video-feedback Intervention to promote Positive Parenting adapted to Autism (VIPP-AUTI): A randomized controlled trial. *Autism, 19*(5), 588–603. doi:10.1177/1362361314537124 PMID:24919961

Pratt, B. M., & Woolfenden, S. (2002). Interventions for preventing eating disorders in children and adolescents. *Cochrane Database of Systematic Reviews*, 2. PMID:12076457

Prior, V., & Glaser, D. (2006). *Understanding attachment and attachment disorders: Theory, evidence and practice*. Jessica Kingsley Publishers.

Prot, S., Gentile, D. A., Anderson, C. A., Suzuki, K., Swing, E., Lim, K. M., ... Liau, A. K. (2014). Long-term relations among prosocial-media use, empathy, and prosocial behavior. *Psychological Science, 25*(2), 358–368. doi:10.1177/0956797613503854 PMID:24335350

Pruess, A. (2018). *The Importance of Setting Family Goals and How to Do It*. Retrieved from https://www.mother.ly/parenting/the-importance-of-setting-family-goals-and-how-to-do-it

Pruess, A. (2019). *The Importance of Setting Family Goals – and How to Do It*. Academic Press.

Pullen, J. (2017). *Renovating a house can be such a nightmare that it leads over 10% of couples to consider divorce*. Retrieved from https://www.businessinsider.com/12-of-couples-consider-divorce-when-they-are-remodeling-their-home-2017-11

Quoidbach, J., Mikolajczak, M., & Gross, J. J. (2015). Positive interventions: An emotion regulation perspective. *Psychological Bulletin, 141*(3), 655–693. doi:10.1037/a0038648 PMID:25621978

Radesky, J. S., Schumacher, J., & Zuckerman, B. (2015). Mobile and interactive media use by young children: The good, the bad, and the unknown. *Pediatrics, 135*(1), 1–3. doi:10.1542/peds.2014-2251 PMID:25548323

Renzaho, A., Green, J., Mellor, D., & Swinburn, B. (2011). Parenting, family functioning and lifestyle in a new culture: The case of African migrants in Melbourne, Victoria, Australia. *Child & Family Social Work, 16*(2), 228–240. doi:10.1111/j.1365-2206.2010.00736.x

Republic of Botswana. (2008). *National Situation Analysis on Orphans and Vulnerable Children in Botswana, Ministry of Local Government Department of Social Services*. Gaborone: Government Printers.

Republic of Botswana. (2009). *Children's Act*. Gaborone: Government Printers.

Republic of Botswana. (2010). *Improving the quality of life in Botswana: National Plan for Orphans and Vulnerable Children 2010-2016*. Gaborone: Ministry of Local Government.

RespectAbility, Fighting Stigmas, Advancing Opportunities. (2018). Retrieved from www.respectability.org

Retnowati, G. M., Agoes Salim, R. Y., & Saleh, A. (2017). Effectiveness of Picture Story Books Reading To Increase Kindness In Children Aged 5-6 Years. *Lingua Cultura, 12*(1), 89–95.

Riopel, L. (2019). *Emotional Intelligence Frameworks, Charts, Diagrams and Graphs*. Retrieved from www.positivepsychology.com

Robinson, K., & Aronica, L. (2015). *Creative Schools: The Grassroots Revolution That's Transforming Education*. New York, NY: Viking Penguin.

Rogers, S. J., & Vismara, L. A. (2008). Evidence-based comprehensive treatments for early autism. *Journal of Clinical Child and Adolescent Psychology*, *37*(1), 8–38. doi:10.1080/15374410701817808 PMID:18444052

Rosen, D. S. (2010). Clinical report—identification and management of eating disorders in children and adolescents. *Pediatrics*.

Rosenbaum, P. L., Armstrong, R. W., & King, S. M. (1986). Improving attitudes toward the disabled: A randomized controlled trial of direct contact versus Kids-on-the-Block. *Journal of Developmental and Behavioral Pediatrics*, *7*(5), 302–307. doi:10.1097/00004703-198610000-00005 PMID:2945833

Rosen, L. D., Lim, A. F., Felt, J., Carrier, L. M., Cheever, N. A., Lara-Ruiz, J. M., ... Rokkum, J. (2014). Media and technology use predicts ill-being among children, preteens and teenagers independent of the negative health impacts of exercise and eating habits. *Computers in Human Behavior*, *35*, 364–375. doi:10.1016/j.chb.2014.01.036 PMID:25717216

Rowe, R., Costello, E. J., Angold, A., Copeland, W. E., & Maughan, B. (2010, November). Developmental pathways in oppositional defiant disorder and conduct disorder. *Journal of Abnormal Psychology*, *119*(4), 726–738. doi:10.1037/a0020798 PMID:21090876

Rozga, A., Hesse, E., Main, M., Duschinsky, R., Beckwith, L., & Sigman, M. (2018). A short-term longitudinal study of correlates and sequelae of attachment security in autism. *Attachment & Human Development*, *20*(2), 160–180. doi:10.1080/14616734.2017.1383489 PMID:28959921

Ruiz-Casares, M., & Heymann, J. (2009). Children home alone unsupervised: Modeling parental decisions and associated factors in Botswana, Mexico, and Vietnam. *Child Abuse & Neglect*, *33*(5), 312–323. doi:10.1016/j.chiabu.2008.09.010 PMID:19477517

Rutgers, A. H., Van Ijzendoorn, M. H., Bakermans-Kranenburg, M. J., Swinkels, S. H., Van Daalen, E., Dietz, C., ... Van Engeland, H. (2007). Autism, attachment and parenting: A comparison of children with autism spectrum disorder, mental retardation, language disorder, and non-clinical children. *Journal of Abnormal Child Psychology*, *35*(5), 859–870. doi:10.100710802-007-9139-y PMID:17505877

Safe, A., Joosten, A., & Molineux, M. (2012). The experiences of mothers of children with autism: Managing multiple roles. *Journal of Intellectual & Developmental Disability*, *37*(4), 294–302. doi:10.3109/13668250.2012.736614 PMID:23171310

Salovey, P., Hsee, C. K., & Mayer, J. D. (1993). *Emotional intelligence and the self-regulation of affect. In Handbook of mental control* (pp. 258–277). Englewood Cliffs, NJ: Prentice Hall.

Salovey, P., & Mayer, J. D. (1990). Emotional intelligence. *Imagination, Cognition and Personality*, *9*(3), 185–211. doi:10.2190/DUGG-P24E-52WK-6CDG

Salvatore, J. E., & Dick, D. M. (2018). Genetic influences on conduct disorder. *Neuroscience and Biobehavioral Reviews*, *91*, 91–101. doi:10.1016/j.neubiorev.2016.06.034 PMID:27350097

Sánchez-Carracedo, D., Neumark-Sztainer, D., & López-Guimera, G. (2012). Integrated prevention of obesity and eating disorders: Barriers, developments and opportunities. *Public Health Nutrition*, *15*(12), 2295–2309. doi:10.1017/S1368980012000705 PMID:22455792

Sanders, M. R. (2008). Triple P-Positive Parenting Program as a public health approach to strengthening parenting. *Journal of Family Psychology*, *22*(4), 506–517. doi:10.1037/0893-3200.22.3.506 PMID:18729665

Sasson, N. J., Lam, K. S., Parlier, M., Daniels, J. L., & Piven, J. (2013). Autism and the broad autism phenotype: Familial patterns and intergenerational transmission. *Journal of Neurodevelopmental Disorders*, *5*(1), 11. doi:10.1186/1866-1955-5-11 PMID:23639131

Scelfo, J. (2016, Apr. 8). Angela Duckworth on Passion, Grit and Success. *The New York Times*. Retrieved from: https://www.nytimes.com/2016/04/10/education/edlife/passion-grit- success.html

Schaaf, C. P., & Zoghbi, H. Y. (2011). Solving the autism puzzle a few pieces at a time. *Neuron*, *70*(5), 806–808. doi:10.1016/j.neuron.2011.05.025 PMID:21658575

Schopler, E. (1994). A statewide program for the treatment and education of autistic and related communication handicapped children (TEACCH). *Child and Adolescent Psychiatric Clinics*, *3*(1), 91–103. doi:10.1016/S1056-4993(18)30517-0

Schuhmann, E. M., Foote, R. C., Eyberg, S. M., Boggs, S. R., & Algina, J. (1998). Efficacy of parent-child interaction therapy: Interim report of a randomized trial with short-term maintenance. *Journal of Clinical Child Psychology*, *27*(1), 34–45. doi:10.120715374424jccp2701_4 PMID:9561935

Schwarz, N. (1990). Feelings as information: Informational and motivational functions of affective states. In *Handbook of motivation and cognition: Foundations of social behavior* (Vol. 2, pp. 527–561). New York: Guilford Press.

Schwichtenberg, A., & Poehlmann, J. (2007). Applied behavior analysis: Does intervention intensity relate to family stressors and maternal well-being? *Journal of Intellectual Disability Research*, *51*(8), 598–605. doi:10.1111/j.1365-2788.2006.00940.x PMID:17598873

Scott-Little, C., Kagan, S. L., & Frelow, V. S. (2006). Conceptualization of readiness and the content of early learning standards: The intersection of policy and research? *Early Childhood Research Quarterly*, *21*(2), 153–173. doi:10.1016/j.ecresq.2006.04.003

Seligman, M. (2004). Can Happiness Be Taught? *Daedalus*, *133*(2), 80–87. doi:10.1162/001152604323049424

SeligmanM. (n.d.). Retrieved from https://www.pursuit-of-happiness.org/history-of-happiness/martin-seligman-psychology/

Seligman, M. E. P., & Csikszentmihalyi, M. (2000). Positive psychology: An introduction. *The American Psychologist*, *55*(1), 5–14. doi:10.1037/0003-066X.55.1.5 PMID:11392865

Seligman, M. E. P., Steen, T. A., Park, N., & Peterson, C. (2005). Positive Psychology Progress: Empirical Validation of Interventions. *The American Psychologist*, *60*(5), 410–421. doi:10.1037/0003-066X.60.5.410 PMID:16045394

Seligman, M., Ernst, R., Gillham, J., Reivich, K., & Linkins, M. (2009). Positive education: Positive psychology and classroom interventions. *Oxford Review of Education*, *35*(3), 293–311. doi:10.1080/03054980902934563

Sewpaul, V. (2013). Inscribed in our blood: Challenging the ideology of sexism and racism. *Affilia*, *28*(2), 116–125. doi:10.1177/0886109913485680

Shelley, T. (2008). *Health psychology* (7th ed.). New York, NY: McGraw Hill.

Sheyholislami, J. (2001). *Critical Discourse Analysis*. Retrieved from http://www.carleton.ca/~jsheyhol/cda.htm

Shiota, M. N., Campos, B., Oveis, C., Hertenstein, M. J., Simon-Thomas, E., & Keltner, D. (2017). Beyond happiness: Building a science of discrete positive emotions. *The American Psychologist*, *72*(7), 617–643. doi:10.1037/a0040456 PMID:29016167

Sigman, M., & Ungerer, J. A. (1984). Attachment behaviors in autistic children. *Journal of Autism and Developmental Disorders*, *14*(3), 231–244. doi:10.1007/BF02409576 PMID:6207163

Silton, N. R., Flannelly, K. J., Milstein, G., & Vaaler, M. L. (2011). Stigma in America: has anything changed?: Impact of perceptions of mental illness and dangerousness on the desire for social distance: 1996 and 2006. *The Journal of Nervous and Mental Disease*, *199*(6), 361–366. doi:10.1097/NMD.0b013e31821cd112 PMID:21629012

Simonoff, E., Elander, J., Holmshaw, J., Pickles, A., Murray, R., & Rutter, M. (2004). Predictors of antisocial personality: Continuities from childhood to adult life. *The British Journal of Psychiatry*, *184*(2), 118–127. doi:10.1192/bjp.184.2.118 PMID:14754823

Siperstein, G. N. (1980). *Development of the Adjective Checklist: An instrument for measuring children's attitudes toward the handicapped* (Unpublished manuscript). University of Massachusetts, Boston, MA.

Siperstein, G. N., & Bak, J. (1977). *Instruments to measure children's attitudes toward the handicapped: Adjective Checklist and Activity Preference List* (Unpublished manuscript). University of Massachusetts, Boston, MA.

Smeets, K. C., Leeijen, A. A., van der Molen, M. J., Scheepers, F. E., Buitelaar, J. K., & Rommelse, N. N. (2015). Treatment moderators of cognitive behavior therapy to reduce aggressive behavior: A meta-analysis. *European Child & Adolescent Psychiatry*, *24*(3), 255–264. doi:10.100700787-014-0592-1 PMID:25138144

Smith, M. (2011). Measures for assessing parenting in research and practice. *Child and Adolescent Mental Health, 16*(3), 158–166. doi:10.1111/j.1475-3588.2010.00585.x

Springer Netherlands Csikszentmihalyi, M., Graef, R., & Gianinno, S. M. (2014). Measuring Intrinsic Motivation in Everyday Life. In *Flow and the Foundations of Positive Psychology* (pp. 113–125). Dordrecht: Springer.

Statistics Botswana. (2011). *Population and housing census 2011, analytical report.* Gaborone: Department of Printing & Publishing Services.

Steele, M., Steele, H., Bate, J., Knafo, H., Kinsey, M., Bonuck, K., ... Murphy, A. (2014). Looking from the outside in: The use of video in attachment-based interventions. *Attachment & Human Development, 16*(4), 402–415. doi:10.1080/14616734.2014.912491 PMID:24972107

Steinberg, L., Lamborn, S. D., Dornbusch, S. M., & Darling, N. (1992). Impact of parenting practices on adolescent achievement: Authoritative parenting, school involvement, and encouragement to succeed. *Child Development, 63*(5), 1266–1281. doi:10.2307/1131532 PMID:1446552

Steiner, A. M., Koegel, L. K., Koegel, R. L., & Ence, W. A. (2012). Issues and theoretical constructs regarding parent education for autism spectrum disorders. *Journal of Autism and Developmental Disorders, 42*(6), 1218–1227. doi:10.100710803-011-1194-0 PMID:21336525

Sternberg, R. J., Conway, B. E., Ketron, J. L., & Bernstein, M. (1981). People's conceptions of intelligence. *Journal of Personality and Social Psychology, 41*(1), 37–55. doi:10.1037/0022-3514.41.1.37

Story, M., Neumark-Sztainer, D., & French, S. (2002). Individual and environmental influences on adolescent eating behaviors. *Journal of the American Dietetic Association, 102*(3), S40–S51. doi:10.1016/S0002-8223(02)90421-9 PMID:11902388

Sucksmith, E., Roth, I., & Hoekstra, R. A. (2011). Autistic traits below the clinical threshold: Re-examining the broader autism phenotype in the 21st century. *Neuropsychology Review, 21*(4), 360–389. doi:10.100711065-011-9183-9 PMID:21989834

Suizzo, M. A., Rackley, K. R., Robbins, P. A., Jackson, K. M., Rarick, J. R., & McClain, S. (2017). The unique effects of fathers' warmth on adolescents' positive beliefs and behaviors: Pathways to resilience in low-income families. *Sex Roles, 77*(1-2), 46–58. doi:10.100711199-016-0696-9

Suldo, S. M., & Huebner, E. S. (2004). The role of life satisfaction in the relationship between authoritative parenting dimensions and adolescent problem behavior. *Social Indicators Research, 66*(1-2), 165–195. doi:10.1023/B:SOCI.0000007498.62080.1e

Tan, L., & Smith, C. L. (2018). *Intergenerational transmission of maternal emotion regulation to child emotion regulation: Moderated mediation of maternal positive and negative emotions. Emotion.* Retrieved from https://slb.mmm.edu:2208/10.1037/emo0000523

Tang, X., Wang, M. T., Guo, J., & Salmela-Aro, K. (2019). Building grit: The longitudinal pathways between mindset, commitment, grit, and academic outcomes. *Journal of Youth and Adolescence, 48*(5), 850–863. doi:10.100710964-019-00998-0 PMID:30788767

Taylor, L. E., Swerdfeger, A. L., & Eslick, G. D. (2014). Vaccines are not associated with autism: An evidence-based meta-analysis of case-control and cohort studies. *Vaccine, 32*(29), 3623–3629. doi:10.1016/j.vaccine.2014.04.085 PMID:24814559

Temperament: Temperamental Effortful Control (Self-Regulation). (n.d.). Retrieved from http://www.child-encyclopedia.com/temperament/according-experts/temperamental-effortful-control-self-regulation

Tessina, T., Smith, R. (2016). *How to Be Happy Partners: Working it out Together.* CreateSpace Independent Publishing Platform.

The Enterprise of the Future. (n.d.). *IBM 2008 Global CEO Study*. Retrieved from http://globalforum.items-int.com/gf/gf-content/uploads/2014/04/ceostudy2008_fullrep.pdf

The Science of a Meaningful Life. (n.d.). Retrieved from https://greatergood.berkeley.edu/

The Science of Happiness – Tal Ben-Shahar. (n.d.). Retrieved from https://positivepsychologynews.com/news/bridget-grenville-cleave/2014080629622

Thios, S. J., & Foster, S. B. (1991). *Changing Preschoolers' Attitudes toward Children with Disabilities.* Paper presented at the Annual Meeting of the American Psychological Association, San Francisco, CA.

Thorndike, E. L. (1920). Intelligence and its uses. *Harper's Magazine.*

Thorndike, R. L., & Stein, S. (1937). An evaluation of the attempts to measure social intelligence. *Psychological Bulletin, 34*(5), 275–285. doi:10.1037/h0053850

Tiet, Q. Q., Huizinga, D., & Byrnes, H. F. (2010). Predictors of resilience among inner city youths. *Journal of Child and Family Studies, 19*(3), 360–378. doi:10.100710826-009-9307-5

Tirri, K., & Husu, J. (2002). Care and Responsibility in 'The Best Interest of the Child': Relational voices of ethical dilemmas in teaching. *Teachers and Teaching, 8*(1), 65–80. doi:10.1080/13540600120110574

Tonn, J. C. (2003). *Mary P. Follett: Creating Democracy, Transforming Management.* New Haven, CT: Yale University Press. doi:10.12987/yale/9780300096217.001.0001

Tough, P. (2012). *How children succeed: Grit, curiosity, and the hidden power of character.* Houghton Mifflin Harcourt.

Tracy, R. L., & Ainsworth, M. D. S. (1981). Maternal Affectionate Behavior and Infant-Mother Attachment Patterns. *Child Development, 52*(4), 1341–1343. doi:10.2307/1129529 PMID:7318528

Trice, H. M., & Beyer, J. M. (1993). *The cultures of work organizations.* Prentice-Hall, Inc.

Trimingham, M. (2010). Objects in transition: The puppet and the autistic child. *Journal of Applied Arts & Health, 1*(3), 251–265. doi:10.1386/jaah.1.3.251_1

Tronick, E. Z. (1989). Emotions and emotional communication in infants. *The American Psychologist, 44*(2), 112–119. doi:10.1037/0003-066X.44.2.112 PMID:2653124

Types of Eating Disorders. (2019). Retrieved from http://www.reelstoriesrealpeople.org/educational-films/types-of-eating-disorders/? gclid=EAIaIQobChMI4NziuN-W4gIVBqSzCh3w9g3qEAAYAyAAEgIx9vD_BwE

U.S. Department of Health and Human Services, National Institute of Mental Health. (2017). *Any anxiety disorder.* Retrieved from https://www.nimh.nih.gov/health/statistics/any-anxiety-disorder.shtml

U.S. Department of Health and Human Services, Substance Abuse and Mental Health Administration. (2017). *Key substance use and mental health indicators in the United States: Results from the 2016 National Survey on Drug Use and Health.* Retrieved from https://www.samhsa.gov/data/sites/default/files/NSDUH-FFR1- 2016/NSDUH-FFR1-2016.pdf - PDF

UNICEF. (2011). *The situation analysis of children and their families in Botswana. Summary Report: Findings and recommendations to policy makers 2010/2011.* Gaborone: UNICEF Botswana Country Office.

Vaillant, G. E. (1992). Ego mechanisms of defense: a guide for clinicans and researchers. American Psychiatric Pub.

Vail, P. (1981). *Emotion: The On Off Switch for learning.* Rosemont, NJ: Modern Learning Press.

Vallerand, R. (2000). Deci and Ryan's Self-Determination Theory: A View from the Hierarchical Model of Intrinsic and Extrinsic Motivation. *Psychological Inquiry, 11*(4), 312–318. Retrieved from http://www.jstor.org/stable/1449629

Van Cauwenberghe, E., Maes, L., Spittaels, H., van Lenthe, F. J., Brug, J., Oppert, J. M., & De Bourdeaudhuij, I. (2010). Effectiveness of school-based interventions in Europe to promote healthy nutrition in children and adolescents: systematic review of published and 'grey' literature. *British Journal of Nutrition, 103*(6), 781-797.

Van Dijk, T. A. (2001). Multidisciplinary CDA: a plea for diversity. In Methods of critical discourse analysis. London: Sage Publications.

Van Dijk, T. A. (1993). Principles of critical discourse analysis. *Discourse & Society, 4*(2), 249–283. doi:10.1177/0957926593004002006

Van IJzendoorn, M. H., Rutgers, A. H., Bakermans-Kranenburg, M. J., Swinkels, S. H., Van Daalen, E., Dietz, C., ... Van Engeland, H. (2007). Parental sensitivity and attachment in children with autism spectrum disorder: Comparison with children with mental retardation, with language delays, and with typical development. *Child Development, 78*(2), 597–608. doi:10.1111/j.1467-8624.2007.01016.x PMID:17381792

Van Ness, P.H. (1999). *Yoga as spiritual but not religious: A pragmatic perspective.* University of Illinois Press.

Van Noorden, T. H. J., Haselager, G. J. T., Cillessen, A. H. N., & Bukowski, W. M. (2014). Empathy and Involvement in Bullying in Children and Adolescents: A Systematic Review. *Journal of Youth and Adolescence*, 1–22.

Vela, J. C., Lu, M.-T. P., Lenz, A. S., & Hinojosa, K. (2015). Positive psychology and familial factors as predictors of Latina/o students' psychological grit. *Hispanic Journal of Behavioral Sciences, 37*(3), 287–303. Retrieved from org.proxy.wexler.hunter.cuny.edu/10.1177/0739986315588917

Vela, J. C., Sparrow, G. S., Whittenberg, J. F., & Rodriguez, B. (2018). The Role of Character Strengths and Importance of Family on Mexican American College Students' Career Decision Self-Efficacy. *Journal of Employment Counseling*, *55*(1), 16–26. doi:10.1002/joec.12070

Vernetti, A., Senju, A., Charman, T., Johnson, M. H., & Gliga, T. (2018). Simulating interaction: Using gaze-contingent eye-tracking to measure the reward value of social signals in toddlers with and without autism. *Developmental Cognitive Neuroscience*, *29*, 21–29. doi:10.1016/j.dcn.2017.08.004 PMID:28939027

Versaci, R. (2001). How Comic Books Can Change the Way Our Students See Literature: One Teacher's Perspective. *English Journal*, *91*(61), 61–67. doi:10.2307/822347

Vess, M. (2012). Warm thoughts: attachment anxiety and sensitivity to temperature cues. *Psychological Science, 23*(5), 472-474. Retrieved from http://www.jstor.org/stable/414899727

Vicedo, M. (2009). The Father of Ethology and the Foster Mother of Ducks: Konrad Lorenz as Expert on Motherhood. *Isis*, *100*(2), 263–291. doi:10.1086/599553 PMID:19653490

Vignes, C., Godeau, E., Sentenac, M., Coley, N., Niavarro, F., & Grandjean, H. (2009). Determinants of students' attitudes towards peers with disabilities. *Developmental Medicine and Child Neurology*, *51*(6), 473–479. doi:10.1111/j.1469-8749.2009.03283.x PMID:19416319

Vik, K., & Rohde, R. (2014). Tiny moments of great importance: The Marte Meo method applied in the context of early mother–infant interaction and postnatal depression. Utilizing Daniel Stern's theory of 'schemas of being with'in understanding empirical findings and developing a stringent Marte Meo methodology. *Clinical Child Psychology and Psychiatry*, *19*(1), 77–89. doi:10.1177/1359104512468286 PMID:23242466

Wagner, M. F., Milner, J. S., McCarthy, R. J., Crouch, J. L., McCanne, T. R., & Skowronski, J. J. (2015). Facial emotion recognition accuracy and child physical abuse: An experiment and a meta-analysis. *Psychology of Violence*, *5*(2), 154–162. Retrieved from https://slb.mmm.edu:2208/10.1037/a0036014

Walker, C. O. (2017). Exploring the contributions of grit and personality in the prediction of self-and other-forgiveness. *Journal of Individual Differences*, *38*(3), 196–202. doi:10.1027/1614-0001/a000236

Wang, Q., Pomerantz, E. M., & Chen, H. (2007). The role of parents' control in early adolescents' psychological functioning: A longitudinal investigation in the United States and China. *Child Development*, *78*(5), 1592–1610. doi:10.1111/j.1467-8624.2007.01085.x PMID:17883450

Wan, M. W., Green, J., Elsabbagh, M., Johnson, M., Charman, T., & Plummer, F. (2012). Parent–infant interaction in infant siblings at risk of autism. *Research in Developmental Disabilities*, *33*(3), 924–932. doi:10.1016/j.ridd.2011.12.011 PMID:22257674

Ward, M. A., Theule, J., & Cheung, K. (2016, October). Parent–child interaction therapy for child disruptive behaviour disorders: A meta-analysis. In *Child & Youth Care Forum* (Vol. 45, No. 5, pp. 675-690). Springer US.

Wechsler, D. (1958). *The measurement and appraisal of adult intelligence*. Academic Press.

Weiss, F. (1998). The Field of Wings, Puppetry as Therapy from an Object Relations Point of View and Incorporating Field Psychology. In A. Robbins (Ed.), *Therapeutic Presence* (pp. 219–243). London: Jessica Kingsley.

Werling, D. M., & Geschwind, D. H. (2013). Sex differences in autism spectrum disorders. *Current Opinion in Neurology*, *26*(2), 146–153. doi:10.1097/WCO.0b013e32835ee548 PMID:23406909

Wetherby, A. M., Woods, J., Allen, L., Cleary, J., Dickinson, H., & Lord, C. (2004). Early indicators of autism spectrum disorders in the second year of life. *Journal of Autism and Developmental Disorders*, *34*(5), 473–493. doi:10.100710803-004-2544-y PMID:15628603

What are Eating Disorders? (2018, August 7). Retrieved from https://www.nationaleatingdisorders.org/what-are-eating-disorders

White, D. (2017). *How to Overcome Relationship Problems After Having a Baby*. Retrieved from https://www.bergencounselingcenter.com/articles/relationship-problems-after-baby/

Wieder, S., & Greenspan, S. I. (2003). Climbing the symbolic ladder in the DIR model through floor time/interactive play. *Autism*, *7*(4), 425–435. doi:10.1177/1362361303007004008 PMID:14678681

Wodak, R. (2001). What CDA is about-a summary of its history, important concepts and its development. In Methods of critical discourse analysis. London: Sage Publications.

Wodak, R. (1999). Critical discourse analysis at the end of the 20th century. *Research on Language and Social Interaction*, *32*(1-2), 185–193. doi:10.1080/08351813.1999.9683622

Woltmann, A. (1951). The Use of Puppetry as a Projective Method in Therapy. In H. Anderson & G. Anderson (Eds.), *Introduction to Projective Techniques* (pp. 606–637). New York: Prentice Hall.

Wright, A., Jorm, A. F., Harris, M. G., & McGorry, P. D. (2007). What's in a name? Is accurate recognition and labelling of mental disorders by young people associated with better help-seeking and treatment preferences? *Social Psychiatry and Psychiatric Epidemiology*, *42*(3), 244–250. doi:10.100700127-006-0156-x PMID:17450404

Wright, S. C., Aron, A., McLaughlin-Volpe, T., & Ropp, S. A. (1997). The extended contact effect: Knowledge of cross-group friendships and prejudice. *Journal of Personality and Social Psychology*, *73*(1), 73–90. doi:10.1037/0022-3514.73.1.73

Yaman, A., Mesman, J., van IJzendoorn, M. H., Bakermans-Kranenburg, M. J., & Linting, M. (2010). Parenting in an individualistic culture with a collectivistic cultural background: The case of Turkish immigrant families with toddlers in the Netherlands. *Journal of Child and Family Studies*, *19*(5), 617–628. doi:10.100710826-009-9346-y PMID:20835387

Zhao, Y. (2012, June 6). *Test Scores vs. Entrepreneurship: PISA, TIMSS, and Confidence*. Retrieved from http://zhaolearning.com/2012/06/06/test-scores-vs-entrepreneurship-pisa-timss-and- confidence/

Zhao, Y. (2017). *What works may hurt: Side effects in Education*. Springer.

About the Contributors

Nava R. Silton, a Developmental Psychologist, received her B.S. from Cornell University in 2002 and her M.A. and Ph.D. from Fordham University in 2009. Silton has worked at Nickelodeon and Sesame Street Workshop and has consulted for Netflix and The Autism Seaver Center. She appears regularly on Fox 5 News and NBC as a Psychological Correspondent. Nava is currently an Associate Professor of Psychology at Marymount Manhattan College. She edited two books pertaining to Disabilities in March 2014 and June 2015, respectively. She released her third on Creativity in the Summer of 2016, her fourth on Relationships and Family Dynamics in the Summer of 2017 and her fifth on Happiness, Kindness and Empathy in 2018. Moreover, Silton created the *Realabilities Educational Comic Book Series Curriculum* and the *Addy & Uno* Off-Broadway Musical, which has run for over 18 months on Theater Row in Manhattan. The comic book series and show intend to fill a significant void in children's media and literature so that individuals with disabilities can see themselves represented positively on-screen, and typical children and adults can become increasingly knowledgeable, sensitive and interested in their peers with disabilities.

* * *

Amanda Anzovino is a summa cum laude graduate of Marymount Manhattan College. She earned a B.A. in Psychology with minors in Forensic Psychology, Social Work, and Sociology. As a Jeannette K. Watson Fellow, Amanda has had multiple internships in the areas of forensic psychology, developmental psychology and social justice non-profits. Furthermore, she has presented numerous research projects at local and regional psychology conferences. As a member of Dr. Nava R. Silton's *Realabilities* research team, Amanda became interested in the topic of emotional intelligence and the impact it can have on all aspects of one's life, including at school, at work, in relationships, and in future success.

Lauren Ashbrook is a recent graduate from Marymount Manhattan College, with two Bachelor of Arts degrees in Psychology and Business. Lauren's undergraduate research has primarily focused on eating disorders and on the negative effects of various marketing techniques on consumers. Lauren currently works at the Healthcare Innovation and Technology Lab (HITLAB), founded by Columbia University's Business and Medical schools. While at HITLAB, she supports all business advisory and organizational functions of the lab. In the future, Lauren hopes to receive a Ph.D. in Health Psychology and to become a researcher and therapist, who specializes in eating disorders.

Valerie Blanchard-McGehee, Ph.D., received her doctorate in higher education, leadership, management, and policy from Seton Hall University. Her dissertation research was in grit, goal setting, and social support, specifically around doctoral completion. Valerie has worked in the fields of education, entrepreneurship, and sales, which eventually lead her to become a client partner at Franklin Covey. While leading the New Jersey sales team, she became a certified facilitator in The Seven Habits of Highly Effective People and in The Seven Habits of Highly Effective Families. Valerie currently resides in Lafayette, Louisiana, where she teaches marketing and sales courses and is the Interim Director of the B.I. Moody College of Business Administration Sales Program. McGehee thrives in an environment where she can teach, network, and bring gritty people together.

Ingrid C. Brussier has been a French international student at Marymount Manhattan College since 2017. She will be graduating with a psychology undergraduate degree in 2021 and has been part of her college's Dean's List for the past two years. Ingrid Brussier is now participating in research and translation projects for Marymount Manhattan College Psychology Department's faculty.

Jacopo De Angelis is a psychologist and Ph.D. candidate at University of Milano – Bicocca, Department of Psychology (Italy). He pursued his Master's Degree at The University of Pavia and then moved to The University of Milano – Bicocca (Italy), Goldsmiths University of London (UK) and The Italian Institute of Technology (IIT) to work as a research assistant. His research interests relate to social cognition and autism. Specifically, his main research interests include: i) the modulatory effects of social and non-social rewards on visual selective attention; ii) the study of pain perception and empathy in individuals with Autism Spectrum Disorder (ASD); iii) the development of interventions aimed at enhancing social attention in individuals with ASD; iv) the development of technology-based diagnostic tools for ASD; v) the study of social attention in parents of children with ASD to increase the knowledge of the Broad Autism Phenotype and to increase the quality of parent-mediated interventions. The relentless challenges of parenting children with ASD has raised Jacopo's interest in the clinical and educational implications of parental strategies in terms of the social and emotional development of ASD children.

Emily Hotez is a project scientist for the Life Course Intervention Research Network at the UCLA Center for Healthier Children, Families & Communities. Dr. Hotez collaborates with the Network on the design, implementation, and evaluation of incubated life course intervention studies and leads a participatory process for developing a life course intervention research agenda for the Network. Prior to her work at the Center, Dr. Hotez served as a research associate at the CUNY Institute for State and Local Governance, conducting research, performance measurement, and data analysis for the MacArthur Foundation's Safety and Justice Challenge. She was also an adjunct assistant professor at Hunter College and Fordham University, where she taught psychology, child development, research methods, and statistics courses and led and collaborated on several participatory research and advocacy initiatives for diverse populations in higher education. Dr. Hotez's previous research has addressed parent-child relationships, autism across the lifespan, and families in poverty. Dr. Hotez's interest in grit stems from her work and collaboration with diverse college students and the numerous findings that link grit to achievement in higher education. Her chapter in the current book merges this interest with her broader interest in child and family development. Dr. Hotez earned her B.A. in psychology from George Washington University and her Ph.D. in developmental psychology from the CUNY Graduate Center.

Jaclyn Kell is currently living in Manhattan, New York, and is completing her Psychological and Public Health studies at Marymount Manhattan College. Her research areas of interest include child development, childhood happiness, and health psychology.

Erika Nolan is a student at Marymount Manhattan College, currently pursuing a Bachelor of Arts degree with a major in Psychology and a double minor in Music and Theater. Erika became interested in the study of attachment throughout various General Psychology Courses during her first semester of college. She then took a Developmental Psychology Course that gave her the opportunity to further delve into attachment theory. In these courses, she learned that infant-parental attachment can have lasting impacts on a child's social life. She was eager to learn what behaviors yield which attachments, and, therefore, began work on her chapter.

Poloko Nuggert Ntshwarang is currently a senior lecturer in the department of Social Work at the University of Botswana. She acquired her Ph.D. in Social Work at the University of KwaZulu-Natal, South Africa. She completed her Masters of Social Work degree (measuring in health) from the University of Utah, U. S.A. in 2004. She also has a Bachelor's of Social Work degree from the University of Botswana, which she acquired in 2001. After completing her studies, Mrs. Ntshwarang worked in health services as a hospital social worker and as a Refugee Health Program Social Welfare officer before joining the University. She has served on several research teams. She has also served on the University of Botswana Research and Activism Project, focusing on young women. She has participated in local, regional and international conferences. She is interested in issues pertaining to social work, especially health, gender issues, and child welfare (with a particularly keen interest in parenting issues). She has published a number of journal articles and book chapters on her areas of interest.

Giulia Perasso is a psychologist and Ph.D. Candidate at the University of Pavia (Italy), where she is currently working at the Department of Brain and Behavioural Science. After obtaining her Master's Degree at the University of Pavia, she worked as a visiting intern researcher at the Centre for Abuse and Trauma Studies (Middlesex University of London, UK). Her research and clinical practice focus on development, in terms of protective and risk factors for psychosocial health. Specifically, her main interests include: i) emotion regulation and difficulties in emotion regulation; ii) parenting; iii) puberty and adolescence. The complex challenges of parenting children with ASD has raised Giulia's interest in highlighting - through Attachment Theory's conceptual framework - the issues and strengths that ASD children's mothers and fathers experience in everyday life.

Patrick Riley is a Senior at Marymount Manhattan College, majoring in Psychology and Public Health. Patrick has served as the Lead Research Assistant on Dr. Nava R. Silton's research team for the past three years and has assisted Dr. Silton in advancing the *Realabilities/Addy & Uno* educational series. Patrick has presented research projects at over a dozen national and regional conferences and has co-authored three publications with Dr. Silton. At Marymount Manhattan College, Patrick is involved on campus, through his various roles as the Psychology Department Student Recruiter, Statistics Teaching Assistant, President of the Psychology Club and Academic Peer Leader. Patrick has completed internships at The Quad Preparatory School, The Child Mind Institute, at Theater Row and at MediaKidz. Through Patrick's coursework and research experiences, he has cultivated interests in the areas of developmental psychology, children's media, LGBTQ+ health, and individuals with disabilities. Patrick looks forward to attending graduate school in the near future and pursuing an advanced degree in developmental psychology.

Odireleng Shehu (Ph.D., MSW) is an Associate Professor in the Department of Social Work at the University of Botswana. She graduated from the University of Utah, USA with a Ph.D. in Social Work. She is currently based in Botswana and teaches courses in the clinical field at the University of Botswana. She has participated in several research studies including, coping strategies for informal caregivers in Botswana, children as victims of violence, parenting of adolescents, and counseling students. She evaluates disability programmes in Botswana, linking alcohol abuse, gender-based violence and HIV/AIDS in Botswana, assessing the magnitude of disability, teenage pregnancy as well as substance use and abuse, and the evaluation of District multi-sectoral AIDS Committee (DMSAC). She has published extensively on issues pertaining to social protection, caregiving, health, and gender-based violence. She has experience working with NGO's, FBO's and communities. She is currently the board chairperson of The Kagisano Women's Shelter.

Stephanie Johan Valencia is an artist at heart and designer by trade. She studied Service Design at Parsons THE New School of Design and Environmental Studies at Eugene Lang College of Liberal Arts. Her studies have produced a body of work concerning the design of services to improve the lives of everyday people through advocacy and co-creation. All of the projects she has pursued have had a common thread of art, science and/or design interlaced in the work. Her work is heavily informed by ethnography and the concept of designing "with" rather than "for." She recently worked at the Henry Hudson School (J.H.S. 125) in the Parkchester section of the Bronx as a teaching artist. There she discovered that the classroom is a teachers' laboratory for creative confidence and a way to introduce and engage students to their very own 'flow states.' She currently works at Apple where she is able to create and redesign service experiences geared towards our technical needs and wants.

Tatiana Valencia was born and raised in Queens, New York and graduated from Marymount Manhattan College (MMC) with a Bachelor's degree in Psychology and Dance with a concentration in Body, Science and Motion. During her time at MMC, Tatiana interned with Dr. Martha Eddy, an exercise specialist and movement therapist. Under her guidance, she successfully completed a Moving for Life Instructor Training Program and is currently teaching gentle aerobics to vulnerable populations around NYC. Her work ethic and passion for helping others through a club on campus called Advocates for Wellness did not go unnoticed. She was soon offered a job at MMC's Counseling and Wellness Center upon graduating from MMC. Her new role as Health Promotion Coordinator allows her to eagerly work on outreach and event planning around topics such as mental health, sleep and healthy personal and interpersonal relationships. She understands that college is an impactful time for students and, therefore, strives to inspire students' awareness of holistic health during this critical period of emerging adulthood. Aside from her work in wellness promotion, Tatiana also enjoys training in commercial dance and in pursuing several dance performance projects.

Index

N

O

P

R

S

T

W

www.ingramcontent.com/pod-product-compliance
Lightning Source LLC
LaVergne TN
LVHW060002031026
849161LV00025B/1331
9781799829409